PCTA
AN INVESTIGATIONAL TOOL AND
A NON-OPERATIVE TREATMENT OF ACUTE ISCHEMIA

Developments in Cardiovascular Medicine

VOLUME 101

PTCA

An Investigational Tool and a Non-operative Treatment of Acute Ischema

edited by

PATRICK W. SERRUYS
Professor of Interventional Cardiology
Cardiac Catheterization Laboratory, Thorax Center,
Erasmus University, Rotterdam, The Netherlands

RÜDIGER SIMON
Professor of Cardiology
Department of Cardiology, University Hospital,
Kiel, F.R.G.

KEVIN J. BEATT
Academic Unit of Cardiovascular Medicine,
Charing Cross and Westminster Hospital,
London, United Kingdom

Kluwer Academic Publishers
DORDRECHT / BOSTON / LONDON

Library of Congress Cataloging in Publication Data

PTCA, an investigational tool and a non-operative treatment of acute
  ischemia/edited by Patrick W. Serruys, Rüdiger Simon, Kevin J.
  Beatt.
        p.   cm.—(Developments in cardiovascular medicine: 101)
  Includes bibliographies.
  ISBN-13:978-94-010-6688-4   e-ISBN-13:978-94-009-0453-8
  DOI: 10.1007/978-94-009-0453-8

  1. Transluminal angioplasty.   2. Coronary heart disease-
Treatment.   I. Serruys, P.W.   II. Simon, Rüdiger, Dr. med.
III. Beatt. Kevin J.   IV. Series: Developments in cardiovascular
medicine: v. 101.
     [DNLM: 1. Angioplasty, Transluminal.   2. Coronary Disease-
therapy. W1 DE997VME v. 101/WG 300 P97445]
  RD598.5.P784   1989
  617.4′ 12059—dc20
  DNLM/DLC
  for Library of Congress   89-15296
ISBN-13:978-94-010-6688-4

Published by Kluwer Academic Publishers,
P.O. Box 17, 3300 AA Dordrecht, The Netherlands.

Kluwer Academic Publishers incorporates
the publishing programmes of
D. Reidel, Martinus Nijhoff, Dr W. Junk and MTP Press.

Sold and distributed in the U.S.A. and Canada
by Kluwer Academic Publishers.
101 Philip Drive, Norwell, MA 02061, U.S.A.

In all other countries, sold and distributed
by Kluwer Academic Publishers Group
P.O. Box 322, 3300 AH Dordrecht, The Netherlands.

Printed on acid-free paper

Foreword

Obstruction of coronary blood flow and the resultant consequences are the center stage pathophysiologic events in cardiology today. The speculations of Jenner, Burns, Heberdin, McKenzie, Prinzmetal and many others had until now been left to observations of isolated tissue and intact animal experimentation. Only with the advent of Gruentzig's technique, which allowed us to 'work safely inside the coronary arteries' are we able to observe the effects of coronary occlusion in living conscious man. PTCA provides not only a therapeutic modality for non-operatively opening coronary obstructions, but has also provided the best model for studying the effects of acute ischemia on the heart. The procedure also lead the way to all other interventional cardiology developments, including modern thrombolysis in the setting of acute myocardial infarction.

In his previous works, Serruys has examined how PTCA can serve as a model for studying acute ischemia. In this book, he and his co-authors discuss the effects of balloon-induced ischemia on the electrocardiographic changes, coronary blood flow dynamics, cardiac muscle metabolism and left ventricular function, as well as measures to counter these effects and provide for reperfusion in unstable angina and acute myocardial infarction. Technology has expanded the 'eyes' of the observer of these events. The authors use many techniques including ECG recording from surface, endocardium, and intracoronary electrodes; angiographic assessment of coronary flow pattern using digital techniques, as well as doppler flow measurements; biochemical assessment of metabolic products stimulated by ischemia; and digital angiographic and echo doppler assessment of left ventricular function.

Observations of ischemia-induced and ischemia relieved using all the 'eyes' available to the investigator in the 'experimental animal' (man) of greatest interest will advance our understanding and quicken the day when ischemia can be reliably controlled. In this book, Serruys and his co-authors have made a significant contribution toward that end.

SPENCER B. KING III, M.D.

Contents

Myocardial metabolism

PART TWO: NON-OPERATIVE TREATMENT OF
          ACUTE ISCHEMIA

List of contributors

J. BERLAND
Service de Cardiologie, Hopital Charles-Nicolle, 1 rue de Germont, 76031 Rouen, France
Chapter 22 co-author: J.C. FARCOT

M.E. BERTRAND
Centre Hospitalier Régional et Universitaire de Lille, Boulevard du Prof. J. Leclercq 59037 Lille Cedex, France
Chapter 14 co-authors: J.M. LABLANCHE, J.L. FOURRIER, A. GOMMEAUX and I. MIRSKY

B. de BRUYNE
Centre de Cardiologie, 24 rue Micheli-du-Crest, 1211 Genève 4, Switzerland,
Chapter 6 co-author: B. MEIER

M. COHEN
Division of Cardiology, Mount Sinai Hospital, One Gustave Levy Place, New York, NY 10029-6547, U.S.A.
Chapter 5

P.J. de FEYTER
Erasmus University, Thoraxcenter, P.O. Box 1738, 3000 DR Rotterdam, The Netherlands
Chapter 23 co-authors: H. SURYAPRANATA and P.W. SERRUYS

M. GRBIC
C.H.U.V., rue du Bugmon, 1011 Lausanne, Switzerland
Chapters 12 and 13 co-author: U. SIGWART

M. HALPERN
C.H.U.V., rue du Bugmon, 1011 Lausanne, Switzerland
Chapter 20 co-author: U. SIGWART

G.R. HEYNDRICKX
O.L.-Vrouwziekenhuis, Moorselbaan 164, 9300 Aalst, Belgium
Chapter 1 co-authors: W. WIJNS and S.F. VATNER

J.W. de JONG
Erasmus University, Thoraxcenter, P.O. Box 1738, 3000 DR Rotterdam, The Netherlands
Chapter 10 co-authors: T. HUIZER, J.A. NELSON, W. CZARNECKI, J.J.R.M. BONNIER and P.W. SERRUYS

R.G. MACDONALD
Victoria General Hospital, 1278 Tower Road, Halifax Nova Scotia, B3H 2Y9 Canada
Chapter 4 co-author: R.L. FELDMAN

M. MARZILLI
Istituto di Fisiologia-Clinica, via Savi 8, 56100 Pisa, Italy
Chapter 3

M.S. NORELL
The London Chest Hospital, Bonner Road, E2 9JX London, U.K.
Chapter 15 co-author: R. BALCON

A.C. PEARSON
Division of Cardiology, St. Louis University, 1325 S. Grand Blvd., St. Louis Mo 63104, U.S.A.
Chapter 17 co-authors: A.J. LABOVITZ, M. KERN and M. VANDORMAEL

P.A. POOLE-WILSON
The Cardiothoracic Institute, 2 Beaumont Street, London W1N 2DX, U.K.
Chapter 8

P.W. SERRUYS
Erasmus University, Thoraxcenter, P.O. Box 1738, 3000 DR Rotterdam, The Netherlands
Chapter 2 co-authors: B. JASKI, F. PISCIONE, F. ten KATE, P. de FEYTER, M. van den BRAND and P.G. HUGENHOLTZ
Chapter 7 co-authors: F. ZIJLSTRA, H.C. REIBER, K. BEATT, G.J. LAARMAN, J. ROELANDT and P.J. de FEYTER
Chapter 9 co-authors: F. PISCIONE, W. WIJNS, J.A.J. HEGGE, E. HARMSEN, M. van den BRAND, P. de FEYTER, P.G. HUGENHOLTZ and J.W. de JONG
Chapter 18 co-authors: F. PISCIONE, W. WIJNS, C. SLAGER, P. de FEYTER, M. van den BRAND, P.G. HUGENHOLTZ and G.T. MEESTER

R. SIMON
Department of Cardiology, University Hospital, 2300 Kiel, F.R.G.
Chapter 21 co-authors: G. HERRMANN, I. AMENDE, G.H. REIL and
P.R. LICHTLEN

M. SIMOONS
Erasmus University, Thoraxcenter, P.O. Box 1738, 3000 DR Rotterdam, The
Netherlands
Chapter 25 co-authors: P.J. de FEYTER and H. SURYAPRANATA

H. SURYAPRANATA
Erasmus University, Thoraxcenter, P.O. Box 1738, 3000 DR Rotterdam, The
Netherlands
Chapter 24 co-authors: P.J. de FEYTER and P.W. SERRUYS

J.M. SUTTON
The University of Michigan, Medical Center, B1 F245 University Hospital, Ann
Arbor, Michigan 48109-0022, U.S.A.
Chapter 26 co-author: E.J. TOPOL

H. TILLMANNS
Ruprecht-Karls-Universität, Bergheimerstrasse 58, 6900 Heidelberg 1, F.R.G.
Chapter 11 co-authors: R. ZIMMERMANN, W.H. KNAP, F. HELUS, P.
GEORGI, B. BRAUCH, F.-J. NEUMANN, S. GIRGENSOHN,
W. MAIER-BORST and W. KÜBLER

C.A. VISSER
Academisch Medisch Centrum, Meibergdreef 9, 1105 AZ Amsterdam, The
Netherlands
Chapter 16 co-authors: J.J. KOOLEN, G.K. DAVID and A.J. DUNNING

A. ZALEWSKI
Thomas Jefferson University Hospital, 111 South 11th Street, Philadelphia, PA
19107, U.S.A.
Chapter 19 co-authors: M. SAVAGE and S. GOLDBERG

PART ONE

An investigational tool

1. Myocardial ischemia

Early adjustment and reversibility

GUY R. HEYNDRICKX, WILLIAM WIJNS and STEPHEN F. VATNER

While the effects of permanent coronary occlusion on the global left ventricular function have been studied for centuries, it is only during the last decade that attention has been focused on the effects of transient ischemia on regional myocardial function. It is now established that intense, transient, regional myocardial ischemia may develop, not only from an imbalance between myocardial metabolic demand but also from a primary reduction in coronary blood flow, arising from either arterial spasm, thrombotic events or platelet aggregation [1]. In addition short ischemic insults are routinely inflicted to the myocardium in patients with coronary artery disease during angioplasty.

The goal of this chapter is to review some pertinent features of transient myocardial ischemia with respect to its effect on regional function: (a) the mechanical response of the myocardium to ischemia during transient episodes of myocardial ischemia, and (b) the reversibility to derangements in myocardial function with reperfusion during brief coronary artery occlusion, insufficient to induce infarction.

Instrumentation techniques for measurements of regional myocardial function in conscious animals

As early as 1698 isolated observations on the effect of acute coronary artery ligation in animals are recorded in the literature [2] but it is not until 1935 that Tennant and Wiggers described in a quantitative manner the sequential changes in myocardial contractions which occur following occlusion of a major coronary artery in dogs using an optical myograph [3]. These authors for the first time documented that within 60 sec of coronary occlusion the ischemic zone changed from a state of active systolic shortening to one of passive systolic elongation. This accurate description of the transient changes occurring upon inducing ischemia were confirmed by several investigators, using a variety of invasive and non invasive techniques in anesthetized, open-chest animals [4–6].

The development of miniature ultrasonic transducers has allowed accurate

P.W. Serruys, R. Simon & K.J. Beatt (eds), Percutaneous Transluminal Coronary Angioplasty. ISBN 0-7923-0346-6.
© *1990 Kluwer Academic Publishers, Dordrecht*

and continuous measurement of regional segment length and wall thickness in anesthetized open-chest animals [7–10], but more importantly has made these measurements routinely possible in conscious animals in which the potential complicating effects of general anesthesia and recent surgery are avoided [11–14]. These devices are implanted in the left ventricular (LV) wall, where they are able to move freely with the surrounding myocardium without interfering with the contraction, providing a more physiological measurement of regional function. Arrays of crystal pairs can be used to measure myocardial function over a sizable region of the left ventricle [11, 13, 15] (Fig. 1). Ultrasonic crystals

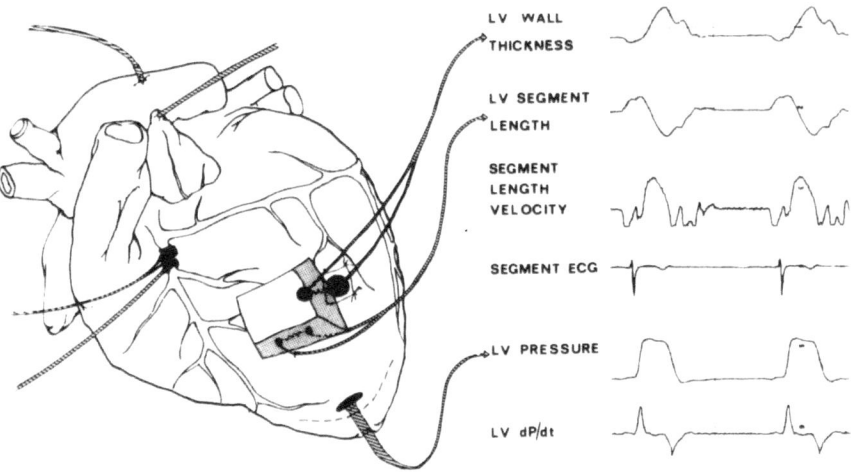

Figure 1. The techniques utilized are shown schematically. Catheters were implanted in the left atrium and aorta to measure pressures and utilize the radioactive microsphere technique. A miniature pressure gauge was implanted in the left ventricle to measure pressure and dP/dt. Miniature electronic transducers were implanted 1–2 cm apart to measure segment length and regional electrocardiograms and across the ventricular wall to measure wall thickness. The endocardial wall thickness transducer was implanted at an angle of 45° to avoid injury to the myocardium between the two transducers. (From Heyndrickx et al, *Am J Physiol* 234: H653 (1978). Reprinted with permission).

implanted in the endocardium and across the myocardial wall have been utilized to measure endocardial segment shortening and wall thickening, respectively [16]. These techniques are superior to other methods to assess regional function. For example, although echocardiography has the potential advantage of being totally atraumatic, this technique suffers a number of shortcomings when it comes to LV regional function analysis. M-mode echocardiography is limited to measurements of wall motion of the posterior wall and septum while two dimensional echocardiography has a much lower resolution for the endocardial surface [17–20].

Relationship between reduction in regional blood flow and myocardial function

Myocardial mechanical function is dependent primarily on its blood supply, since arteriovenous oxygen extraction is near-maximal in the normal heart and anaerobic reserves are minimal [21]. Accordingly, it is generally recognized that reduction in myocardial blood flow results in impaired mechanical function. Furthermore, since myocardial function is the result of a delicate balance between supply and demand, even maintained arterial inflow in the face of augmented myocardial metabolic demand might cause reduction in myocardial function. Earlier studies in open-chest preparations used either less sensitive measures of regional myocardial function [22–24] or a less sensitive indicator of regional myocardial blood flow [22–25]. Weintraub et al [26] observed in anesthetized, open-chest dogs a sigmoidal relationship between regional blood flow measured with radio-active microspheres and endocardial segment length shortening, such that large reduction in blood flow are required to give significant reductions in shortening. Vatner has recently addressed the question of flow-function relationship during acute graded levels of coronary stenosis in conscious dogs [14]. Regional endocardial segment shortening was measured by the ultrasonic dimension technique and correlated with endocardial blood flow measured by the radioactive microsphere technique. The endocardium was chosen as the site for these measurements because myocardial ischemia tends to be most severe in subendocardial regions [27–29]. An excellent correlation between segment shortening and regional blood flow was obtained using an exponential function (Fig. 2). Significant impairment in function was found with only 10 to 20% reductions in blood flow. Severe reduction in blood flow was required to reduce function completely. In segment exhibiting paradoxical systolic lengthening, blood flow was reduced by 90% from control levels. In segments exhibiting only akinesia blood flow was also significantly reduced (-80%) but less so than in segments with paradoxical motion. These data indicate that small reductions in blood flow can significantly impair function, but severe reductions in flow are required to eliminate shortening, indicating sensitive coupling between blood flow and endocardial segment shortening.

Considerable controversy surrounds the question of whether a significant zone of intermediate ischemia surrounds the central ischemic zone. A number of studies have supported the concept of a zone of intermediate ischemia based on analysis of myocardial blood flow [30–31]. However, analysis of tissue containing an admixture of ischemic and nonischemic myocardium would yield intermediate reductions in blood flow. Other studies, in which efforts were made to minimize or account for admixture of ischemic and nonischemic tissue, showed a sharp interface between ischemic and nonischemic tissue without a significant zone of intermediate ischemia [32–33]. Thus, it appears that under many conditions after acute coronary artery occlusion, normally perfused myocardium can exist adjacent to severely ischemic tissue. In a study of conscious dogs Cox and Vatner measured endocardial segment shortening in segments subtending severely ischemic and adjacent, normally perfused myocardium [34]. Surprisingly, rather

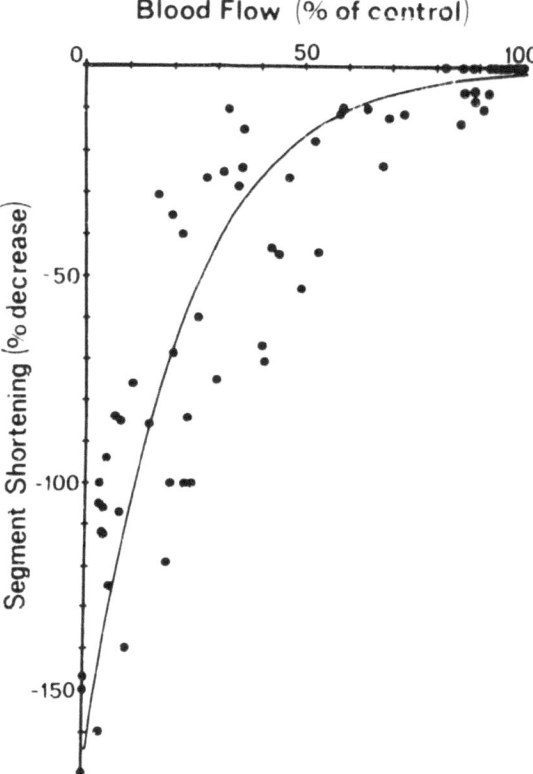

Figure 2. The curvilinear relationship between percentage of decreases in regional segment length (SL) shortening (ordinate) are plotted against decreases in regional myocardial blood flow (BF) as percentage of control. (From Vatner SF *Circulation Research* 47: 201 (1980). Reproduced with permission).

than exhibiting a magnitude of segment shortening intermediate between that observed in ischemic and remote nonischemic myocardium, these segments exhibited severe dysfunction indistinguishable from that in homogeneously ischemic segments in the central ischemic zone. In homogeneously nonischemic segments adjacent to the ischemic zone, shortening was reduced by approximately 50%, supporting the concept that myocardial dysfunction extends beyond the ischemic zone [35, 36]. That is, there is a divergence in the expected close correlation between blood flow and function that occurs at the ischemic 'border', with greater reduction in function than would be expected from measurement of myocardial blood flow.

Adjustment to global LV ischemia

Since reduction in blood flow in one coronary artery induces regional changes in myocardial functon, which differs in various portions of the left ventricle, alteration in performance observed with regional myocardial ischemia may reflect not only the behaviour of the ischemic myocardium but also some interaction of the adjacent normally perfused myocardium on the ischemic segments. On the other hand, if the ventricle were homogeneously ischemic, such interaction would be eliminated and only the direct effect would be exhibited.

Global myocardial ischemia obtaind by occluding the left main coronary artery in dogs to obtain homogeneous flow reduction of 80% produces striking hemodynamic effects. The progressive impairment in systolic shortening is accompanied by a large increase in end-diastolic pressure and a dramatic fall in LV dP/dt (Fig. 3) [37]. Three important observations from these experiments

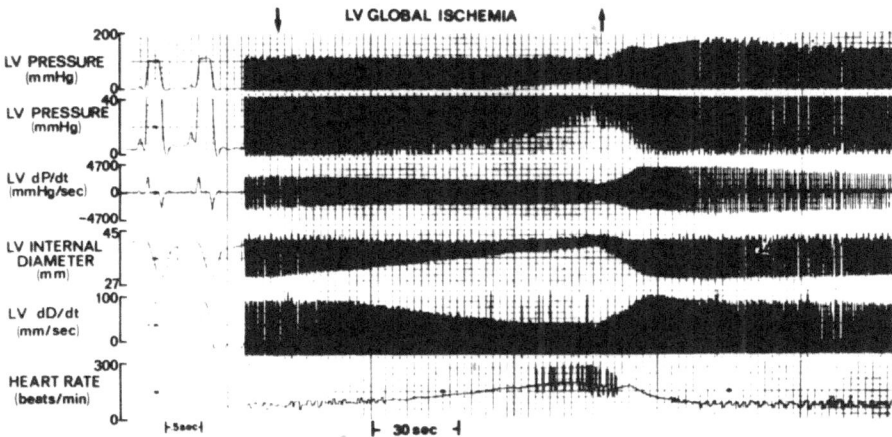

Figure 3. A typical recording of left ventricular (LV) pressure, end diastolic pressure, dP/dt, internal diameter, dP/dt (velocity) and heart rate in a conscious dog is shown for an experiment of global LV ischemia. The period of constriction of the left main coronary artery is indicated by the arrows. Note the dissociation between the extent and rate of shortening early during ischemia and the overshoot in function upon reperfusion (From Pagani et al, *Circulation Research* 43: 83 (1978). Reproduced with permission).

should be noted: First, there is only a slight increase in end diastolic diameter, even at the point of maximum function impairment despite large increases in filling pressure which indicate that the Frank-Starling mechanism plays little role during acute left heart failure. Secondly, the loss of function during the development of ischemia is characterized by a dissociation between shortening on the one hand and velocity of shortening on the other hand. Velocity declines later in time and to a lesser degree than both shortening and work. This observation supports the concept as proposed by several investigators that the maximum velocity of shortening of the unloaded muscle and the force generated by the cardiac muscle may be dependent upon different mechanisms with different time constants, suggesting that early ischemia might shorten the duration of active state while affecting its intensity only slightly. Finally, upon reperfusion LV function not only returned to control levels but is characterized by a transient significant overshoot in function.

Adjustment to regional myocardial ischemia

Brief periods of acute myocardial ischemia induce complex dynamic changes in regional myocardial performance (Fig. 4). Following abrupt occlusion of

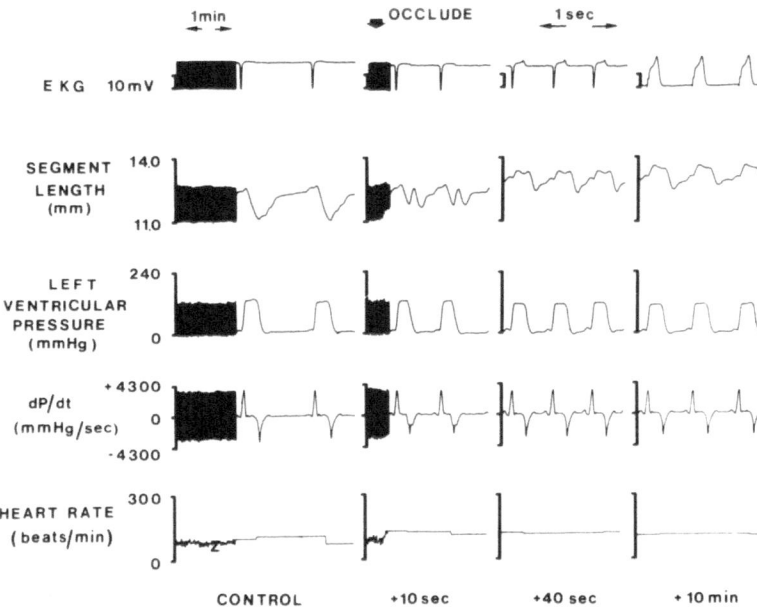

Figure 4. Tracings of intramyocardial ECG, segment length, left ventricular pressure, dP/dt and heart rate during control, during coronary occlusion at 10, 40 sec and 10 min. Arrow indicates the time of occlusion. With the onset of ischemia there is an early systolic lengthening followed by late systolic shortening ('W' phenomenon). At 40 min active shortening is abolished and replaced by passive systolic expansion. The peak rate of LV pressure decay (dP/dt) is reduced and delayed at 10 sec to return to preocclusion level when holosystolic expansion is complete. Note the late intramyocardial ECG changes. (From Heyndrickx et al, *Coronary Heart Disease.* 3th International Symposium. Ed. Kaltenbach et al, Georg Thieme Publishers, Stuttgart 1978. Reproduced with permission).

a coronary artery, the earliest observed change in severely ischemic segments is a small late systolic lengthening, followed by a late secondary shortening of the ischemic segment, beginning with a few beats after the onset of ischemia [8, 38–41], presumably as the result of a diminished duration of contraction with hypoxia [40, 42]. Therefore, the ischemic segment would transiently reach its end diastolic length immediately after closure of the aortic valve, only to shorten again when ventricular pressure fell. A progressive reduction in the duration and extent of shortening occurs until there is a paradoxical holosystolic lengthening of the ischemic segment by 30 to 60 sec after occlusion [8, 37, 38, 41], which persists as long as the occlusion is maintained. These changes are associated with an increase in end diastolic length of the ischemic segment [8, 37, 38, 41]. The decline in the velocity of segment shortening lags several seconds behind the decline in shortening, not being manifested up to 10 to 15 seconds after the onset of ischemia, when shortening is already reduced [37] (Fig 5). This is consistent

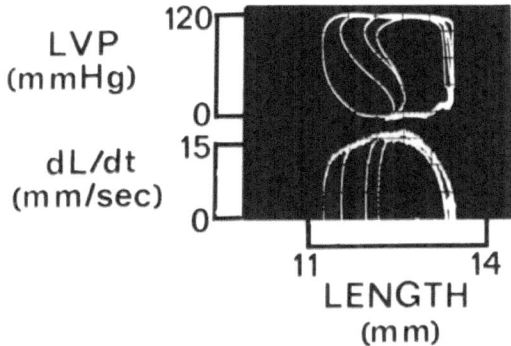

Figure 5. Recordings of pressure-length loops at the top and length-velocity relations (phase-plane plot) at the bottom for one LV segment before occlusion (outer loop) and at 5, 10 and 15 sec into the induction of regional myocardial ischemia. Note the marked disparity between the reduction in extent and rate of shortening during the onset of ischemia (From Pagani et al, *Circulation Research* 43: 83 (1978). Reproduced with permission).

with experiments in isolated isometrically contracting papillary muscle, which showed that the rate of force generated was less sensitive to hypoxia than the amount of force generated [43].

Coincident with these transient changes in the ischemic segment motion, peak rate of left ventricular pressure fall i.e.: negative dP/dt was reduced as much as 40% before returning to preocclusion levels as soon as the ischemic segment lost complete active shortening. This abnormality in LV relaxation occurred as a result of asynchronous systolic contraction of the ischemic segments. Once the ischemic segments was bulging paradoxically and the asynchrony in contraction had disappeared, global LV relaxation is less abnormal.

Pressure-length loops derived from instantaneous plots of left ventricular pressure and epicardial [39–40] or subendocardial [37–38] segment length have been used to provide an index of regional myocardial work, (Fig. 6). Within seconds after the onset of regional ischemia, the morphology of the pressure-length loop changes as a consequence of late systolic lengthening followed by additional

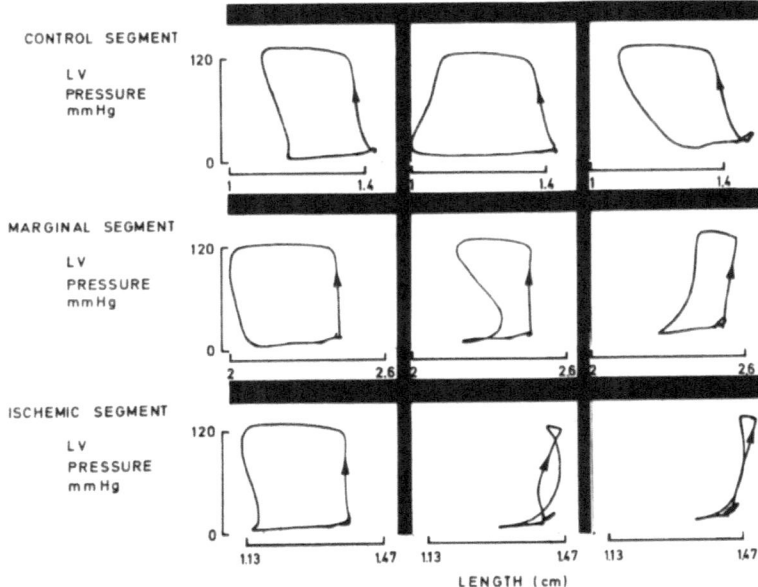

Figure 6. Pressure-length loops of the three segments: A) the control state, B) early after coronary occlusion (about 10 sec) and C) the steady state during coronary occlusion (about 2 min). In A the normal loops rotate counterclockwise. In B, reduced systolic shortening and a marked lengthening during the isovolumetric relaxation phase are apparent in the marginal and ischemic segments; this is more marked and gives rise to a figure-of-eight inscription of the loop in the ischemic segment, and the late systolic length is larger than that at end diastole. Also in B, the control segment shows a relatively normal shortening pattern until late in systole, then additional shortening occurs coincident with the lengthening in the other two segments; thus unloading is apparent in the control segment. In C, during the fall in LV pressure, both ischemic and marginal segments shorten, whereas the control segment lengthens. Work (the area within the loop) in the ischemic zone is near zero. (From Theroux et al, *Circulation* 43: 302 (1976). Reproduced with permission).

shortening, thereby reducing the area of the pressure-length loop even before overall systolic shortening is reduced. The late systolic shortening coincides with lengthening in the non-ischemic segment, suggesting either an unloading effect allowing prolonged active tension to express shortening when LV pressure has decreased, or a passive recoil effect. This temporary asynchronous contraction is reflected, as mentioned earlier by a temporary decrease in LV negative dP/dt. With the further reduction in shortening during the ejection phase, the loop assumes a crescent shape with an area approaching zero, a reduction significantly greater than expected from the reduction in shortening [37]. Within 30 sec of the onset of profound ischemia the segment exhibits holosystolic lengthening with the development of a clockwise pressure-length loop [38–40] (as opposed to the normal counterclockwise loop), implying that the mechanical energy is being dissipated into the ischemic segment. Changes in systolic wall thickening paralleled changes in segment shortening: as the extent and velocity of systolic shortening diminished, the degree and velocity of wall thickening decreased proportionally [16]. By 30 to 60 sec after coronary artery occlusion, when systolic segment shortening was replaced by holosystolic bulging, systolic wall thining was observed. In an elegant study, performed during PTCA of a coronary graft in a patient in which radiopaque epicardial markers had been implanted at the time of previous cardiac surgery, Jaski and Serruys, using biplane cineradiography for epicardial wall motion analysis observed identical transient changes in regional wall motion abnormality during myocardial ischemia induced upon balloon inflation, as observed in the experimental animal model [44].

Effects of reperfusion

After brief coronary artery occlusion a transient overshoot of regional function above preocclusion levels has been observed after reperfusion in anesthetized [43] and in conscious animals [37]. With release of a 100 sec occlusion this transient overshoot was characterized by increases in regional stroke work as reflected by the area of the pressure-length loop, as well as the extent and velocity of shortening [37]. The overshoot was not dependent on adrenergic mechanisms, but was prevented by inhibiting reactive hyperemia. When this restriction to reperfusion was released, the delayed reactive hyperemia was accompanied by a delayed overshoot in function. When reactive hyperemia was prevented by even longer coronary artery constriction following release of coronary occlusion, an overshoot in regional function above preocclusion levels is not observed.

When perfusion is restored within 20 min after the onset of ischemia, regional flow, electrocardiograms as well as regional function eventually returned to normal without permanent functional deficit. The oxygen debt incurred during the ischemic period will be repaid rapidly though the reactive hyperemic response lasts for several minutes, and its duration is roughly proportionally to the time of ischemia. It has been recognized for some time that after brief periods of myocardial ischemia (< 20 min) there is a rapid normalization of regional blood flow and electrocardiographic changes i.e.: ST-segment elevation (Fig. 7). From these observations one might predict that regional mechanical function also normalizes rapidly. This, however, was not the case. We observed, in conscious dogs, that ischemic segments exhibiting paradoxical or absent motion during a 5 min of coronary artery occlusion exhibited gradual return of regional endocardial function as well as LV wall thickening over the next 6 hr following coronary artery reperfusion [11] (Fig. 8). End diastolic segment length remained elevated and segment shortening and velocity of shortening were depressed at 2 hr and did not return completely to preocclusion levels until 6 hr after reperfusion. A 15 min occlusion resulted in derangement of function measured in terms of segment shortening [11] and wall thickening [16] which was even greater and more prolonged (Fig. 9). Evidence exists for several potential mechanisms for this prolonged dysfunction after brief periods of ischemia, termed

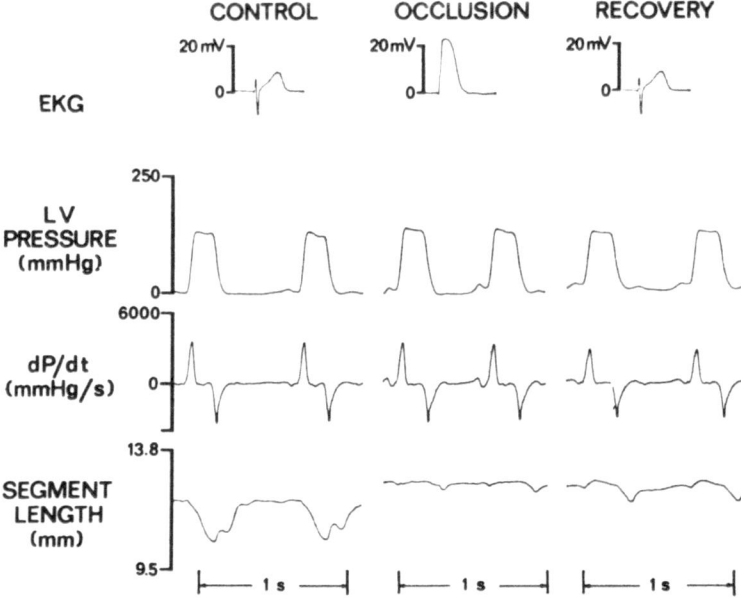

Figure 7. Effects of a 5 min left circumflex coronary occlusion on LV pressure dP/dt and segment length in the ischemic zone along with the electrogram from the ischemic zone (top). During coronary occlusion (middle panel) intense ischemia reflected by substantial ST segment elevation correlates well with impaired function in the ischemic zone, 5 min after release of occlusion, reperfusion and repayment of coronary flow debt (right panel), the electrogram is again completely normal, but regional function is still markedly deranged, i.e., the ischemic segment is expanding paradoxically during systole. (From Heyndrickx GR et al, *J Clin Invest* 56: 978 (1975). Reprinted with permission).

the 'stunned myocardium' [45]. In one study, endocardial blood flow remained significantly depressed 3 hr after reperfusion, following a 15-min occlusion in conscious dogs [16]. Another potential mechanism is impaired purine metabolism for prolonged periods of time after brief coronary artery occlusion [46–48]. Recent evidence however suggest that the 'stunned myocardium' is rather a problem of energy utilization and not of energy supply [49].

During the first few minutes of reperfusion after a 15-min occlusion, systolic segment shortening and wall thickening have been shown to be higher than that measured over the next few hours, paralleling the reactive hyperemic response [16–50], but still slightly lower than preocclusion control. Examining the effects of reperfusion on regional diastolic properties of the ischemic left ventricle, Hess et al [51] found that wall stiffness decreased significantly by 1 to 2 min after a 2-min partial or complete occlusion. Interestingly, after a 2- to 3-min complete occlusion in conscious dogs, Theroux et al [38] observed recovery of systolic function in ischemic segments within 2 min, but abnormal late shortening occurred during isovolumic relaxation in these segments for up to 45 min after release of the occlusion coinciding with an increase in the time constant of left

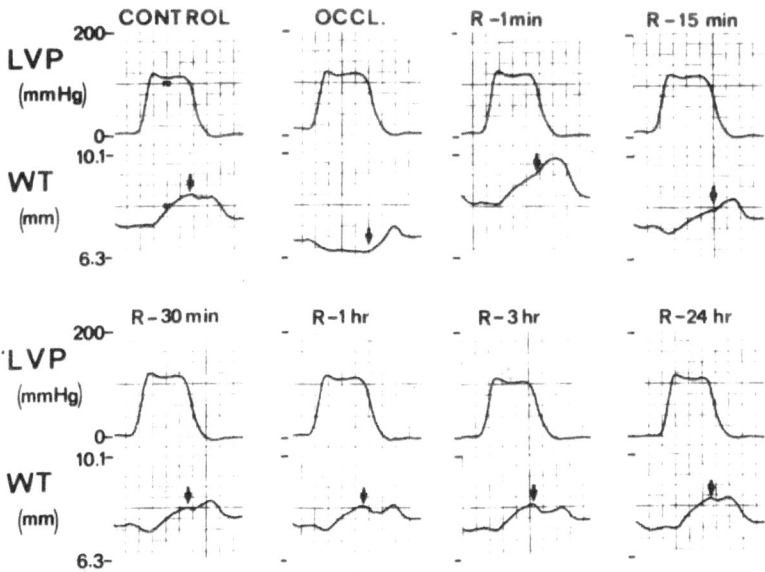

Figure 8. Tracings of left ventricular pressure (LVP) and wall thickness (WT) during control, during a 15 minute coronary occlusion, and at 1, 15 and 30 min, 1, 3 and 24 hr after reperfusion. Arrows denote end-systole. Peak systolic wall thickening was absent during occlusion, significantly prolonged early during reperfusion and significantly diminished up to the 24 hr recording. Complete return to normal for the wall thickness phasic waveform indicates the stability of the measurement and that no permanent damage had occurred. (From Heyndrickx GR et al, *Am J Physiol* 234: H653 (1978). Reproduced with permission.)

ventricular pressure decay suggesting persistent impairment of relaxation. Forrester et al [40] found a similar pattern after occlusions of varying durations.

The effects of repeat ischemia on the still unrecovered myocardium was recently studied by Lange et al [52]. These investigators sought to determine whether recurrent ischemia results in cumulative myocardial damage with subsequent stepwise decrease in regional function. They found that, although functional baseline is depressed after a first 15 min occlusion compared to control, the degree of functional recovery is similar during each reperfusion period after these consecutive occlusions. Increasing the number of ischemic episodes and shortening the length of reperfusion periods may ultimately lead to distinct area of subendocardial necrosis and evidence of irreversible ultrastructural damage as shown by Geft et al [54] suggesting that repetitive ischemic insults, which alone do not result in permanent cellular damage might eventually reach the limit of ischemic tolerance. On the other hand, repeat short occlusions of 5 min with ample reperfusion time (more than 30 min) in conscious dogs was shown to induce full development of functional collateral circulation after an average of 200 brief episodes of ischemia [53].

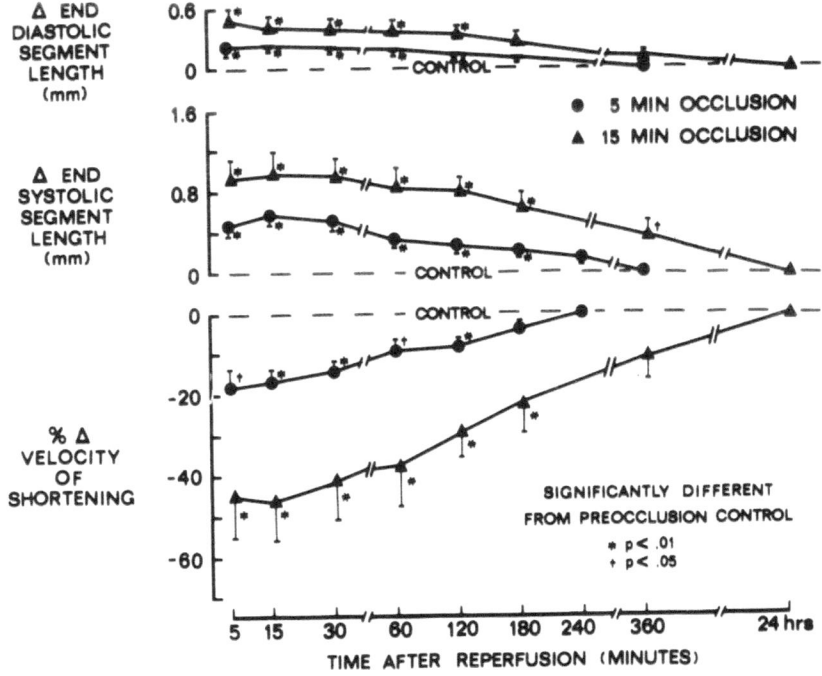

Figure 9. The prolonged recovery times for end-diastolic and end-systolic segment length and velocity of shortening after 5-min (circles) and 15-min (triangles) occlusions are compared. Recovery times from 5 min to 24 hr after reperfusion are shown. Values that were significantly different from control are shown by the asterisk (p < 0.01) and cross (p < 0.05). (From Heyndrickx GR et al, *J Clin Invest* 56: 978 (1975). Reprinted with permission).

Coronary artery stenosis versus coronary artery occlusion

The majority of experiments studying the reversibility of myocardial ischemia have been conducted in animals in which ischemia was induced either by a single episode of coronary artery occlusion of less than 20 min duration or by repetitive episodes of coronary artery occlusion [3, 8, 11, 14, 16, 37, 41, 48]. Less information is available concerning the myocardial adaptation to less severe oxygen deprivation as occurs with severe coronary artery stenosis [68].

We have recently observed that the myocardium subserved by a critical coronary artery stenosis, severe enough to abolish regional systolic function in the ischemic segment for one hour, displays upon reperfusion the same characteristics of stunned myocardium as observed after short episodes of total coronary artery occlusion: i.e. a prolonged depression of systolic contractile function for more than 24 hr. Full recovery of mechanical function with time is the rule, with no histologic evidence for myocardial necrosis despite a small but significant release of creatine kinase [65, 66]. This is at variance with what is observed after complete coronary artery occlusion of the same duration which results in some degree of permanent damage despite full reperfusion [27]. One may hypothetize that the persistance of some residual antegrade flow, although insufficient to maintain normal systolic contraction, nevertheless allows for washout of toxic metabolites and thereby preserves the potential for full recovery. Matsuzaki et al have previously demonstrated that a less severe coronary artery stenosis which only reduced sysolic wall thickening by 50 to 70% but maintained for 5 hr resulted also in prolonged moderate regional dysfunction for several days. In this model however considerable infarction of the posterior papillary muscle was observed [68]. These observations may be relevant to clinical situations such as unstable angina and its treatment.

To further characterize the metabolic alteration of the myocardium recovering from ischemia during the period of reperfusion, positron emission tomography (PET) was performed for metabolic imaging using C-11-palmitate (CPA) and 2-F fluorodeoxyglucose (FDG). We observed in this model that postischemic dysfunction is associated with a decrease in the fraction of exogenous CPA undergoing immediate oxidation as well as a decrease in its oxidation rate (Fig. 10). In addition, peak CPA uptake is slightly reduced despite normal oxygen and tracer delivery at the time of the PET study. A concomitant increase in FDG uptake suggests that stunned myocardium adapts with a shift in substrate utilization from free fatty acids to carbohydrates. This metabolic hallmark of

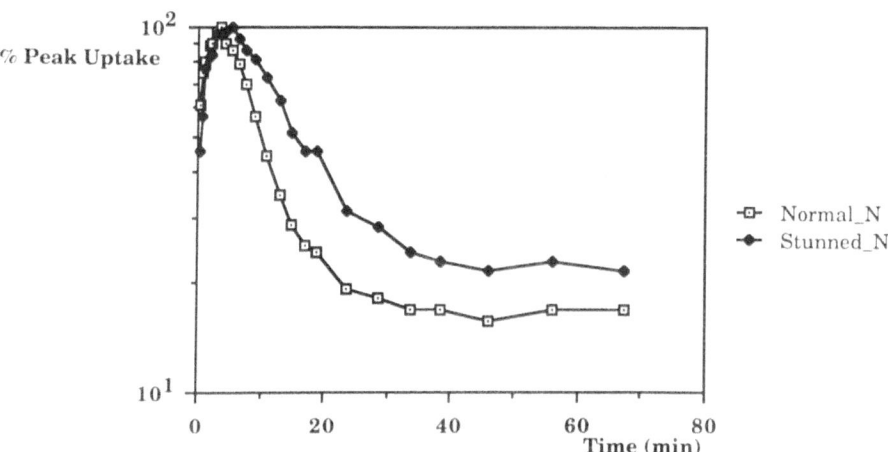

Figure 10. Time activity curves from C-11-palmitate tissue kinetics analysed by biexponential least square curve-fitting techniques are compared for normal zone (□) and stunned zone (♦) 12 hr after restoration of coronary flow to the myocardium, previously subjected to ischemia by 1 hr severe coronary artery stenosis. The halftime of early rapid phase is significantly prolonged from 3.7 min for normal zone to 8.5 min for the stunned zone, demonstrating a prolonged impairment in handling exogenous free fatty acids for energy utilization.

ongoing ischemia seems to persist for much longer periods than the ischemic process itself and is associated with prolonged postischemic dysfunction. The recovery of systolic mechanical function in the stunned zone is paralleled by normalization of CPA handling as reflected by CPA kinetics [67].

Enzyme leakage from ischemic myocardium

In clinical practice, demonstration of elevated plasma creatine kinase (CK) enzyme activity has been used as an important criterion for diagnosing myocardial infarction. This stems from the assumption that once cellular enzyme starts leaking from myocardial cells as the result of altered cellular permeability, the cellular injury has reached a stage of irreversible damage [55, 56]. In addition enzymatic estimation of infarct size experimentally as well as clinically, is based on the premise that release of enzymes from ischemic myocardium reflects irreversible injury.

Recent experiments performed in conscious baboons demonstrate that short periods (15 min) of coronary artery occlusion, which do not result in demonstrable myocardial necrosis or permanent derangement in regional myocardial function, are associated with a significant increase in plasma CK as well as in MB CK (Fig. 11). The peak increases in plasma total CK and MB CK activity occurred at 9.3 and 4.3 hr, respectively. The shorter time to peak activity for MB CK may be due to the shorter half life of MB CK as compared to total CK [57].

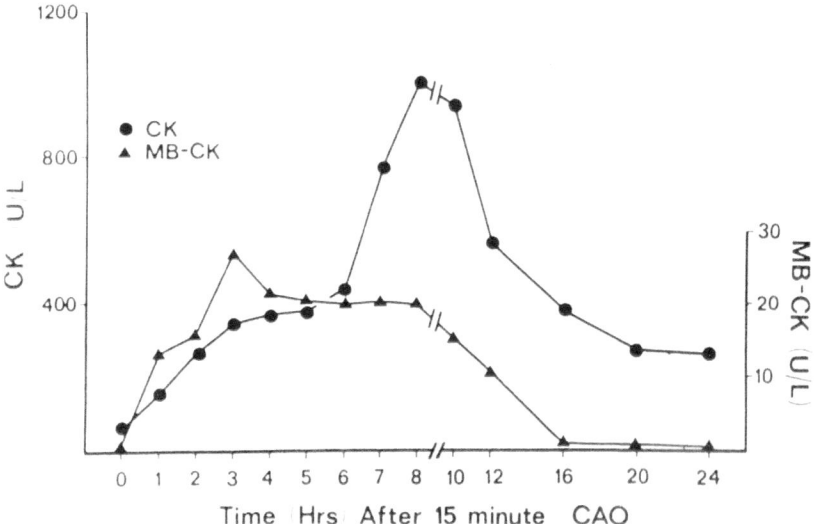

Figure 11. Time course of serial plasma total CK (circles) and CK MB isoenzyme (triangles) curves after 15 min coronary artery occlusions (CAO). (From Heyndrickx GR et al, *J Am Coll Card* (1985) in press. Reproduced with permission).

A similar plasma CK increase was observed in a different model of ischemia and reperfusion in conscious dogs i.e. a 1 hr critical coronary artery stenosis severe enough to abolish systolic contractile function [65, 66].

It was surprising to note that no early peak plasma enzyme activity was noted with the onset of reperfusion at 15 min as is systematically observed with reperfusion after coronary artery occlusions of longer duration (1 to 3 hr) in dogs [58]. This would suggest that either the brief ischemic insult or the insult of the reperfusion resulted in a derangement of membrane permeability, which was gradual in onset and although reversible, slow to recover. The finding that adenosine triphosphate (ATP) and the adenine nucleotide pool remained depressed for a prolonged period after a 15 min occlusion [46 – 48] suggests that the integrity of cellular membranes, which requires high energy phosphate, is still impaired long after the ischemic insult is over. A recent study by Piper et al [60] showed that there is a gradual release of cytosolic enzymes from reversibly injured myocardial cells in culture, which is also consistent with our results in conscious baboons. It is also conceivable that the enzymes, released from myocardial cells, are preferentially drained by the lymphatic channels, which have a relatively low flow rate and therefore delay the appearance of enzyme in the blood [61]. Our results, however, are at variance with the data presented by Ahmed et al [56], who demonstrated that short episodes of ischemia (< 30 min) in conscious dogs did not result in elevated plasma MB CK activity or histologic evidence of myocardial necrosis. However, there are several important consequences due to differences in the species studied. Species differences in resistance to ischemia have been demonstrated by Hearse et al (62). In addition, the percent of MB isoenzyme activity in the heart varies among species. In dogs, the MB fraction accounts for approximately 2 to 3% of total CK; whereas, according to Yasmineh et al [63], the MB fraction accounts for approximately 17% in baboons. With the techniques utilized in our experiments, the MB fraction in the baboon heart was determined to be 9% of the total CK. However, since no MB CK was found in skeletal muscle of the baboon, we expected that MB CK measured in the blood samples after transient myocardial ischemia arose from the heart. It is also important to note that the reduction in blood flow was more intense and homogenously distributed across the myocardial wall in the baboon compared to dogs. However, a recent study by Michael et al also found CK release in the cardiac lymph in conscious dogs after brief coronary artery occlusions, insufficient to induce necrosis [64]. Thus, it appears that all episodes of transient myocardial ischemia which occur with elevation of MB CK in the blood do not result in myocardial infarction. The clinical implications of these findings are extremely important, since it has been suggested, but not proven that this phenomenon can also occur in patients with transient myocardial ischemia.

Reperfusion injury

The concept, that restoring both adequate coronary perfusion and oxygenation to ischemic myocardial cells, which have retained their potential for full functional recovery, may induce substantial injury, has gained wide acceptance [69–72]. Among several important observations that have been accumulated in recent years in support of this thesis, the formation of high concentration of oxygen free radicals at the time of reperfusion and the calcium overload induced by reperfusion have been proposed as major mechanisms to explain the additional functional impairment inflicted to the myocardium upon reperfusion. The actual demonstration of high concentration of oxygen free radicals upon reperfusion by nuclear magnetic resonance as well as the beneficial effect of 0_2 scavengers on the mechanical recovery of the stunned myocardium points towards a cause-effect relationship. In addition, the concept of calcium overload seems real in the light that reperfusion with low calcium concentration prevents myocardial stunning. It is not clear yet whether the production of oxygen free radicals and the calcium overload are two distinct unrelated mechanisms for creating reperfusion injury. In addition, the clinical relevancy of reperfusing injury in the light of the undisputable beneficial effect of early reperfusion is still a matter of debate.

Summary

Myocardial contractile function is sensitive even to minor alterations in coronary blood flow. An excellent correlation is found between reduction of flow and decrease in segment length shortening. Acute cessation in blood flow in a major coronary artery induces a particular sequence of events whereby active systolic shortening is replaced by passive elongation in the ischemic segment. This functional deficit occurs gradually over time and is initially characterized by delayed and reduced extent of systolic shortening of the ischemic segment resulting in a temporary asynchronous contraction, affecting early left ventricular relaxation profoundly. A short ischemic insult to the myocardium, of less than 20 min duration, as a consequence of a temporary acute reduction in coronary blood flow, severe enough to abolish active regional systolic shortening has a significant and prolonged stunning effect on the myocardium. Despite an immediate functional rebound in the ischemic zone upon reperfusion, probably due to local mechanisms, complete recovery of systolic shortening is delayed and requires several hours. This period of prolonged functional impairment is associated with a decrease in free fatty acid utilization by the myocardial cells in favor for increased carbohydrate utilization. In addition, although cellular integrity is disrupted for quite some time allowing creatine kinase to egress from myocardial cells, no permanent damange is observed after brief episodes of myocardial ischemia. The features characterizing stunned myocardium have recently been observed in a model of less severe myocardial ischemia, induced by prolonged coronary artery stenosis rather than total coronary artery occlusion.

References

1. Maseri A, Chierchia S, Kaski JC (1985) Mixed angina pectoris. *Am J Cardiol* 56:30E
2. See G Bochefontaine et Roussy (1881) Arrêt rapide des contractions rhythmiques des ventricules cardiaques sous l'influence de l'occlusion des artères coronaires. *Comptes Rendus* 92:86
3. Tennant R, Wiggers CJ (1935) The effect of coronary occlusion on myocardial contraction *Am J Physiol* 112:351
4. Sayen JJ, Sheldon WF, Peirce G; Kuo PT (1958) Polarographic oxygen, the epicardial electrocardiogram, and muscle contraction in experimental acute regional ischemia of the left ventricle. *Circ Res* 6:779
5. Tatooles CJ, Randall WC (1961) Local ventricular bulging after acute coronary occlusion. *Am J Physiol* 210:451
6. Schelbert HR, Covell JW, Burns JW, Maroko PR, Ross J Jr (1971) Observations on factors affecting local forces in the left ventricular wall during acute myocardial ischemia. *Circ Res* 29:306
7. Bugge-Asperheim B, Leraand S, Kiil F (1969) Local dimensional changes of the myocardium by ultrasonic technique. *Scand J Clin Lab Invest* 24:361
8. Theroux P, Franklin D, Ross J, Jr Kemper WS (1974) Regional myocardial function during acute coronary artery occlusion and its modification by pharmacologic agents in the dog. *Circ Res* 35:896
9. Gallagher KP, Kumada T, Koziol JA, McKown MD, Kemper WS Ross J, Jr (1980) Significance of regional wall thickening abnormalities relative to transmural myocardial perfusion in anesthetized dogs. *Circulation* 62:1266
10. Gallagher KP, Osakada G, Hess OM, Koziol JA, Kemper WS Ross J, Jr (1982) Subepicardial segmental function during coronary stenosis and the role of myocardial fiber orientation. *Circ Res* 50:352
11. Heyndrickx GR, Millard RW, McRitchie RJ, Maroko PR, Vatner SF (1975) Regional myocardial function and electrophysiological alterations after brief coronary artery occlusion in conscious dogs. *J Clin Invest* 56:978
12. Sasayama S, Franklin D, Ross J, Jr, Kemper WS McKnown D (1976) Dynamic changes in left ventricular wall thickness and their use in analyzing cardiac function in the conscious dog. A study based on a modified ultrasonic technique. *Am J Cardiol* 38:870
13. Roan P, Scales F, Saffer S, Buja M, Willerson JT (1979) Functional characterization of left ventricular segmental responses during the initial 24 h and 1 wk after experimental canine myocardial infarction. *J Clin Invest* 64:1074
14. Vatner SF (1980) Correlation between acute reduction in myocardial blood flow and function in conscious dogs. *Circ Res* 47:201
15. Ross J, Jr, Franklin D (1976) Analysis of regional myocardial function, dimensions and wall thickness in the characterization of myocardial ischemia and infarction. *Circulation* 53 (Suppl I):1–88
16. Heyndrickx GR, Baig H, Nellens P, Leusen I, Fishbein MC, Vatner SF (1978) Depression of regional blood flow and wall thickening after brief coronary occlusions. *Am J Physiol* 234:H653
17. Kerber RE, Abboud EM (1973) Echocardiographic detection of regional myocardial infarction. An experimental study. *Circulation* 47:997
18. Kerber RE, Marcus ML; Ehrhardt J, Wilson R, Abboud EM (1975) Correlation between echocardiographically demonstrated segmental dyskinesis and regional myocardial perfusion. *Circulation* 52:1097
19. Lieberman AN, Weiss JL, Jugdutt BI, Becker LC, Bulkley BH, Garrison JG, Hutchins GM, Kallman CA, Weisfeldt ML (1981) Two-dimentional echocardiography and infarct size: Relationship of regional wall motion and thickening to the extent of myocardial infarction in the dog. *Circulation* 65:739
20. Wyatt HL, Meerbaum S, Heng MK, Rit J, Gueret P, Corday E (1981) Experimental evaluation of

the extent of myocardial dyssynergy and infarct size by two-dimensional echocardiography. *Circulation* 63:607

21. Feigl E (1983) Coronary Physiology. *Physiol Rev* 1–203
22. Banka VS, Bodenheimer MM, Helfant RH (1977) Relation between progressive decrease in regional coronary perfusion and contractile abnormalities. *Am. J. Cardiol* 40:200
23. Waters DD, Daluz PL, Wyatt HL, Swan HJC, Forrester JS (1977) Early changes in regional and global left ventricular function induced by graded reductions in regional coronary perfusion. *Am J Cardiol* 39:537
24. Wyatt HL, Forrester JS, Tyberg JV, Goldner S, Logan SE, Parmley WW, Swan HJC (1975) Effect of graded reductions in regional coronary perfusion on regional and total cardiac function. *Am J Cardiol* 36:185
25. Stowe DF, Mathey DG, Moores WY, Glantz SA, Townsend RM, Kabra P, Chatterjee K, Parmley WW, Tyberg JV (1978) Segment stroke work and metabolism depend on coronary blood flow in the pig. *Am J Physiol* 234:H597
26. Weintraub WS, Hattori S, Agarwal JB, Bodenheimer MM, Banka VS, Helfant RH (1981) The relation between myocardial blood flow and contraction by myocardial layer in the canine left ventricle during ischemia. *Circ Res* 48:430
27. Lavallee M, Cox D, Patrick TA, Vatner SF (1983) Salvage of myocardial function by coronary artery reperfusion 1, 2 and 3 hours after occlusion in conscious dogs. *Circ Res* 53:235
28. Salisbury PF, Cross CE, Rieben PA (1963) Acute ischemia of the inner layers of the ventricular wall. *Am Heart J* 66:650
29. Buckberg GD, Fixler DE, Archie JP (1972) Experimental subendocardial ischemia in dogs with normal coronary arteries. *Circ Res* 30:67
30. Becker LC, Ferreira R, Thomas M (1973) Mapping of left ventricular blood flow with radioactive microspheres in experimental coronary artery occlusion. *Cardiovasc Res* 7:391
31. Jugdutt BI, Hutchins GM, Bulkley BH, Becker LC (1979) Myocardial infarction in the conscious dog: Three-dimensional mapping of infarct, collateral flow and region at risk. *Circulation* 60:1141
32. Hirzel HO, Sonnenblick EH, Kirk ES (1977) Absence of a lateral border zone of intermediate creatine phophokinase depletion surrounding a central infarct 24 hours after acute coronary occlusion in the dog. *Circ Res* 41:673
33. Murdock RH, Harlan DM, Morris JJ, Pryor WW, Jr, Cobb FR (1983) Transitional blood flow zones between ischemic and nonischemic myocardium in the awake dog. Analysis based on distribution of the intramural vasculature. *Circ Res* 52:451
34. Cox DA, Vatner SF (1982) Myocardial function in areas of heterogeneous perfusion after coronary artery occlusion in conscious dogs. *Circulation* 66:1154
35. Melin J, Becker LC, Kallman C, Weisfeldt ML, Weis JL (1982) Impaired thickening of non-ischemic myocardium during acute regional transmural ischemia in the dog. *Circ* 66 II:1,n
36. Gallagher KP, Gerren RA, Stirling MC, Choy M, Schlafer M, Buda AJ (1985) Systolic wall thickening at the lateral margins of ischemic myocardium in conscious dogs. *Circ* III:67
37. Pagani M, Vatner SF, Baig H, Braunwald E (1978) Initial myocardial adjustments to brief periods of ischemia and reperfusion in the conscious dog. *Circ Res* 43:83
38. Theroux P, Ross J, Jr, Franklin D, Kemper WS, Sasayama S (1976) Regional myocardial function in the conscious dog during acute coronary occlusion and responses to morphine, propranolol, nitroglycerin and lidocaine. *Circulation* 53:302
39. Tyberg JV, Forrester JS, Wyatt HL, Goldner SJ, Parmley WW, Swan HJC (1974) An analysis of segmental ischemic dysfunction utilizing the pressure-length loop. *Circulation* 49:748
40. Forrester JS, Wyatt HL, DaLuz PL, Tyberg JV, Diamond GA, Swan HJC (1976) Functional significance of regional ischemic contraction abnormalities. *Circulation* 54:64
41. Kumada T, Karliner JS, Pouleur H, Gallagher KP, Shirato K, Ross J, Jr (1979) Effects of coronary occlusion on early ventricular diastolic events in conscious dogs. *Am J Physiol* 237:H542
42. Weigner AW, Allen GJ, Bing OHL (1978) Weak and strong myocardium in series: Implications for segmental dysfunction. *Am J Physiol* 235:H776

43. Tyberg JV, Yeatman LA, Parmley WW, Urschel CW, Sonnenblick EH (1970) Effects of hypoxia on mechanisms of cardiac contraction. *Am J Physiol* 218:1780
44. Jaski BE, Serruys PW (1985) Epicardial wall motion and left ventricular function during coronary graft angioplasty in humans. *J Am Coll Cardiol* 6:695–700
45. Braunwald E, Kloner RA (1982) The stunned myocardium: Prolonged, postischemic ventricular dysfunction. *Circulation* 66:1146
46. Fox AC, Reed GE, Meilman H, Silk BB (1979) Release of nucleotides from canine and human hearts as an index of primary ischemia. *Am J Cardiol* 43:52
47. De Boer LWV, Ingwall JS, Kloner RA, Braunwald E (1980) Prolonged derangements of canine myocardial purine metabolism after a brief coronary artery occlusion not associated with anatomic evidence of necrosis. *Proc Natl Acad Sci USA* 77:5471
48. Swain JL, Sabina RL, McHale PA, Greenfield JC, Jr, Holmes EW (1982) Prolonged myocardial nucleotide depletion after brief ischemia in the open-chest dog. *Am J Physiol* 242:H818
49. Schaper W, Backwald A (1985) Hoffmeister HM, 'Stunned Myocardium' is a problem of energy utilization and not of energy supply. *Circulation* 72:III–19
50. Tomoda H, Parmley WW, Fujimura S, Matloff JM (1971) Effects of ischemia and reoxygenation on regional myocardial performance of the dog. *Am J Physiol* 221:1718
51. Hess OM, Osakada G, Lavelle JF, Gallagher KP, Kemper WS, Ross J, Jr (1983) Diastolic myocardial wall stiffness and ventricular relaxation during partial and complete coronary occlusions in the conscious dog. *Cir Res* 52:387
52. Lange R, Ware J, Kloner RA (1984) Absence of a cumulative deterioration of regional function during three repeated 5 or 15 minute coronary occlusions. *Circulation* 69:400
53. Shimokawa H, Tomoike H, Nabeyama S, Yamamoto H, Nakumara H (1983) A new aspect of collateral development with repeated brief coronary occlusion in conscious dogs. *Circulation* 68:III–306
54. Geft IL, Fishbein MC, Ninomiya K, Hashide J, Chaux E, Yano J, Y-Rit J, Genov T, Shell W, Ganz W (1980) Intermittent brief periods of ischemia have a cumulative effect and may cause myocardial necrosis. *Circ* 66:1150
55. Sobel BE, Shell WE (1972) Serum enzyme determination in the diagnosis and assessment of myocardial infarction. *Circ* 45:472
56. Ahmed SA, Williamson JR, Roberts R, Clarck SE, Sobel BE (1976) The association of increased plasma MB CPK activity and irreversible ischemic myocardial injury in the dog. *Circ* 54:187
57. Lang H, Wurzburg V (1982) Creatine kinase, an enzyme of many forms. *Clin Chem* 28:1439
58. Vatner SF, Baig H, Manders WT, Maroko PR (1978) Effects of coronary artery reperfusion on myocardial infarct size calculated from creatine kinase. *J Clin Invest* 61:1048
59. Reimer KA, Hill ML, Jennings RB (1981) Prolonged depletion of ATP and of the adenine nucleotide pool due to delayed resynthesis of adenine nucleotides following reversible myocardial ischemic injury in dogs. *J Mol Cell Cardiol* 13:299
60. Piper HM, Schwartz P, Spahr R, Hutter JF, Spiekermann PG (1984) Early enzyme release from myocardial cells is not due to irreversible cell damage. *J Mol Cell Cardiol* 16:385
61. Feola M, Glick G (1975) Cardiac lymph flow and composition in acute myocardial ischemia in dogs. *Am J Physiol* 229:44
62. Hearse DJ, Humphrey SM, Garlick PB (1976) Species variation in myocardial enzyme release, glucose protection and reoxygenation damage. *J Mol Cell Cardiol* 8:329
63. Yasmineh WG, Pyle RB, Hanson NQ, Hultman BK (1976) Creatine kinase isoenzymes in baboon tissues and organs. *Clin Chem* 22:63
64. Michael MH, Hunt JR, Weilbaecher D, Perryman MB, Roberts R, Lewis RM, Entman ML (1985) Creatine kinase and phosphorylase in cardiac lymph: coronary occlusion and reperfusion. *Am J Physiol* 248 (*Heart Circ Physiol* 17):H350
65. Heyndrickx GR, Van Rostenberghe H, Vantrimpont P, Wijns W (1987) Time course of recovery from segmental akinesia produced by a one hour critical coronary artery stenosis in conscious dogs. *Circulation* 76 (Suppl IV):337

66. Heyndrickx GR, Wijns W, Vogelaers D, Melin J (1988) One hour of critical coronary artery stenosis: a new model of stunned myocardium. *Eur Heart J* 9 (Suppl 1):23

67. Wijns W, Melin JA, Keyeux A, Bol A, Michel C, Cogneau M, Heyndrickx GR (1987) Metabolic imaging in canine myocardium stunned by one hour critical coronary artery stenosis. *Circulation* 76 (Suppl IV):115

68. Matsuzaki M, Gallacher KP, Kemper SW, White F, Ross J, Jr (1983) Sustained regional dysfunction produced by prolonged coronary stenosis: gradual recovery after reperfusion. *Circulation* 68:170–182

69. Weisfeldt ML (1987) Reperfusion and reperfusion injury. *Clin Res* 35:13–20

70. Braunwald E, Kloner RA (1985) Myocardial reperfusion: a double-edged sword. *J Clin Invest* 76:1713–1719

71. Nayler WG, Elz JS (1986) Reperfusion injury: laboratory artifact or clinical dilemma? *Circulation* 74:215–221

72. Bolli R (1988) Oxygen-derived free radicals and postischemic myocardial dysfunction ('stunned myocardium'). *J Am Coll Cardiol* 12:239–249

2. Early changes in wall thickness and epicardial wall motion during percutaneous transluminal coronary angioplasty in man

Similarities with in-vitro and in-vivo model

PATRICK W. SERRUYS, BRIAN JASKI, FEDERICO PISCIONE, FOLKERT TEN KATE, PIM DE FEYTER, MARCEL VAN DEN BRAND and PAUL G. HUGENHOLTZ

Introduction

Previously, our laboratory has reported the dynamic endocardial wall motion and myocardial wall thickness changes accompanying acute coronary occlusion in patients undergoing transluminal angioplasty (PTCA) [1, 2]. In these studies, the motion of the region of ischemic myocardium was characterized by the early appearance of a late systolic outward expansion followed by an early diastolic inward contraction. We refer to this biphasic motion as the 'W' phenomenon due to its morphologic characteristics, transient duration, and frequency of appearance in studies of endocardial and wall thickness motion during regional ischemia. Similar types of wall motion abnormalities have been described with acute ischemia in animals [1, 2, 4] and in chronic ischemia in man [8, 9]. Since phasic wall motion can, in general, be encountered whenever spatial or temporal nonuniformities in regional contraction or relaxation in the left ventricle exist, the specific etiology of this pattern during acute ischemia is uncertain.

Recently, we had the opportunity to extend these observations by evaluating the changes in wall thickness and epicardial length-pressure changes accompanying acute coronary vascular occlusion in a patient undergoing PTCA of a coronary artery bypass graft in whom pairs of epicardial wall markers had been placed at the time of the original cardiac surgery.

Echocardiographic changes in wall thickness

Continuous M-mode echocardiogram at the chordal level of the left ventricle was obtained immediately before, during, and after balloon occlusion of the stenosis. A total of five separate dilatations of the stenosis were carried out. The echocardiograms during the fifth dilatation is shown (Fig. 1). Continuous ECG, high-fidelity tip manometer, left ventricular pressure and its derivative (dp/dt), Vmax, time constant during early (Tau$_1$) and late (Tau$_2$) relaxation were recorded and computed [13]. Coronary sinus-great cardiac vein flow measure-

P.W. Serruys, R. Simon & K.J. Beatt (eds), Percutaneous Transluminal Coronary Angioplasty. ISBN 0-7923-0346-6.
© *1990 Kluwer Academic Publishers, Dordrecht*

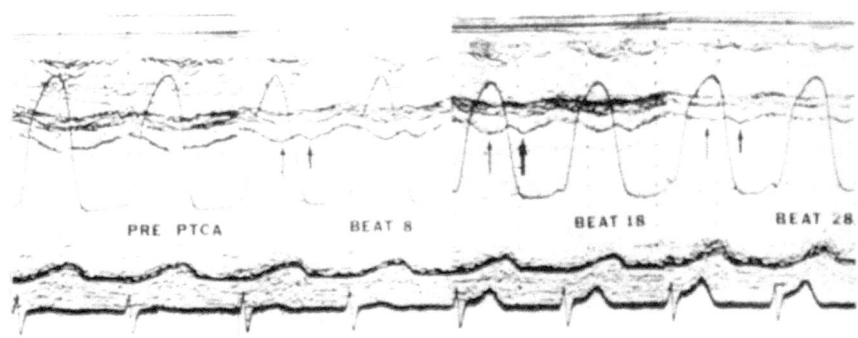

Figure 1. M-mode echocardiographic and left ventricular pressure pulse patterns before (PRE PTCA) and after (POST PTCA) percutaneous transluminal coronary angioplasty of left anterior descending coronary artery. Normal systolic wall thickening becoming less prominent (long arrow) while early diastolic notch (thick arrow) becoming more prominent during PTCA, and disappearing after PTCA.

ments before, during occlusion, and after release of balloon inflation were carried out in a manner similar to our earlier experience [9]. Coronary lactate measurements from great cardiac vein and aorta were also made during these periods (Table 1).

Table 1. Hemodynamic measurements before and at 8th, 18th and 28th heartbeats during transluminal occlusion.

	Before occlusion	During occlusion		
		Beat 8	Beat 18	Beat 28
RR interval msec	764	776	792	792
LVP mmHg	138	130	126	128
LVEDP mmHg	5	8	14	20
dp/dt mmHg	1364	1038	1003	1085
Vmax	46.3	40.4	35.9	32.4
−dP/dt mmHg	1935	1011	1207	1309
Tau$_1$ msec	39	66	54	58
Tau$_2$ msec	25	27	36	44
GCVF ml/min	87	56	52	57
			109[a]	
Lactate (GCV)	+0.06		−1.32[a]	

Abbreviations; LVP = peak left ventricular pressure; LVEDP = left ventricular end-diastolic pressure; +dP/dt = peak positive rate of change of LVP; Vmax = theoretical maximum velocity of the contractile element; −dP/dt = peak negative rate of change of LVP during isovolumic relaxation; Tau$_1$ = time constant of relaxation during the early phase (40 msec) of relaxation; Tau$_2$ = time constant of relaxation during late phase (4 msec–80 msec after aortic valve closure); GCVF = great cardiac vein flow; GCV-A = great cardiac vein aorta lactate gradient.

[a] Measurement taken during reactive hyperemia.

With balloon occlusion of the anterior descending coronary artery at the site of stenosis, there was decrease in systolic thickening in the septum with appearance of a prominent notch in early diastole associated with increase in left ventricular end-diastolic and end-systolic dimensions after the seventh beat following occlusion. At the 28th beat, systolic motion in the septum was absent. The only motion in the septum occurred early in diastole. There was pronounced decrease in the end-diastolic thickness of the septum at beat 28. The LV pressure decreased noticeably after beat 15 associated with the appearance of an a wave. Simultaneously ECG record showed ischemic changes beginning at beat 16, which become progressively more pronounced until release of the occlusion. No arrhytmias were noted during occlusion or after release of balloon inflation. The earliest hemodynamic alteration was a prolongation in early relaxation, which became apparent after the 6th beat. Following release of balloon inflation at beat 45, the echocardiographic parameter returned to baseline at beat 79, while LV pressure returned to baseline at beat 74.

Changes in epicardial wall motion

The patient described in this report is a 47 year old male who presented with severe symptoms of exertional chest pain in 1975. Angiographic evaluation showed significant stenose of the left main, left anterior descending, and right coronary arteries and he underwent cardiac surgery with a single bypass graft placed to each of the left anterior descending, obtuse marginal, and posterior descending vessels. At the time of surgery, the patient was entered into a prospective study assessing the use of epicardial wall markers for longterm assessment of graft patency and left ventricular function as previously described [4]. Recurrent symptoms in January, 1984 led to angiography that revealed the presence of a severe distal stenosis of the left anterior descending bypass graft, occlusion of the obtuse marginal bypass graft, and a high grade stenosis of the distal circumflex, in addition to the lesions previously identified (Fig. 2). The right coronary artery was filled by a patent bypass graft and gave collaterals to the left anterior decending. Right anterior oblique left ventricular angiography showed a mildly enlarged left ventricle (end-diastolic volume index, $116 \, ml/ml^2$) with anteroapical and inferior hypokinesis and a global ejection fraction of 0.50. The patient gave informed consent to the investigational part of the angioplasty of the left anterior descending bypass graft stenosis procedure. The patient's oral medications of beta blockers and calcium antagonists were not discontinued before the procedure.

An 8F tip manometer pigtail catheter (Millar Instruments; Houston) was advanced into the left ventricle. PTCA was performed with a 4.2 mm balloon through a 9F Judkins guiding catheter (Schneider, Zurich) with up to 12 atmospheres of pressure applied. Following three dilatations with a total occlusion time of 105 s, the stenotic pressure gradient decreased from 46 to 9 mmHg and a complete resolution of the angiographic narrowing was achieved

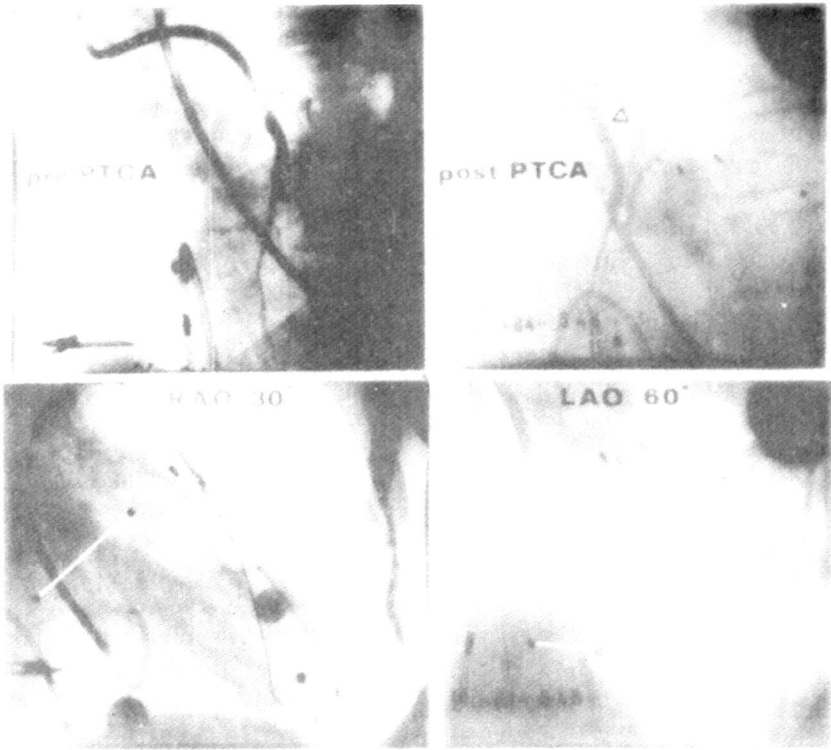

Figure 2. Angiograms of left anterior descending bypass graft stenosis and markers before and after dilatation.

(a)   Before dilatation angiogram shows severe stenosis of the distal bypass graft. The ring markers are located in the vascular territory of the bypass graft. Bead and bar marker pairs are also present.

(b)   After dilatation, angiogram shows total elimination of bypass graft stenosis.

(Fig. 2). Then, biplane cameras were positioned for a final investigational occlusion (additional occlusion time of 50 s). Distal perfusion pressure during the investigational occlusion was 26 mmHg.

Regional marker motion

Absolute marker separation was determined from radiopaque markers implanted during surgery on the epicardium in each bypassed region as previously described [4]. Markers were placed in pairs 2 cm apart and located from 0–3 cm distal to each coronary anastomosis transverse to the long axis of the heart (Fig. 2). Synchronized biplane cine-films (50 frames/sec) at 30° right anterior oblique and 60° left anterior oblique were performed before the placement of the angioplasty catheter (control), during the first 8 s of the investigational occlusion (5 min following the preceding dilatation), 40 s after the onset of occlusion, and 3 min post-occlusion. Absolute distances between markers for each marker pair were determined on all frames using a calibration grid. Correction for x-ray and optical distortion was performed to give true anatomic dimension. In order to reduce high frequency spatial noise, raw marker length data was filtered with a digital nearest neighbor averaging algorithm. L max and L min were defined as the maximal and minimal marker separation. The shortening fraction calculated between these two points (SF max,%) was calculated as (L max-L min)/L max.

Analysis of pressure-derived indexes during systole and diastole

Left ventricular pressure was digitized at 250 samples/s. Left ventricular peak systolic and end-diastolic pressure, peak negative dP/dt, peak positive dP/dt, and the relationship between dP/dt/pressure and pressure linearly extrapolated to pressure $= O$ (V_{max}, the maximal velocity of the contractile element), were computed for each measured beat as previously described [5].

Relaxation parameters were also computed for each beat from peak negative dP/dt to the previous left ventricular end-diastolic pressure using the semilogarithmic model $P(t) = P_o e^{-t/T}$ with P_o the pressure at peak negative dP/dt when a true exponential decay is present and T the time constant of relaxation or the time for the best fit pressure curve to fall from P_o to $.37 \times P_o$[11]. In addition, to assess asynchronous relaxation, a biexponential fit for isovolumic relaxation was determined characterized by two exponential time constants [3]: the fit for the first 40 msec (n = 8 samples), T_1; and the fit after the first 40 msec (n = 4 samples), T_2. When data was fit to single time constant derivative or nonlinear best fit exponential models with pressure offsets [14], derived fits differed significantly from actual data points so only the semilogarithmic analyses were used.

Results

Each pair of markers was located on a characteristically different part of the ventricle. The markers in the left anterior descending artery distribution (rings) were in the post-stenotic territory and showed the most dynamic changes with occlusion (Figs 3 and 4). The second marker pair (beads), distal to the occluded bypass graft on the obtuse marginal, was located in a region that showed initial paradoxical motion (similar to the late occlusion motion in the post-stenotic territory) and was unaffected by the occlusion. The final pair of markers (bars), located in the left circumflex artery distribution, exhibited an initially abnormal and complex motion that became paradoxical during coronary occlusion. The

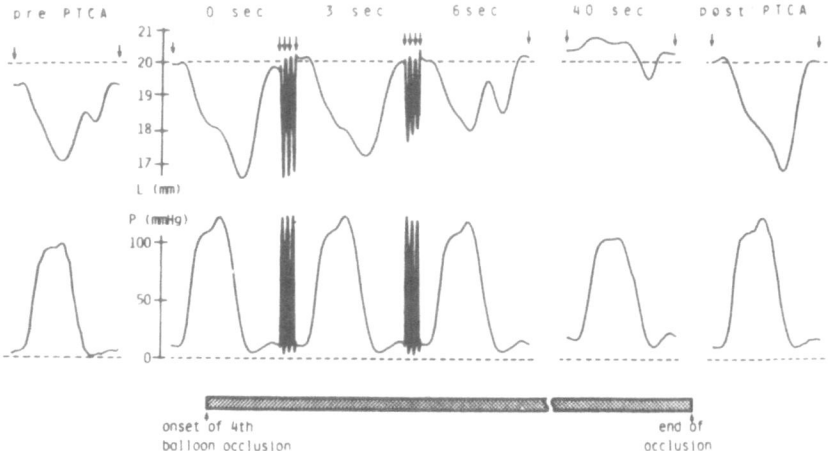

Figure 3.   Changes in epicardial marker pair shortening in region of bypass graft and left ventricular pressure with graft occlusion. Preceding PTCA, marker pair showed abnormal late systolic lengthening and early diastolic lengthening. Similar changes were evident in beats 6–8 after occlusion (see text) (the 'W' phenomenon).

marker pair of interest in the post-stenotic territory was further analyzed and so only data from its region is presented.

Changes in regional epicardial wall motion

In this transiently ischemic zone, epicardial wall motion before the PTCA procedure showed a biphasic systolic shortening pattern (Figs 2 and 3) similar to what we refer to as the 'W' phenomenon. At the time of onset of the investigational occlusion, epicardial wall motion had significantly changed with loss of this biphasic 'W' pattern. With coronary occlusion, the earliest change in shortening occurred at beat 4 after the onset of occlusion, manifest as a decrease in the shortening fraction from 17.2 to 16.8%. Beats 6 through 8, again manifest the late systolic to early diastolic 'W' pattern as before PTCA, however at a higher initial segment length. Fractional shortening decreased further to 11.9% secondary to a decrease in L min. During these first seconds of ischemia, the extent of shortening, but not the early systolic velocity of shortening, dL/dt, was affected (Fig. 5). Initial segment shortening persisted beyond peak negative dP/dt and thus occurred during isovolumic relaxation. With early ischemia, early diastolic shortening following late systolic lengthening occurred after the onset of peak negative dP/dt and during isovolumic relaxation up to the minimal diastolic pressure. During late occlusion (40 s after onset), the ischemic zone showed a paradoxical lengthening throughout systole beyond the point of initial

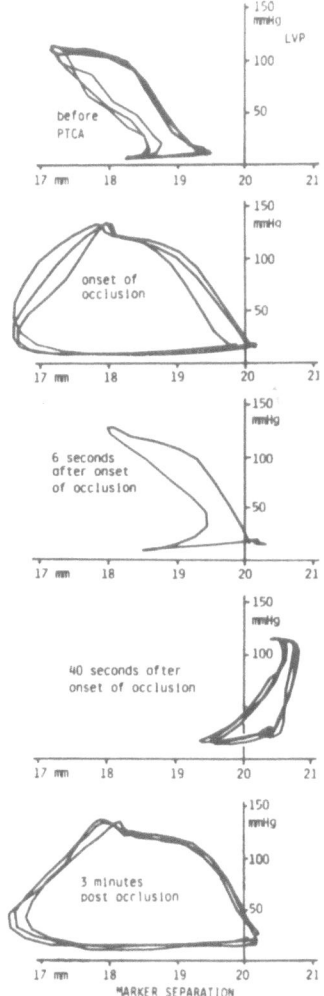

Figure 4. Changes in epicardial pressure length relationships with graft occlusion. Pressure epicardial marker pair distance relationships are shown for the preceding PTCA, the onset of occlusion, 6 s of occlusion, 40 s of occlusion, and post-occlusion; 3 consecutive beats are shown for all except the 1 beat at 6 s of occlusion. Early changes in epicardial pressure length relations are exemplified by the curves after 6 s of occlusion. Paradoxial systolic expansion is evident after 40 s of occlusion. Post occlusion curve returns to that immediately preceding occlusion.

end-diastolic length followed by an early diastolic shortening below the level of end-diastolic length. Post-PTCA ischemic zone wall motion returned to its onset morphology with a fractional shortening of 17.8% (Figs 3 and 4). The diastolic pressure curve was shifted upward and to the right during occlusion.

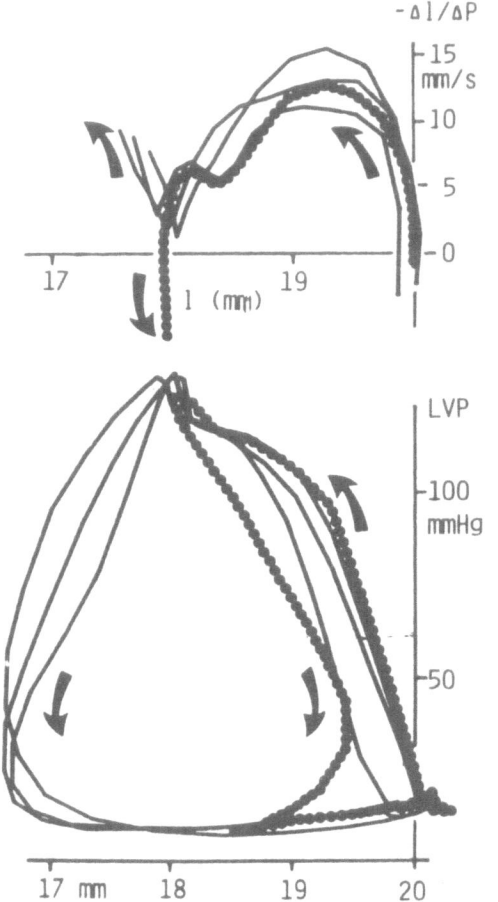

Figure 5. Early changes in pressure velocity and pressure length relationships with graft occlusion. The early change in epicardial shortening is characterized by a decrease in the extent of shortening with a preservation in the velocity of shortening. Onset of occlusion beats in solid lines, 6 s after occlusion beat in dots.

Changes in global left ventricular function

Heart rate did not change during the occlusion. Peak + dP/dt and peak systolic pressure gradually decreased accompanied by a rise in left ventricular minimum and end diastolic pressure. Peak − dP/dt also decreased during the occlusion accompanied by a change in its isovolumic pressure fall such that it was better characterized by a biexponential model of relaxation (Table 2).

Discussion

The time course and magnitude of changes in global parameters of left ventricular function following coronary occlusion in this patient are similar to those previously reported in patients undergoing PTCA of an isolated stenosis of a native coronary artery [1]. Progressive and gradual decreases in parameters of systolic function accompanied very early changes in the rate of left ventricular pressure decay. The biexponential approximation of the isovolumic pressure fall is consistent with an asynchrony of regional myocardial contraction or relaxation [3]. Changes in parameters of isovolumic pressure fall were most pronounced during the first half of occlusion and slightly less at the end of occlusion. In this case, the earliest change in epicardial wall motion was a decrease in the extent of shortening while velocity of early shortening was maintained. These results are similar to the earliest changes of motion of left ventricular mid-wall ultrasonic crystals during ischemia in conscious dogs as reported by Pagani et al [6]. In contrast, Forrester et al observed isovolumic systolic lengthening of mercury-in-silastic epicardial length gauges accompanying the onset of decreases in the extent of shortening in anesthetized dogs [7]. Our findings, in a conscious patient are similar to those reported by Pagani and not Forrester.

After 40 s of ischemia, despite paradoxic lengthening throughout systole, early diastolic shortening was still observed consistent with a markedly diminished yet persistent tension becoming manifest only after a decline in the load imposed upon the region by the remainder of the effectively contracting ventricle. Post-occlusion regional function returned to the appearance of wall motion at the onset of occlusion.

Early wall motion changes during acute ischemia

Frist et al [8] demonstrated that the decline of tension is prolonged during hypoxia in euthermic cat papillary muscle preparations. Tyberg et al [9] simulated the effects of asynchronous contraction and relaxation by analyzing a pair of hypoxic and normal papillary muscles in series. Phasic changes in individual tension length relations in both muscles were observed.

Weigner et al [10] extended these observations by simulating normal papillary muscle with a computer-controlled tension generator in series with a hypoxic papillary muscle. A biphasic pattern of motion of the hypoxic muscle was observed analogous to the 'W' phenomenon in the regionally ischemic zone in the intact left ventricle (Fig. 6). The early lengthening phase of the hypoxic muscle was attributed to a premature onset of force decline and the second late shortening phase was ascribed to either a persisting contractile force of the muscle or a manifestation of stored force from elastic recoil of previously stretched passive muscle elements.

During graded acute myocardial ischemia in dogs, Smalling et al [11] observed

Table 2.   Global left ventricular function during transluminal angioplasty.

	Beat	Preceding R-R interval (msec)	LV Sys mmHg	LV EDP mmHg	+dP/dt mmHg/sec
Onset	−2	760.0	133.0	17.0	1293.0
of	−1	760.0	133.0	17.0	1269.0
occlusion	0	764.0	133.0	17.0	1305.0
	1	764.0	132.0	16.0	1276.0
	2	768.0	133.0	17.0	1258.0
	3	772.0	134.0	17.0	1268.0
	4	780.0	133.0	18.0	1275.0
	5	772.0	133.0	18.0	1275.0
	6	772.0	129.0	16.0	1190.0
	7	768.0	129.0	18.0	1177.0
	8	768.0	128.0	18.0	1197.0
	9	768.0	124.0	18.0	1148.0
	10	760.0	120.0	18.0	1147.0
	11	752.0	115.0	16.0	1096.0
	12	752.0	117.0	18.0	1063.0
	13	760.0	116.0	18.0	1065.0
	14	748.0	114.0	18.0	1051.0
	15	744.0	111.0	16.0	1021.0
40 seconds of		724.0	115.0	24.0	940.0
occlusion		724.0	114.0	23.0	977.0
Post		756.0	134.0	20.0	1295.0
occlusion		752.0	132.0	20.0	1297.0

Abbreviations: LV sys: left ventricular systolic pressure; LVEDP left ventricular end-diastolic pressure; $\pm$ dP/dt: peak positive or negative left ventricular dP/dt: T, T_1, T_2: time constants of relaxations for mono- and bi-exponential models. Vmax; velocity of contractile element extrapolated to 0 pressure.

a biphasic expansion and contraction in both endocardial wall motion and myocardial wall thickening. These changes were attributed to both a loss of the early diastolic distending force of coronary pressure (the 'erectile' effect) and to a persistent contraction of the ischemic zone during early diastole.

In summary, the late systolic lengthening and early diastolic shortening in epicardial wall motion following acute coronary occlusion is most likely secondary to the early onset of tension decline in the ischemic region, however, with tension persisting secondary to a prolonged rate of decline. Early diastolic contraction may be secondary to passive elastic rebound forces with or without the contribution of persistent active tension. The absence of the 'erectile' properties of coronary blood flow may allow more pronounced early diastolic shortening. The relationship of these mechanical events to the intracellular biochemical events of activation and relaxation is unknown.

Vmax sec^{-1}	−dP/dt mmHg/sec	T msec	T$_1$ msec	T$_2$ msec
39.1	−1162.0	−56.0	−70.0	−47.0
39.1	−1154.0	−60.0	−75.0	−49.0
40.1	−1114.0	−61.0	−77.0	−48.0
39.3	−1141.0	−59.0	−76.0	−49.0
38.6	−1120.0	−60.0	−76.0	−50.0
38.1	−1133.0	−60.0	−78.0	−51.0
39.1	−1127.0	−61.0	−75.0	−51.0
37.7	−1106.0	−62.0	−75.0	−52.0
38.2	−1160.0	−59.0	−74.0	−50.0
38.4	−1139.0	−64.0	−78.0	−56.0
37.3	−1109.0	−66.0	−79.0	−56.0
37.0	−1087.0	−66.0	−80.0	−56.0
37.1	−1058.0	−66.0	−81.0	−54.0
37.6	− 990.0	−66.0	−84.0	−53.0
36.5	− 982.0	−69.0	−90.0	−58.0
34.5	− 960.0	−71.0	−95.0	−58.0
35.5	− 902.0	−69.0	−95.0	−56.0
37.2	− 891.0	−66.0	−96.0	−52.0
24.4	− 867.0	−71.0	−89.0	−60.0
24.3	− 894.0	−70.0	−89.0	−58.0
41.4	−1087.0	−64.0	−80.0	−55.0
39.4	−1110.0	−61.0	−77.0	−50.0

Wall motion abnormalities in chronic ischemia

A possible relationship between the resting wall motion abnormalities with chronic ischemia and those transiently observed during acute ischemia is suggested by the similarity in the regional pressure length relationships preceding PTCA to beats 7–9 following occlusion. Regional epicardial wall motion in this ischemic zone was certainly improved following the first three dilatations although this immediate effects should not be equated to the sustained improvement in systolic and diastolic function following PTCA reported by others [12, 13]. Sasayama et al [14] recently demonstrated an inward motion of left ventricular ischemic segments accompanied by an outward motion of normal segments during isovolumic relaxation in patients with chronic angina. This motion was attributed to both a persisting contractile activity and elastic recoil of

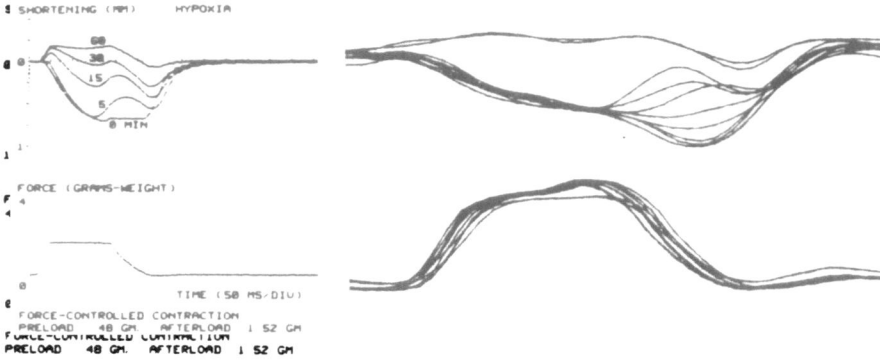

Figure 6. (a)   Left hand sided panel: Interaction between a muscle subjected to hypoxia for 60 min (length record in upper panel) and a 'normal' muscle (force record in lower panel). The earliest change is a premature onset of lengthening (5 min) and as hypoxia progress, there is less total shortening; by 60 min the hypoxia muscle demonstrates 'systolic' lengthening which coincides with the period of force development in the normal muscle. During the period of force decline (normal muscle, below), the hypoxic muscle manifests late systolic shortening.

(b)   Right hand sided panel: Beat by beat changes in epicardial marker pair shortening in region of bypass graft and left ventricular pressure with graft occlusion. Within 6–8 beats after occlusion, marker pair showed abnormal late systolic lengthening and early diastolic shortening. Paradoxical systolic expansion is evident after 40 s of occlusion.

passive elements within the ischemic muscle. In these patients, however, a late systolic expansion of ischemic segments preceding early diastolic contraction was not observed.

Whether a relationship exists between abnormal left ventricular relaxation and left ventricular rapid diastolic filling is uncertain. In patients with coronary artery disease, a prolongation of the monoexponential time constant of relaxation has been shown to correlate with an increase in minimal left ventricular pressure and inversely correlate with early diastolic ventricular inflow rate and inflow volume [15, 16]. Increases in the time constant of isovolumic relaxation have also been associated with increases in the left ventricular diastolic constant of elastic chamber stiffness during both acute coronary occlusion [17] and exercise induced angina [18].

References

1. Serruys PW, van den Brand M, Meij S, Slager C, Schuurbiers JCH, Hugenholtz PG, Brower RW (1984) Left ventricular performance, regional blood flow, wall motion, and lactate metabolism during transluminal angioplasty. *Circulation* 70:25–36
2. Das SK, Serruys PW, van den Brand M, Domenicucci S, Vletter WB, Roelandt J (1983) Acute echocardiographic changes during percutaneous coronary angioplasty and their relationship to coronary blood flow. *J Cardiovasc Ultrasonogr* 2:269–271
3. Brower RW, Meij S, Serruys PW (1983) A model of asynchronous left ventricular relaxation predicting the bi-exponential pressure decay. *Cardiovasc Res* 17:482–488

4. Serruys PW, Brower RW, Ten Katen HJ, Bom AH, Hugenholtz PG (1981) Regional wall motion from radiopaque markers after intravenous and intracoronary injections of nifedipine. *Circulation* 63:584–591

5. Meester GT, Bernard N, Zeelenberg C, Brower RW, Hugenholtz PG (1975) A computer system for real time analysis of cardiac catheterization data. *Cathet Cardiovasc Diagn* 1:112–132

6. Pagani M, Vatner S, Brig H, Braunwald E (1978) Initial myocardial adjustments to brief periods of ischemia and reperfusion in the conscious dog. *Circ Res* 43:83–91

7. Kumada T, Karliner JS, Pouleur H, Gallagher KP, Shirato K, Ross J (1979) Effects of coronary occlusion on early ventricular diastolic events in conscious dogs. *Am J Phys* 237:H542–549

8. Frist WH, Palacios I, Powell WJ (1978) Effect of hypoxia on myocardial relaxation in isometric cat papillary muscle. *J Clin Invest* 1218–1224

9. Tyberg JV, Parmley WW, Sonnenblick EH (1969) In-vitro studies of myocardial asynchrony and regional hypoxia. *Circ Res* 25:569–579

10. Wiegner AW, Allen GJ, Bing OHL (1978) Weak and strong myocardium in series: implications for segmental dysfunction *Am J Phys* 235:H776–783

11. Smalling RW, Kelley KO, Kirkeeide RL, Gould KL (1983) Comparison of early systolic and diastolic regional function during regional ischemia in chronically instrumented canine model. *J Am Coll Card* 2:263–269

12. Kent KM, Bonow RO, Rosing DR, Ewels CJ, Lipson LC, McIntosh CC, Bacharach S, Green M, Epstein SE (1982) Improved myocardial function during exercise after successful percutaneous transluminal coronary angioplasty. *N Engl J Med* 306:441–446

13. Bonow RO, Kent KM, Rosing DR, Lipson LC, Bacharach SL, Green MV, Epstein SE (1982) Improved left ventricular diastolic filling in patients with coronary artery disease after percutaneous transluminal coronary angioplasty. *Circulation* 66:1154–1167

14. Sasayama S, Nonogi H, Fujita M, Sakurai T, Wakabayashi A, Kawai C, Eiho S, Kuwahara M (1984) Analysis of asynchronous wall motion by regional pressure length loops in patients with coronary artery disease. *J Am Coll Card* 4:256–267

15. Fioretti P, Brower R, Meester GT, Serruys PW (1980) Interaction of left ventricular relaxation and filling during early diastole in human subjects. *Am J Card* 46:197–203

16. Piscione F, Serruys PW (1985) Asynchrony in regional filling dynamics as a consequence of uncoordinated segmental contraction during transluminal coronary angioplasty. *J Am Coll Card* (abstract) 7:II-57

17. Serruys PW, Wijns W, Grimm J, Slager C, Hess OM (1984) Effects of repeated transluminal occlusions during angioplasty on global and regional left ventricular chamber stiffness. *Circulation* (abstract) 70:II-348

18. Carroll JD, Hess OM, Hirzel HO, Krayenbrehl HP (1983) Dynamics of left ventricular filling at rest and during exercise. *Circulation* 68:59–67

3. Early mechanical changes associated with coronary artery occlusion

MARIO MARZILLI

Introduction

Myocardial contraction is strictly dependent upon adequate blood supply. In fact, myocardial ischemia causes immediate impairement of myocardial contractile performance that manifests as changes in left ventricular wall dimensions, depression of systolic wall thickening, changes in left ventricular end-diastolic wall thickness, local ventricular bulging, or changes in subepicardial and subendocardial intramural pressures [1–7].

After release of brief coronary occlusions a transient regional left ventricular hyperfunction is observed [6, 8–11]; conversely, longer coronary occlusions cause a persistent dysfunction despite reperfusion, a condition known as 'stunned myocardium' [9, 12–14].

In man, transient myocardial ischemia secondary to reversible coronary occlusion occurs during episodes of vasospastic angina and during balloon inflation in PTCA procedures [15–17]. In both circumstances, alterations of regional left ventricular function similar to what described in animal models have been observed.

However, the time course of the mechanical changes associated with brief ischemic events, the transmural distribution of these ischemic changes and the sensitivity of different exploring tools in identifying the changes have not been clearly assessed.

This investigation intended to explore the effects of very brief coronary occlusions on the contractile performance of the subendocardial and subepicardial layers of the left ventricular free wall in an open chest dog preparation in order to obtain information useful to the understanding of the mechanical events associated with percutaneous coronary angioplasty.

Materials and methods

The study has been performed in five open chest anesthetized dogs. After left thoracotomy, the heart was exposed in a pericardial cradle and the proximal left

P.W. Serruys, R. Simon & K.J. Beatt (eds), Percutaneous Transluminal Coronary Angioplasty. ISBN 0-7923-0346-6.
© *1990 Kluwer Academic Publishers, Dordrecht*

anterior descending coronary branch was dissected free from surrounding tissue and instrumented with an electromagnetic flow probe (Biotronex Laboratory) and an occluding snare. Two pairs of sonomicrometers (Schuessler and Ass.) were positioned in the myocardium perfused by the left anterior descending coronary branch. One pair was placed 8–10 mm deep, along the minor axis of the left ventricle; the second pair was positioned 2–4 mm deep parallel to the direction of the superficial fibers. Two custom-made miniature pressure trasducers (Millar) were positioned in the same area, at 2 and 8 mm depth respectively. The position of the pressure and length probes within the territory perfused by the left anterior descending coronary branch was assured at the end of each experiment by visual inspection after dye injection into the coronary and only data from dogs with correct positioning of all probes were accepted for analysis. Left ventricular and aortic pressures were also recorded by catheter-tip manometers.

Pressure, length, flow, and ECG signals were recorded on paper at various speeds (Electronics for Medicine-Honeywell VR12).

After instrumentation, the preparation was allowed to stabilize for 15 min and the baseline values were recorded. Recordings were repeated before, during, and after 30 sec complete coronary occlusion obtained by pulling the coronary snare. Reperfusion was produced by releasing the snare.

In subsequent occlusions the coronary snare was pulled for 5, 15, 30, 45, and 60 sec. Intervals of 10–15 mins were left between two consecutive occlusions.

Experimental results are given as mean $\pm$ standard error of the mean. A t-test was used to assess the difference between all pairs of comparable data.

Results

Regional function after 30 sec coronary occlusion

Occlusion of the left anterior descending coronary branch caused a contractile dysfunction of the depending myocardium manifested by reduction of intra-myocardial pressure and of systolic segment shortening (Fig. 1). After 30 sec of ischemia, systolic subendocardial pressure had decreased from $186 + 12$ to 120 ± 9 mmHg ($p < 0.001$) and subepicardial pressure from 89 ± 9 to 58 ± 1 mmHg ($p < 0.001$) (Fig. 2). End-diastolic segment length had increased from 9.2 ± 0.7 to 10.2 ± 0.8 mm ($p < 0.01$) in the subendocardium and from 9.7 ± 0.6 to 10.7 ± 0.8 mm ($p < 0.02$) in the subepicardium and in both layers systolic shortening had been substituted by lengthening.

Left ventricular pressure, aortic pressure, and heart rate were not significantly modified after 30 sec coronary occlusion compared to control.

Effects of longer and shorter occlusions

Changes of regional intramyocardial pressure and segment length were not simultaneous. Reduction of systolic intramyocardial pressure occurred immed-

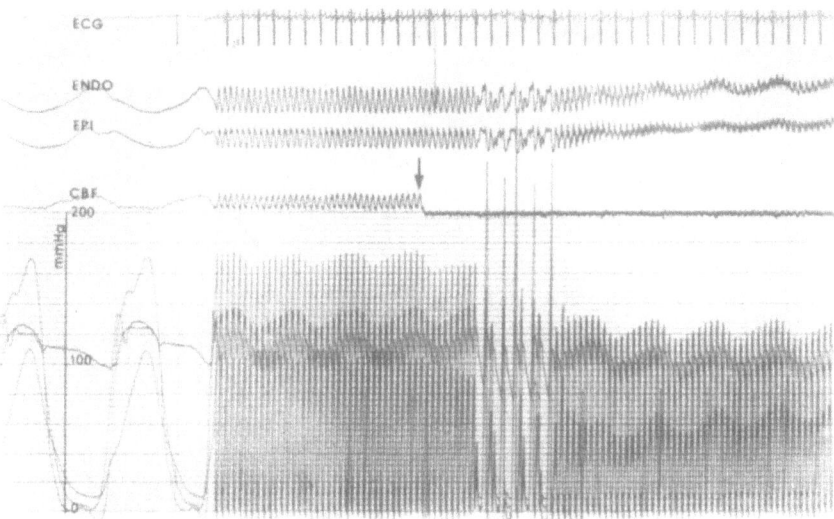

Figure 1. Effect of coronary occlusion upon regional myocardial contractile functon. Continuous recording at high (left) and low (right) paper speed before and after the closure of the coronary snare (arrow). Equisensitive and superimposed tracings of subendocardial intramural pressure, left ventricular pressure, aortic pressure, and subepicardial intramural pressure in the lower part of the figure.
Abbreviations: ECG = electrocardiogram lead II; ENDO = subendocardial segment length; EPI = subepicardial segment length; CBF = coronary blood flow.

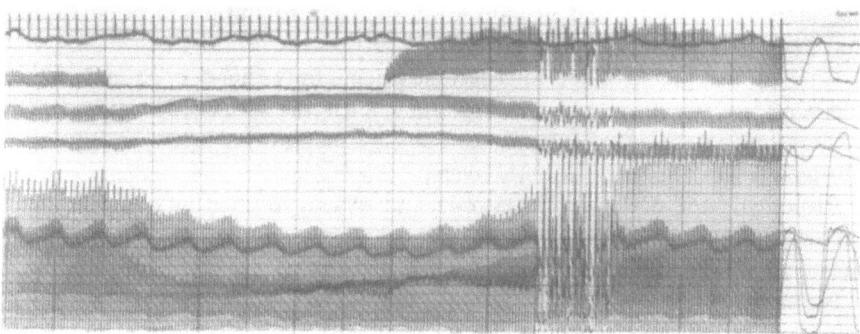

Figure 2. Effect of 30 sec coronary occlusion upon regional myocardial function. Continuous recording at low (left) and fast (right) paper speed during a 30 sec coronary occlusion. Tracings sequence from top to bottom as in Fig. 1.

iately after the pulling of the coronary snare, whereas changes in systolic segment shortening became appreciable only after 5–6 sec. That is to say that in the initial 10–12 heart beats following coronary occlusion, intramyocardial pressure showed a progressive decrease, while systolic segment shortening appeared

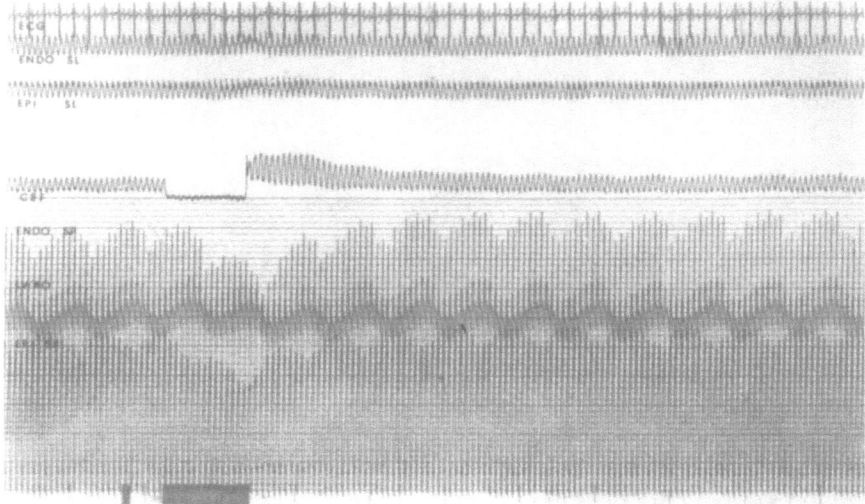

Figure 3.   Effect of a 5 sec coronary occlusion on regional myocardial function.
Abbreviations: ECG = electrocardiogram lead II; ENDO SL = subendocardial segment length; EPI
SL = subepicardial segment length; CBF = coronary blood flow; ENDO SP = subendocardial
intramural pressure; LV/AO = left ventricular and aortic pressure; EPI SP = subepicardial intramural
pressure.

unchanged (Fig. 3). At the end of a 5 sec coronary occlusion, systolic intramyocardial pressure was $18 \pm 3\%$ lower than control and subepicardial pressure was $21 \pm 6\%$ lower than control. After 15 sec coronary occlusion, intramyocardial pressures were $25 \pm 3\%$ and $30 \pm 4\%$ lower than control in the subendocardium and in the subepicardium respectively.

Changes in regional dimensions became evident only after 5–6 sec, and, at the end of a 15 sec occlusion, end-diastolic segment lengths were $8 \pm 2\%$ and $6 \pm 1\%$ greater than control in the subendocardial end subepicardial layers, and systolic shortening was abolished in both layers.

Prolonging the occlusion time to 45 and 60 secs resulted in no additional decrease in intramyocardial pressure and in no further deterioration of regional shortening compared to a 30 sec coronary closure.

No time difference was observed in pressure and/or length changes between the superficial and deeper layers, modifications of both signals occurring simultaneously across the left ventricular wall.

Discussion

Coronary angioplasty requires the temporary closure of a major coronary branch. The ischemia resulting from the manouvre causes regional wall dysfunction.

In this study, an animal model was utilized to identify the time of appearance of regional dysfunction, to assess the relative sensitivity of different measuring techniques, and to compare the contractile behaviour of the superficial and deep layers of the left ventricular free wall.

The observations of this study suggest that mechanical changes associated with a sudden coronary closure occur simultaneously in subendocardial and subepicardial muscle and that the earliest manifestation of myocardial ischemia are detectable from the intramyocardial pressure signal. The reduction of intramyocardial pressure consistently preceeded the changes in segment length of 5–6 sec. This delay between pressure and length changes suggest that force development and dimensional changes may be dependent upon different mechanisms with different time constants, as observed in isolated cardiac muscle [18]. The persistence of a reduced but appreciable intramyocardial pressure when systolic shortening was completely abolished suggests that a rythmic contractile activity is present in 'akinetic' muscle and that no dimensional changes can be appreciated because the force of contraction is to weak to overcome left ventricular pressure [6]. The persistence of a contractile activity in non-perfused muscle merit further studies to confirm this observation, to establish for how long this activity can persist, and to investigate its possible role in the pathogenesis of the ischemic damage.

Subendocardial layers are commonly regarded as being more sensitive to ischemia than superficial layers. In contrast with this opinion, in this study the contractile changes associated with coronary occlusion occurred simultaneously in both layers and were of similar magnitude.

In this animal model of transient myocardial ischemia, left ventricular and aortic pressures were scarcely sensitive to regional ischemia, but it should be considered that more sofisticated analysis such as calculation of dP/dt and time constant T, would certainly increase the possibility to detect ischemia from central hemodynamics.

In reference to PTCA this study suggests that occlusions from 30 to 60 sec produce mechanical alterations of similar severity. Considering that measurement of intramyocardial pressure could be performed only during intra-operative PTCA associated with open chest surgery, this study suggests that the most practical tools to detect regional myocardial ischemia are those capable to detect changes in wall dimensions and movements, such as mono- and bi-dimensional echocardiography that can be expected to detect ischemic changes as early as 10 sec after coronary closure.

The presence of collaterals and/or of non-viable myocardium in the depending territory could affect the pattern and time course of the mechanical response to coronary occlusion and this should be considered in transferring these information from the experimental model to man.

Echocardiografic monitoring of regional myocardial function seems the most appropriate technique to assess the effects of repeated coronary occlusions and to evaluate pharmacologic and/or hemodynamic interventions aimed at 'myocardial protection'; an objective of paramount importance if inflation time should be prolonged to several minutes in order to reduce restenosis rate, as recently suggested.

References

1. Goldstein S, De Jong JW (1974) Changes in left ventricular wall dimensions during regional myocardial ischemia. *Am J Cardiol* 34:56
2. Tennant ER, Wiggers CJ (1935) The effect of coronary occlusion on myocardial contraction. *Am J Physiol* 112:351
3. Theroux P, Franklin D, Ross J Jr, Kemper WS (1974) Regional myocardial function during acute coronary artery occlusion and its modification by pharmacologic agents in the dog. *Circ Res* 35:896
4. Theroux P, Ross J Fr, Franklin D, Kemper WS, Sasayama S (1976) Regional myocardial function in the conscious dog during acute coronary occlusion and responses to morphine, propranolol, nitroglicerine, and lidocaine. *Circulation* 53:302
5. Vatner SF (1980) Correlation between acute reductions in myocardial blood flow and function in conscious dogs. *Circ Res* 47:201
6. Tatooles CJ, Randall WC (1961) Local ventricular bulging after acute coronary occlusion. *Am J Physiol* 201:451
7. Sabbah HN, Stein PD (1982) Effect of acute regional ischemia on pressure in the subepicardium and subendocardium. *Am J Physiol* 242:H240
8. Marzilli M, Levantesi D, Sabbah HN, Taddei L, Dalle Vacche M, Stein PD (1984) Regional myocardial systolic function. Effects of coronary occlusion and reperfusion. *G It Cardiol* 14/11:1052
9. Egeblad H, Haunso S, Amtorp O (1982) Regional dynamic behaviour of the canine myocardium following brief ischemia: wall thickness, wall thickening, and blood flow. *Cardiovasc Res* 16:249
10 Newman WH, Mathur PP, Walton RP (1975) Cathecolamines and local rebound in left ventricular contractile force after release of coronary artery occlusion. *Cardiovasc Res* 5:81
11. Pagani M, Vatner SF, Baig H, Braunwald E (1978) Initial myocardial adjustments to brief periods of ischemia and reperfusion in the conscious dog. *Circ Res* 43:83
12 Heyndrickx GR, Millard RW, McRitchie RJ, Maroko PR, Vatner SF (1975) Regional myocardial functional and electrophysiological alterations after brief coronary artery occlusion in conscious dogs. *J Clin Invest* 56:978
13. Heyndrickx GR, Baig H, Nellens P, Leusen I, Fishbein MC, Vatner SF (1978) Depression of regional blood flow and wall thickening after brief coronary occlusions. *Am J Physiol* 234:H653
14. Kloner RA, DeBoer LWV, Darsee JR, Ingwall JS, Hale S, Tumas J, Braunwald E (1981) Prolonged abnormalities of myocardiam salvaged by reperfusion. *Am J Physiol* 241:H591
15. Distante A, Rovai D, Picano E, Moscarelli E, Palombo C, Morales MA, Michelassi C, L'Abbate A (1984) Transient changes in left ventricular mechanics during attacks of Prinzmetal's angina: a B-mode echocardiographic study. *Am Heart J* 108:440
16. Das SK, Serruys PW, van den Brand M, Domenicucci S, Vletter WB, Roelandt J (1983) Acute echocardiografic changes during percutaneous coronary angioplasty and their relationship to coronary blow flow. *J Cardiovasc Ultrasonography* 2:269
17. Alam M, Kahja F, Brymer J et al (1986) Echocardiografic evaluation of left ventricular function during coronary artery angioplasty. *Am J Cardiol* 57:20–25
18. Julian FJ, Moss RL (1976) The concept of active state in striated muscle. *Circ Res* 38:53

4. Coronary angiographic and hemodynamic determinants of ST-segment response to acute coronary occlusion

ROBERT G. MACDONALD and ROBERT L. FELDMAN

The direction and magnitude of electrocardiographic (ECG) ST-segment response to acute coronary occlusion are highly variable. Factors to be considered are the extent and viability of the myocardium supplied by the coronary artery undergoing occlusion, the extent of collateral circulation to the coronary bed distal to the occlusion and the duration of coronary occlusion. Reversible ST-segment elevation is generally considered to reflect transmural myocardial ischemia and ST depression to reflect non-transmural or subendocardial ischemia [1–2]. Hemodynamic and angiographic observations in humans and animal models of coronary artery spasm have suggested that ST-segment elevation reflects either total coronary occlusion in the absence of developed collateral circulation of subtotal occlusion with or without an increase in myocardial oxygen demand [3–6].

Using coronary angioplasty as a model for acute coronary occlusion [7], we evaluated the ST-segment response to occlusion in a series of patients undergoing angioplasty for standard clinical indications. By monitoring the ECG, systemic, left ventricular and coronary pressures and coronary venous blood flow, important predictors of direction of ST-segment response were documented [8].

Patient selection

We selected patients with a severe narrowing in the proximal left anterior descending artery amenable to PTCA, and no important narrowing in other locations. Patients in whom left ventriculography demonstrated more than mild hypokinesis of the anterior wall were excluded. All patients gave informed consent to allow insertion of additional catheters necessary for measurement of coronary venous blood flow and to undergo the research protocol.

Medications

Before PTCA all vasoactive medications were discontinued except in three patients in whom it was considered clinically inappropriate. All patients were

P.W. Serruys, R. Simon & K.J. Beatt (eds), Percutaneous Transluminal Coronary Angioplasty. ISBN 0-7923-0346-6.
© *1990 Kluwer Academic Publishers,*

given ASA 325 mg orally for a minimum of two days before the procedure. No nitroglycerin was given until the research portion of the PTCA procedure was completed.

Angioplasty procedure and measurements

Angioplasty was performed via the Judkins technique using USCI balloon catheters, through which distal coronary pressure could be reliably measured. A balloon flotation catheter was inserted from the femoral vein to record left ventricular filling pressure (pulmonary capillary wedge pressure). A modified coronary sinus thermodilution catheter (dual thermistor Pepine catheter, Webster Laboratories) was inserted from a brachial vein for measurement of great cardiac vein blood flow and its position was confirmed by contrast venography [9]. Surface ECG leads I, II, V_2 and V_5 were monitored and recorded.

Several balloon inflations were first performed to dilate the lesion and minimize the transstenotic pressure gradient. Any ischemia which occurred with the initial inflations was allowed to resolve and a series of balloon inflations was then performed to assess the sequence and nature of ECG and hemodynamic changes produced by LAD occlusion. An example of such a sequence is shown in Fig. 1. During each recording, measurements were made at baseline and then during coronary occlusion just prior to balloon deflation. Individual recordings were separated by more than five minutes to allow ischemia to resolve and parameters to return to baseline. The following parameters were evaluated: Aortic, distal coronary and left ventricular filling pressures, great cardiac vein flow and ST-segment response to ischemia. Leads I, V_2, V_5 were considered to reflect the anterior region and only changes in these leads were reported.

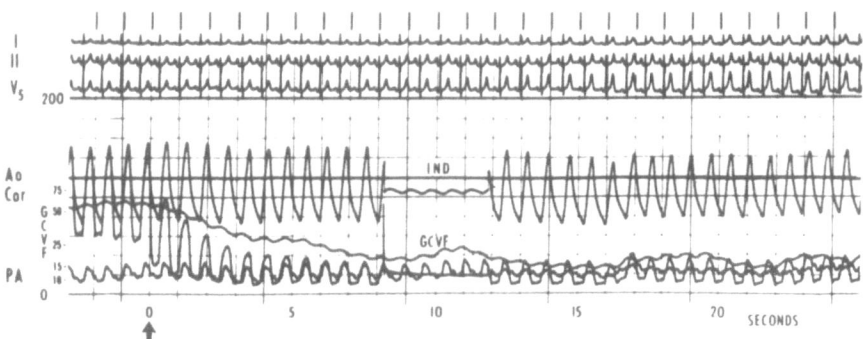

Figure 1. A continuous recording demonstrating the time course of development of ischemia following acute occlusion of the left anterior descending artery. Coincident with occlusion (time 0) there is an abrupt decline in great cardiac vein flow (GCVF) and distal coronary pressure (COR). Aortic (AO) and pulmonary artery (PA) pressures remain relatively unchanged. By 20 sec after occlusion there is evidence of ischemia on ECG manifested by ST elevation leads I to V_5.

ST-segment shifts from baseline were measured with handheld calipers. New ST-segment depression or elevation of 1 mm or greater, measured 80 msec from the J point, was considered significant. We developed an index of collateral resistance calculated as the ratio of the difference between mean aortic and distal coronary pressure and great cardiac vein blood flow during occlusion [7].

Angiography

Coronary and left ventricular angiography were performed in the usual fashion not more than three weeks prior to PTCA. Coronary angiography was performed in multiple views with and without preadministration of nitroglycerin. Measurements were made by handheld calipers on a traced magnified image of the view showing the stenosis at greatest severity. Traced images were coded to allow measurement in a 'blind fashion'. Stenosis severity was expressed as percent diameter reduction.

Presence of collateral filling of the LAD was assessed prior to PTCA. Collaterals were graded only present or absent and no attempt was made to quantitate the degree of collateral filling. Angiographic evaluation of recruitment of collaterals at the time of LAD dilation was not performed.

Results

In some of our patients, balloon occlusion of the LAD did not produce chest pain or ECG or hemodynamic evidence of ischemia despite prolonged inflations. These were generally patients with a total occlusion or a very severe stenosis with well developed collateral supply before PTCA. For the purpose of analysis we selected only those patients who, during LAD occlusions, developed either ST depression or elevation ⩾ 1 m volt from baseline. Patients were then divided into those with ST elevation (group I) and ST depression (group II). The group mean values for hemodynamic parameters during occlusion are shown in Table 1. Heart rate, aortic pressure, double product and left ventricular filling pressure were similar, indicating no difference in myocardial oxygen demand during LAD occlusion between the two groups. The group with ST elevation, however, had lower distal coronary pressure (coronary wedge pressure) and residual great cardiac vein flow and higher calculated collateral resistance during LAD occlusion. These are all indices of poorer collateral perfusion as compared to patients with ST depression during LAD occlusion.

Angiographic correlates

When the angiographic findings before PTCA for the two groups were compared (Table 2), two important findings were evident. First, the group with ST elevation

Table 1. Mean hemodynamic values in patients with ST elevation vs ST depression during LAD coronary artery occlusion.

	ST ↑	ST ↓
Heart rate (beats/min)	78 ± 16	79 ± 12
Aortic pressure (mmHg)	107 ± 17	108 ± 16
Double product (mmHg) beats/min × 10^{-2})	107 ± 33	114 ± 30
Distal coronary pressure (mmHg)	25 ± 8	41 ± 16*
LVFP (mmHg)	19 ± 9	20 ± 9
Residual GCVF (ml/min)	33 ± 14	51 ± 22*
Collateral resistance (mmHg/ml/min)	3.1 ± 2.1	1.5 ± 0.8*

*p < 0.05
LVFP = Left ventricular filling pressure.
GCVF = Great cardiac vein flow.

during coronary occlusion had less severe LAD stenosis before PTCA than the group with ST depression (69 ± 15% vs 88 ± 10%, (p < 0.005). Second, patients with ST depression were more likely to have angiographically demonstrable collaterals prior to PTCA (6 of 9 vs 0 of 16, p < 0.01). These angiographic data also supported the concept of better collateral supply in the patients with ST depression during coronary occlusion. As expected, from previous studies [10–11] patients with more severe stenosis were more likely to have angiographically visible collaterals before PTCA.

Discussion

In summary, this model for studying the responses to acute coronary occlusion provides important information on parameters used to evaluate ischemia in clinical settings. By monitoring the ECG, coronary venous blood flow and other hemodynamic parameters, the relation between stenosis severity, collateral blood flow and degree of ischemia during coronary occlusion is better understood. Some patients will tolerate prolonged coronary occlusion at the time of angioplasty without developing angina, ECG changes or any other evidence of myocardial ischemia. These patients generally have a very severe coronary stenosis before PTCA and angiographic evidence of well established collateral circulation to the myocardial region supplied by the artery undergoing dilation. We now recognize prospectively that such patients are at very low risk for ischemic complications at the time of angioplasty and in the event of acute occlusion following angioplasty [12].

This model, used in the study described above, has demonstrated a relation between the direction of ST-segment response to acute coronary occlusion and the presence or absence of collateral circulation.

Table 2. Individual angiographic values obtained before coronary angioplasty

Patient	EF (%)	LAD stenosis (%)	Visible collaterals to LAD
Group I (ST elevation)			
1	58	53	0
2	51	82	0
3	60	82	0
4	50	51	0
5	58	86	0
6	62	72	0
7	60	51	0
8	65	78	0
9	50	73	0
10	50	51	0
11	65	71	0
12	74	58	0
13	52	47	0
14	64	77	0
15	75	90	0
16	63	86	0
Group II (ST depression)			
1	68	75	0
2	60	99	+
3	68	87	0
4	70	99	+
5	60	89	+
6	45	99	+
7	65	75	0
8	58	86	+
9	61	84	+

EF = ejection fraction; LAD = left anterior descending artery.

In patients with ST elevation during coronary occlusion there was no angiographic evidence of preexisting collateral circulation distal to the stenosis dilated. The coronary stenosis in these patients tended to be less severe, marking collateral development before PTCA less likely. It is possible that small amounts of 'recruitable' collateral blood flow occurred during coronary occlusion in these patients but it was inadequate to prevent ischemia such that ST elevation developed on the surface ECG. The measured residual great cardiac vein flow during occlusion in these patients was, on average, lower than in those with ST depression in keeping with less collateral blood flow to the anterior left ventricular region. The overlap in values between patients from the two groups reflects the imprecision of the venous flow technique and the possibility that some

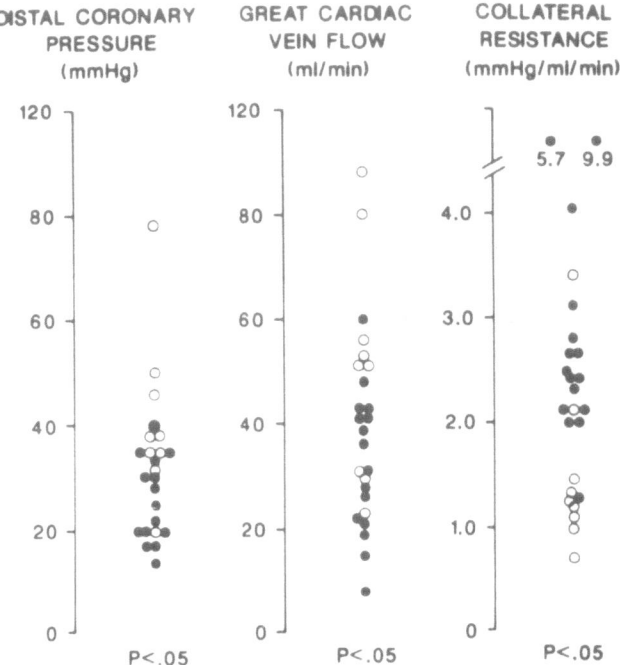

Figure 2. Individual patient values for distal coronary pressure, residual great cardiac vein flow and calculated collateral resistance during LAD occlusion in patients with ST elevation (●) vs ST depression (○). Although overlap in values occurs between groups, statistically significant group differences in each parameter are noted.

great cardiac venous drainage may come from other regions (e.g. circumflex obtuse marginal distribution) in some patients. Measurement of distal coronary occlusion pressure (wedge pressure) has been shown to be a good predictor of the presence or absence of collaterals [13, 14] and in this study was consistent with the coronary venous flow and angiographic data. In patients with ST elevation, the coronary occlusion pressure was lower suggesting poorly developed collaterals.

In the patients who developed only ST-segment depression during coronary occlusion, we found more severe preexisting coronary stenosis, a high prevalence of preexisting collaterals, and high residual great cardiac vein flow values coupled with high coronary occlusion pressures. These data suggested better collateral development prior to occlusion results in less ischemia during occlusion in the presence of comparable indices of myocardial oxygen demand.

The above findings are consistent with previous studies in humans with coronary spasm [3, 4] and provide further insight into why patients with total coronary occlusion associated with coronary spasm or non-Q-wave MI do not always develop ST elevation. With repeated episodes of coronary spasm or the gradual development of a severe fixed stenosis followed by thrombotic occlusion, collaterals may develop, limiting the degree of ischemia such that ST depression rather ST elevation is seen on the ECG recording during pain.

Quantitation of ischemia: surface versus intracoronary ECG

The model used in our studies has relied on the surface electrocardiogram to quantitate ischemia. We used surface ECG leads I, V_2 and V_5 to represent the anterior myocardial region supplied by the LAD. We have assumed that ST-segment elevation reflects more severe and extensive ischemia than ST-segment depression as this has been suggested by many animal and clinical models [1–3]. It is possible that some of our patients with ST depression may have demonstrated ST elevation by a more sensitive monitoring technique such as the intracoronary ECG. In previous studies the intracoronary ECG has been shown to be more likely to demonstrate ST elevation than the surface ECG, particularly when less than 12 leads are monitored [15]. There is some question as to whether all cases of ST elevation on the intracoronary ECG are associated with any physiologic changes compatible with ischemia. Monitoring of myocardial lactates, left ventricular filling pressures, wall motion changes and other more sensitive indices of myocardial ischemia would improve the reliability of the model in evaluating ischemia. Radiolucent ECG leads and wires are now available for placement on the precordium such that the 12 lead ECG can be monitored without interfering with radiographic visualization of the coronary arteries or PTCA equipment. It could be argued that the intracoronary ECG has little clinical value over this system for routine PTCA.

Use of the model in evaluating drug therapy

This model of acute coronary occlusion, by analyzing both indices of myocardial oxygen demand and collateral blood supply, can be used to evaluate effects of cardioactive drugs in treating acute ischemia. By measuring the above hemodynamic parameters during repeated coronary occlusions before, and after intravenous administration of different agents, the effect on acute ischemia can be evaluated. The time to development and magnitude of ischemia may be favorably or adversely affected by certain agents. Using this model, we have evaluated nitrates, beta blockers and calcium antagonists during angioplasty [16–18] and the results have often influenced our clinical practice. Demonstration of beneficial effects of intravenous beta blockade during angioplasty has led us to continue beta blockers in our patients until after successful PTCA and to administer beta blockers intravenously prior to PTCA in many patients with rapid resting heart rates secondary to nitrates or nifedipine. With a lower myocardial oxygen demand, more prolonged balloon inflations can then be tolerated.

Conclusion

In conclusion, we have described an angioplasty model for studying the effects of acute coronary occlusion on myocardial ischemia. We have shown that the ST-segment response to coronary occlusion is determined by the presence or absence of collateral circulation. This study and others using this model have also provided insight into medications used to treat acute ischemia and factors which predict the likelihood of ischemia during acute occlusion complicating failed PTCA.

References

1. Ekmekci A, Toyoshima H, Kwoczynski JK, Nagaya T, Prinzmetal M (1961) Angina Pectoris, IV. Clinical and experimental difference between ischemia with S–T elevation and ischemia with S–T depression. *Am J Cardiol* 7:412–26
2. Timogiannakis G, Amende I, Martinez E, Thomas M (1974) ST segment deviation and regional myocardial blood flow during experimental partial coronary artery occlusion. *Cardiovascular Research* 8:469–477
3. Maseri A, Severi S, De Nes M, L'Abbate A, Chierchia S, Marzilli M, Ballestra AM, Parodi O, Biagini A, Distante A (1978) 'Variant' Angina: One aspect of a continuous spectrum of vasospastic myocardial ischemia. Pathogenetic mechanisms, estimated incidence and clinical and coronary arteriographic findings in 138 patients. *Am J Cardiol* 42:1019–33
4. Yasue H, Omote S, Takizawa A, Masao N, Hyon H, Nishida S, Horie M (1981) Comparison of coronary arteriographic findings during angina pectoris associated with S–T elevation or depression. *Am J Cardiol* 47:539–46
5. De Servi S, Specchia G, Angoli L (1979) Coronary artery spasm of different degrees as cause of angina at rest with ST segment depression and elevation. *British Heart J* 42:110–112
6. De Servi S, Specchia G, Ardissino D, Falcone C, Mussini A, Angoli L, Bramucci E, Marinoni GP, Gavazzi A, Bobba P (1980) Angiographic demonstration of different pathogenetic mechanisms in patients with spontaneous and exertional angina associated with S–T segment depression. *Am J Cardiol* 45:1285–92
7. Feldman RL, Pepine CJ (1984) Evaluating of coronary collateral circulation in conscious humans. *Am J Cardiol* 53:1233–38
8. Macdonald RG, Hill JA, Feldman RL (1986) ST segment response to acute coronary occlusion: Coronary hemodynamic and angiographic determinants of direction of ST segment shift. *Circulation* 5:973–79
9. Pepine CJ, Mehta J, Webster WW Jr., Nichols WW (1978) In vivo validation of a thermodilution method to determine regional left ventricular blood flow in patients with coronary disease. *Circulation* 58:795–802
10. MacArthur AE, Mathur VS, Hall RJ, Massumi GA, Garcia E, De Castro CM (1985) Collateral circulation in coronary artery disease. *Am J Cardiol* 55:58–60
11. Goldberg HL, Goldstein J, Borer JS, Collins MB, Moses JW, Ellis G, with the technical assistance of Quiroz R (1983) Determination of the angiographic appearance of coronary collateral vessels: The importance of supplying and recipient arteries. *Am J Cardiol* 51:434–39
12. Rentrop KP, Thornton JC, Feit F, Van Buskirk M (1988) Determinants and protective potential of coronary arterial collaterals as assessed by an angioplasty model. *Am J Cardiol* 61:10, 677–684
13. Probst P, Zangl W, Pachinger O (1985) Relation of coronary arterial occlusion pressure during percutaneous transluminal coronary angioplasty to presence of collaterals. *Am J Cardiol* 55:1264–69
14. Meier B, Luethy P (1984) Coronary wedge pressure as predictor of recruitable collateral arteries. *Circulation* 2 (abstracts) 70:II

15. Friedman PL, Shook TL, Kirshenbaum JM, Selwyn AP, Ganz P (1986) Value of the intracoronary electrocardiogram to monitor myocardial ischemia during percutaneous transluminal coronary angioplasty. *Circulation* 74:2, 330–39
16. Feldman RL, Joyal M, Conti R, Pepine CJ (1984) Effect of nitroglycerin on coronary collateral flow and pressure during acute coronary occlusion. *Am J Cardiol* 54:958–63
17. Feldman RL, Macdonald RG, Hill JA, Limacher MC, Conti RC, Pepine CJ (1986) Effect of propranolol on myocardial ischemia occurring during acute coronary occlusion. *Circulation* 73:4, 727–33
18. Feldman RL, Macdonald RG, Hill JA, Pepine CJ (1987) Effect of nicardipine on determinants of myocardial ischemia occurring during acute coronary occlusion produced by percutaneous transluminal coronary angioplasty. *Am J Cardiol* 60:267–70
19. Yamagishi M, Kuzuya T, Kodama K, Nato S, Tada M (1985) Functional significance of transient collaterals during coronary artery spasm. *Am J Cardiol* 56:407–12
20. Tada M, Yamagishi M, Kodama K, Kuzuya T, Nanto S, Inoue M, Abe H (1983) Transient collateral augmentation during coronary arterial spasm associated with ST-segment depression. *Circulation* 67:693–98
21. Takeshita A, Koiwaya Y, Nakamura M, Yamamoto K, Torii S (1982) Immediate appearance of coronary collaterals during ergonovine-induced arterial spasm. *Chest* 82:3
22. Burns RJ, Bar-Shlomo B-Z, McLaughlin PR (1982) Functional collaterals in coronary artery spasm. *CMAJ* 127: September 1

5. Dynamic appearance of collaterals during coronary occlusion and their impact on electrocardiographic changes and wall motion abnormalities

MARC COHEN

Introduction

Patients with coronary artery disease undergoing elective percutaneous trans-luminal coronary angioplasty (PTCA), provide a model for prospective evaluation of the dynamic and functional significance of the coronary collateral circulation in human subjects. By using a second arterial catheter for contrast injections of the contralateral coronary artery and the left ventricle, during angioplasty balloon inflation (the model for sudden controlled coronary artery occlusion), the degree of collateral circulation to the dilated artery during balloon occlusion can be characterized and correlated with the impact of sudden coronary occlusion on ventricular function. In addition, the changes observed in collateral filling and ventricular function, can then be correlated with changes seen on a 12 lead electrocardiogram (ECG), obtained during balloon occlusion. Using this model, which we developed in the cardiac catheterization laboratory [1, 2], we prospectively persued three aims: (1) To study the capacity of the collateral circulation to acutely augment its filling after sudden total coronary occlusion, (2) To study the capacity of the different degrees of collateral filling seen *during* coronary occlusion to limit myocardial ischemia, and (3) To assess the usefulness of the surface 12 lead ECG in predicting the location and extent of wall motion abnormalities.

Methods

Study patients

The study patients were selected from consecutive patients undergoing elective PTCA of either the left anterior descending or the right coronary artery. Criteria for inclusion were: (1) History of angina pectoris, and no previous transmural myocardial infarction, (2) Normal segmental and global left ventricular function, and (3) Coronary arteriography revealing a right dominant coronary system and

P.W. Serruys, R. Simon & K.J. Beatt (eds), Percutaneous Transluminal Coronary Angioplasty. ISBN 0-7923-0346-6.
© *1990 Kluwer Academic Publishers, Dordrecht*

single vessel coronary disease in either the right coronary (RCA), or the left anterior descending (LAD) artery. Using the CASS coronary anatomy nomenclature (3), lesions in the RCA had to be within segments 1–3, and lesions within the LAD artery had to be within segments 12 or 13. These segments correspond to proximal and mid coronary lesions. Patients with circumflex artery angioplasty were excluded because of the lack of a well established method for quantifying the extent of posterior wall motion abnormalities. Patients with the following characteristics were excluded: (1) History of hypertension (diastolic pressure above 90 mm Hg), additional non-coronary cardiac disease, chronic obstructive lung disease, anemia, bleeding diathesis, angina at rest compatible with intermittent coronary spasm, (2) Peripheral vascular disease compromising arterial access, or renal insufficiency, and (3) Baseline ECG showing pathologic Q waves, left ventricular hypertrophy, bundle branch block, or ST segment deviation of greater than 0.5 mV. Patients were informed of the need for additional catheters and additional contrast injections and consented.

The baseline (prior to PTCA), clinical and angiographic characteristics, of the 23 patients reported on below are as follows. There were 18 males and 5 females with a mean age of 57 ± 8 yr. The mean duration of symptoms was 5.2 ± 7.9 months. Twelve patients had left anterior descending lesions dilated and 11 had right coronary lesions dilated. The mean grade of collateral filling was 0.5 ± 0.8.

Cardiac catheterization and angioplasty protocol

The principles of our coronary angioplasty premedications, hemodynamic monitoring, guiding and balloon dilatation catheter systems have been described in previous publications [1, 2, 4].

Medications and catheter systems. All patients received the following medications prior to the catheterization: Dipyridamole, aspirin, and oxazepam. In the catheterization laboratory, just prior to insertion of the catheters, nifedipine 10 mgs sublingually were given followed by a continuous intravenous infusion of nitroglycerin titrated to maintain the mean arterial pressure between 80 and 100 mm Hg.

A standard balloon angioplasty guiding catheter was advanced via the right brachial or femoral artery. Balloon dilatation catheters and guide wires of variable sizes were used as clinically indicated. A 5 French right or left Judkins coronary arteriography catheter (Cook) and a 5 Fr pigtail catheter (Cook) were sequentially advanced through a 5 Fr sheath placed in the left femoral artery. The 5 French coronary catheters were used to inject the contralateral artery (the right if the lesion was in the LAD or the left coronary artery if the lesion was in the RCA). The 5 Fr pigtail catheter was used for left ventriculography.

Hemodynamics and electrocardiography. Simultaneous aortic, peripheral coronary artery, and left ventricular pressure were measured using fluid filled tubing and Statham P23ID pressure transducers. Heart rate was calculated from a Honeywell Electronics for Medicine recording console. Standard 12 lead ECG's were recorded at 25 mm/sec paper speed using a Hewlett Packard 4700A Pagewriter model which acquires all 12 leads within 10 secs. Precordial leads were monitored using X-ray transparent electrodes. Recordings were made during held end-expiration, with a standardization of $1.0\,mV = 1.0\,cm$. ST segment elevation, ST sgment depression, R-wave amplitude, and the corrected QT interval (QT_c), were measured on all ECG tracings [4]. ST segment elevation above baseline (as defined by two consecutive P-R segments) was measured to the closest 0.5 mm, 0.02 sec after the J point [5]. ST segment depression was measured to the closest 0.5 mm, 0.08 sec after the J point. The magnitude of ST segment elevation in each lead showing elevation was measured and summed over the 12 leads. The total number of leads showing ST segment elevation was also calculated. ST segment depression greater than or equal to 0.5 mm below the baseline, 0.08 sec after the J point in any lead was considered significant.

R wave amplitude was measured to the closest 0.5 mm, as the vertical distance from the preceding P-R interval to the peak of the R wave. The sum of R wave amplitudes in all 12 leads was calculated. The sum of R wave amplitudes in only those leads with ST segment elevation during ischemia was also noted. The QT interval was measured to the closest 0.02 sec, in each of the 12 leads and using the Bazett's formula [6], was expressed as the QT_c interval. In each ECG, the longest QT_c interval and the sum of the 12 QT_c interval's, was calculated.

All ECG measurements were made blinded to the clinical and ventriculographic impact of balloon inflation. In five randomly chosen patients, two consecutive baseline ECG's were recorded prior to PTCA in order to assess the intrinsic variability of our measurements. The difference between the two measurements of sum of ST segment elevation, sum of R wave amplitudes, QT_c interval, and sum of the 12 QT_c interval's for each of the five patients was analyzed and the standard deviation about the mean value of the differences was calculated. Intrinsic variability was described as $\pm 2SD$: Sum of ST elevation varied by ± 0.5 mm. Sum of R wave amplitude varied by ± 7.6 mm. QT_c interval varied by ± 0.04 seconds, and the sum of the 12 QT_c intervals varied by ± 0.6.

Grading of collaterals and angiography. The severity of coronary stenosis was evaluated by measuring the percent reduction in lumen diameter from a magnified image of the cine-arteriogram [7]. The grading scale used to quantify the extent of collateral channel filling has been described and validated in a previous publication [1]. In brief: Grade 0 = no visible filling of any collateral channels, grade 1 = filling by means of collateral channels of side branches of the vessel being dilated but without any dye reaching the epicardial segment of that vessel, grade 2 = partial filling via collateral channels of the epicardial sement of the vessel being dilated, and grade 3 = complete filling of the vessel being dilated. Examples of the different grades of collaterals observed before and during balloon inflation are seen in Figs 1 and 2.

The Diasonics/Fischer digital subtraction imaging system was used for

A. Pre TCA

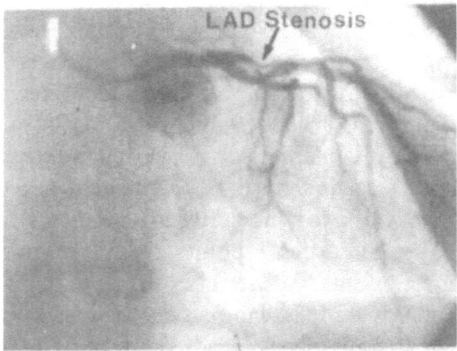

B. Pre TCA, coll grade = O

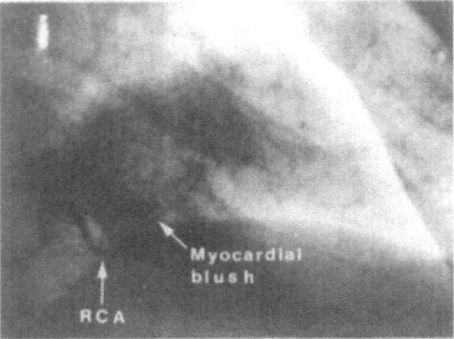

C. During TCA, coll grade = 2

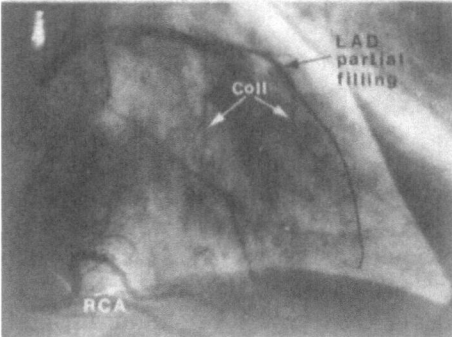

Figure 1.   Example of a change in collateral filling from grade 0 to grade 2 during balloon inflation in patient #02: Panel A. Prior to angioplasty (Pre-TCA), there is a 90% stenosis in the proximal left anterior descending (LAD). Panel B. There are no visible collaterals originating from the right coronary artery (RCA). Panel C. During balloon inflation, Grade 2 collaterals (Coll), are seen partially filling the epicardial segment of the LAD.

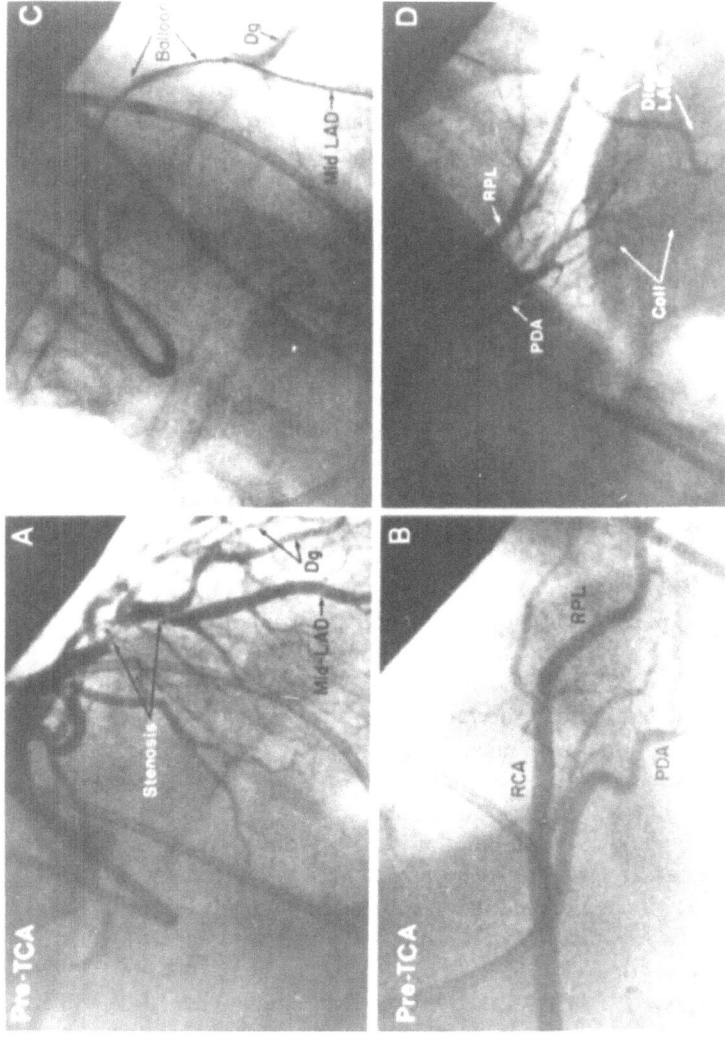

Figure 2. Example of a change in collateral filling from grade 0 to grade 3 during balloon inflation in patient #17: Panel A. Prior to angioplasty (Pre-TCA), there is a 95% stenosis in the proximal left anterior descending (LAD) near the origin of a diagonal (Dg) branch. Panel B. There are no visible collaterals originating from the posterior descending artery (PDA). Panels C and D. During balloon inflation, Grade 3 collaterals (Coll), are seen originating from the posterior descending artery and completely filling the mid and distal LAD and the diagonal branch. RCA = right coronary artery; RPL = right posterolateral.

creation and analysis of the left ventricular images obtained from injection of 40 ccs of Renografin 38% contrast directly into the left ventricle in the 20° right anterior oblique view. The extent of segmental wall motion abnormalities precipitated by balloon inflation, was quantified using the radial axis model of Ingels et al. [8, 9], in which radial shortening less than 2 standard deviations below the mean value for a normal population defined a 'hypocontractile segment'. The 'percent hypocontractile perimeter', was defined as the length of the hypocontractile segment divided by the total ventricular perimeter (in diastole), excluding the aortic and mitral valves. Since the area of myocardium in jeopardy was different for each patient, (depending on the vessel dilated and the location of the stenosis), an additional parameter of the extent of segmental wall motion abnormalities seen during inflation was measured, the 'percent hypocontractile perimeter of the area at risk'. This variable was defined as the length of the hypocontractile segment, (as measured above), divided by the length of the ventricular perimeter *at risk*. The segment at risk was measured starting at the proximal end of the angioplasty balloon and extending as far as the epicardial segment of the vessel being dilated.

Study protocol. Cycle 0, Baseline Pre PTCA: A 12-lead ECG was obtained followed by arteriograms of the contralateral artery using the 5 Fr coronary catheter. Thereafter, the 5 Fr pigtail was advanced into the left ventricle, pressures recorded and a left ventriculogram was obtained. After the pigtail catheter was withdrawn to the descending aorta, multiple views of the stenosed vessel being dilated were obtained through the guiding catheter and the deflated angioplasty balloon was guided through the lesion. Routine PTCA proceeded with two therapeutic inflations. Just prior to deflating the balloon during the second inflation, an injection was made through the guiding catheter to document the absence of any flow around the inflated balloon and the absence of any intracoronary collateral filling. Several minutes after recovery from these initial inflations three additional inflations were performed during which the 'study', variables were measured.

Cycle 1: The pigtail catheter was advanced into the left ventricle. Immediately prior to and throughout balloon inflation simultaneous aortic, left ventricular, and distal coronary artery pressure were continuously recorded as well as a rhythm strip. At 30 secs into balloon inflation a simultaneous 12-lead ECG was recorded. At 40 sec the inflation was terminated and 3 min of recovery elapsed before proceeding with cycle 2.

Cycle 2: At 30 sec into the next balloon inflation a simultaneous 12-lead ECG was recorded. At 40 sec a left ventriculogram was acquired. The balloon was immediately deflated followed by 3 min of recovery.

Cycle 3: The pigtail catheter was removed and a 5 Fr arteriography catheter was placed in the contralateral artery. At 30 sec into balloon inflation a simultaneous 12-lead ECG was repeated. At 40 sec an arteriogram of the contralateral artery was obtained.

Cycle 4: After removing the balloon catheter, one final injection of the contralateral artery was made. Examples of the ECG's and left ventriculograms obtained before and during inflation in two patients are shown in Figs 3 and 4.

Statistics. All continuous variables are presented as the mean $\pm$ the standard deviation. The measurements recorded during Cycle 0 will were considered control values. The values referred to for heart rate and pressure during cycles 1–3 are those measured at 35 seconds into inflation. The examination of differences between the control cycle and intervention cycles involved one-way analysis of variance and the paired t-test. The nonparametric statistic, the Spearman rank correlation coefficient, was used to test the relation between collateral grade, (measured on an ordinal scale 0–3), and the variables measuring the extent of myocardial ischemia. The analyses correlating the ECG with the wall motion abnormalities involved dividing the study population into 12 patients with LAD artery dilatation and 11 patients with RCA dilatation. Each group was analyzed separately. The relationship between the electrocardiographic variables; (1) sum of ST segment elevation, and (2) magnitude of ST segment elevation in V_2 or Lead III, to the percent hypocontractile perimeter was best fitted by applying a second order polynomial equation and a correlation coefficient was calculated. The relationship between the electrocardiographic variable, number of leads with ST

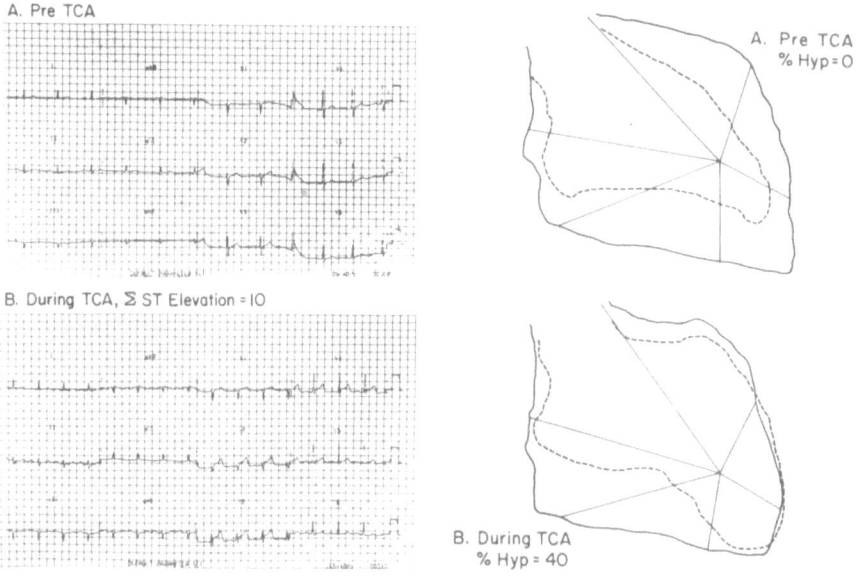

Figure 3. Panel A, from left to right, the pre angioplasty (Pre TCA) ECG and left ventriculogram respectively for patient #20. Panel B, from left to right, the ECG and left ventriculogram during balloon inflation (During TCA). In comparison to the pre TCA ECG, the recording during balloon inflation reveals a sum of ST elevation = 10 mm. In comparison to the normal pre TCA left ventriculogram (%Hyp=0), the ventriculogram during balloon inflation reveals hypocontractility involving 40% of the left ventricular perimeter (%Hyp=40). %Hyp = percent hypocontractility.

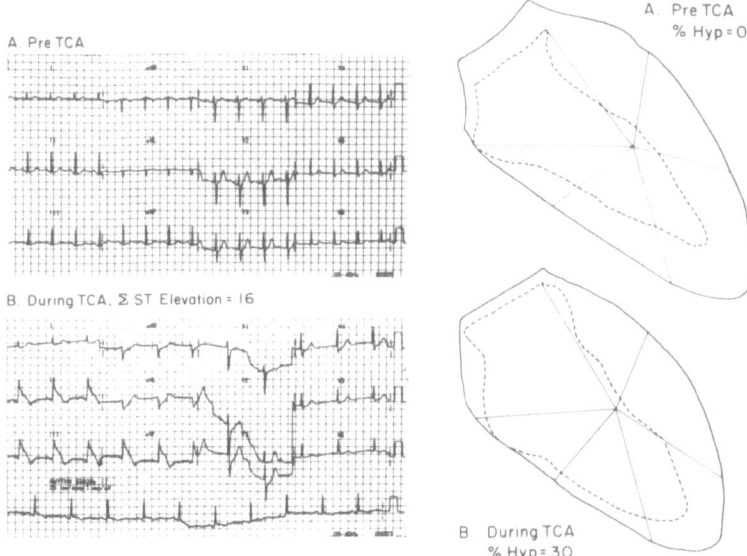

Figure 4. Panel A, from left to right, the Pre angioplasty ECG and left ventriculogram respectively for patient #16. Panel B, from left to right, the ECG and left ventriculogram during balloon inflation. In comparison to the pre TCA, the recording during balloon inflation reveals a sum of ST elevation = 16 mm. In comparison to the normal pre TCA left ventriculogram (%Hyp = 0), the ventriculogram during balloon inflation reveals hypocontractility involving 30% of the left ventricular perimeter (%HYP = 30).

segment elevation, to the percent hypocontractile perimeter, was assessed by the Spearman rank correlation coefficient. Probability (p) values greater than or equal to 0.05 were considered non-significant (NS).

Results

Changes in collateral filling during coronary occlusion (Fig. 5). Baseline arteriography of the contralateral vessels immediately prior to passage of the angioplasty balloon, revealed a mean grade of collateral filling of 0.5 ± 0.8. During balloon inflation, there was a significant increase in the mean grade of collateral filling to 1.7 ± 1.0 (p = 0.01). Nineteen of the 23 patients improved their collateral filling by at least one grade. Seven of the 23 patients improved by at least 2 grades. Six patients who originally had no visible collaterals increased their collateral fillings to grade 2 or 3. Arteriography, after the stenosis was dilated and the balloon removed, revealed no visible collateral channels to the dilated vessel in any patient.

Hemodynamics. No significant changes were observed in heart rate, mean aortic

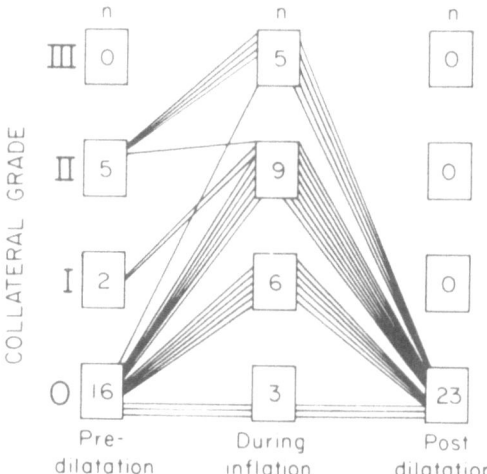

Figure 5. Change in grade of collateral filling arising from the contralateral coronary artery before, during and after balloon occlusion (cycle 0, 3, 4).

pressure, or in the product of heart rate and peak systolic aortic pressure. In contrast, left ventricular end-diastolic pressure increased slightly but significantly, from 11.3 ± 2.8 mm Hg (cycle 0), to 13.7 ± 4.2 and 14.0 ± 3.4, (cycle 2 and 3) ($p = 0.04$).

Indices of myocardial ischemia with reference to collateral filling. Sudden coronary occlusion by the angioplasty balloon resulted in significant myocardial ischemia as assessed by the percent hypocontractile perimeter, and by the sum of ST segment elevation. New wall motion abnormalities were observed during the cycle 2 left ventriculogram in nineteen of 23 patients. The wall motion ranged from 5–40% of the left ventricular perimeter. Three patients had no new wall abnormalities. There was a weak association between the percent hypocontractile perimeter and the grade of collateral filling during cycle 0 ($r = -0.50$). A highly significant correlation however, was observed between the percent hypocontractile perimeter assessed during cycle 2, and the grade of collateral filling assessed during cycle 3 ($r = -0.85$) (Fig. 6). In addition, a close correlation was also observed between the percent hypocontractile perimeter at risk and the grade of collateral filling during cycle 2 ($r = -0.81$).

Nineteen out of 23 patients developed new ST segment elevation greater than 0.5 mm as compared to their baseline ECG. One patient developed isolated ST segment depression and the remaining 3 patients had no ECG changes at 30 sec into inflation. There was a weak association between the sum of ST segment elevation and the grade of collateral filling during cycle 0 ($r = -0.40$). A highly significant correlation however, was observed between the sum of ST segment elevation during balloon inflation (cycle 2), and the grade of collateral filling during inflation cycle 3 ($r = -0.87$) (Fig. 7).

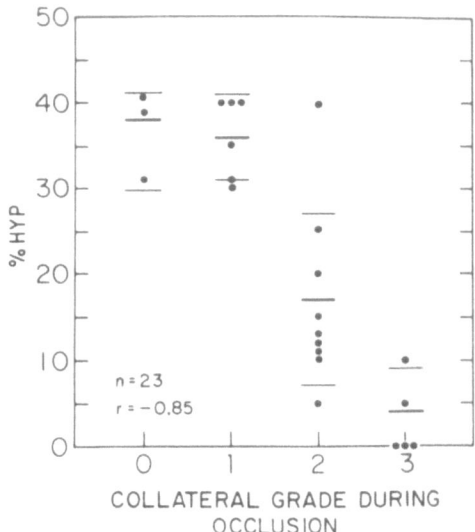

Figure 6. The relation between the grade of collaterals during coronary occlusion, (abscissa), and the percent hypocontractile perimeter, (%Hyp) (ordinate).

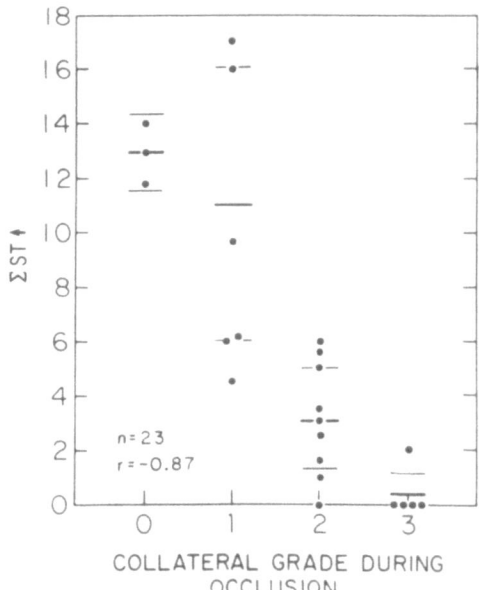

Figure 7. The relation between the grade of collaterals during coronary occlusion, (abscissa), and the sum of ST segment elevation, (ΣST↑) (ordinate).

Fourteen of the 23 patients developed their typical anginal pain during each balloon inflation (Table 1). The time of onset of pain ranged from 24 to 40 secs after the beginning of the balloon inflation. Nine of the 23 patients experienced no angina during the inflation cycles. These 9 patients had either grade 2 or 3 collaterals. All of the patients with only grade 0 or 1 collaterals experienced angina within 40 seconds.

Electrocardiographic detection of the presence and location of new wall motion abnormalities. The number of patients experiencing changes in their ST segments or T waves is depicted in Table 2, according to LAD versus RCA dilatation. Sixteen of the 19 patients, who developed new wall motion abnormalities, developed acute ST segment elevation greater than 0.5 mm compared to their baseline ECG. In contrast, only 13 of these 19 patients manifested ST segment depression. In 2 patients, with mid RCA lesions and hypocontractile segments of only 3 and 5%, the only ST or T segment change observed was isolated ST segment depression in the inferior leads. In one other patient, with a mid RCA lesion and a hypocontractile segment of only 5%, no ECG changes were observed. Four patients had no new wall motion abnormalities. None of these patients, had any ST or T wave changes. None of the 21 patients had significant T wave changes in the absence of ST segment shifts. Comparing ST segment or T wave changes, acute ST segment elevation was the most sensitive ECG indicator of new asynergy; Sensitivity = 85%, specificity = 100%, predictive value = 100%.

Among the 19 patients with new asynergy, 10 had anterior wall and 7 had inferior wall asynergy. All 10 of the 10 patients with new anterior wall asynergy experienced ST segment elevation in lead V_2 equal to or greater than 0.5 mm (see Table 2). No other lead was more sensitive in localizing new anterior wall asynergy. One patient, however, had a greater magnitude of ST segment elevation in lead V_3, than in V_2, but both leads demonstrated ST segment elevation. Among the 7 patients with new inferior wall motion abnormalities, 5 of the 7 experienced ST segment elevation in leads II and III equal to or greater than 0.5 mm. Lead AVF was less sensitive.

Changes in the R wave amplitude and QT intervals between the baseline cycle

Table 1. Relation of the collateral grade during balloon inflation, to the development of anginal pain during balloon inflation

	Collateral grade	
Pain	0 or 1	2 or 3
no	0	9
yes	9	5

Table 2. Number of patients with ST segment or T wave shifts in each lead

Artery occluded	1	AVL	V_1	V_2	V_3	V_4	V_5	V_6	II	III	AVF
				ST elevation							
LAD (n = 12)	2	5	6	10	9	7	3	1	0	0	0
RCA (n = 11)	0	0	0	0	0	0	0	1	6	6	5
				ST depression							
LAD (n = 12)	0	0	0	0	0	0	1	1	5	5	5
RCA (n = 11)	2	4	0	4	5	2	2	1	1	2	2
				T wave changes							
LAD (n = 12)	1	4	1	2	2	2	2	3	3	5	3
RCA (n = 11)	2	2	0	1	1	0	1	0	3	3	3

LAD = left anterior descending artery; RCA = right coronary artery.

Table 3. Changes in R wave amplitude and QT intervals

A. *R wave amplitude during baseline (R_0) cycle, and inflation cycle (R_4) in patients with new hypocontractility*

LAD occlusion (n = 10)   RCA occlusion (n = 9)

Sum of R waves in all 12 leads
1. Sum of $R_0 = 79.2 \pm 27.9$ 1. Sum of $R_0 = 76.6 \pm 14.0$
2. Sum of $R_4 = 75.0 \pm 28.2$ 2. Sum of $R_4 = 75.1 \pm 15.6$

Sum of R waves in leads with ST elevation
1. Sum of $R_0 = 34.9 \pm 24.5$ 1. Sum of $R_0 = 20.2 \pm 15.3$
2. Sum of $R_4 = 30.0 \pm 23.6$ 2. Sum of $R_4 = 18.9 + 13.0$

B. *QT_c interval during baseline (QT_{c0}) and inflation cycle (QT_{c4}) in patients with new hypocontractility*

LAD occlusion (n = 10)   RCA occlusion (n = 9)

Sum of QT_c in all 12 leads
1. Sum of $QT_{c0} = 4.5 \pm 0.13$ 1. Sum of $QT_{c0} = 4.70 \pm 0.16$
2. Sum of $QT_{c4} = 4.80 \pm 0.33*$ 2. Sum of $QT_{c4} = 4.80 \pm 0.19*$

QT_c in lead with longest QT_c
1. $QT_{c0} = 0.44 \pm 0.03$ 2. $QT_{c0} = 0.46 \pm 0.03$
2. $QT_{c4} = 0.48 \pm 0.04*$ 2. $QT_{c4} = 0.47 \pm 0.03$

*p less than 0.05 compared to baseline cycle using the paired t-test.
LAD = left anterior descending artery; RCA = right coronary artery.

and the inflation cycle were analyzed in those patients with new asynergy (see Table 3). No significant difference was observed between the sum of R wave amplitudes on the inflation cycle ECG compared to the baseline ECG. When this analysis was carried out summing the R waves only in those leads in which there was ST elevation there was still no significant change in the sum of R wave amplitude during coronary occlusion. In contrast, both groups of patients experienced a significant prolongation in the sum of the QT_c interval, during ischemia (Table 3). When one compared only the lead with the longest QT_c interval, before and during balloon occlusion, only the patients with LAD dilatations demonstrated a significant prolongation in the longest QT_c interval during ischemia.

Electrocardiographic correlation to extent of new wall motion abnormalities (Figs. 8–10). Three ECG parameters utilizing ST segment elevation were analyzed to assess the correlation between the ECG and the extent of the new hypocontractile segment. Using a second order polynomial equation to describe the relation between the sum of ST elevation and percent hypocontractility, a highly significant correlation was observed for LAD as well as for RCA occlusion, $(r = 0.96)$ and $(r = 0.89)$ respectively (Fig. 8). Since the prior analysis revealed that lead V_2 and lead III were the most sensitive leads for anterior and inferior asynergy respectively, we analyzed the relation between the magnitude of ST segment elevation in only one lead, (lead V_2 or lead III), and percent hypocontractile segment. A significant correlation was observed for V_2 $(r = 0.92)$ and lead III $(r = 0.90)$ (Fig. 9). Lastly, there was a significant correlation between the total number of leads with ST segment elevation and the percent hypocontractile perimeter, (Spearman rank $r = 0.77$ for the LAD artery, and $r = 0.92$ for the RCA) (Fig. 10).

Discussion

Our studies, using the angioplasty model described above, constitute the first prospective analyses of the role of collaterals in fixed isolated coronary disease in which the major study variables are known prior to as well as during the controlled coronary artery occlusion. In addition, we selected patients in whom

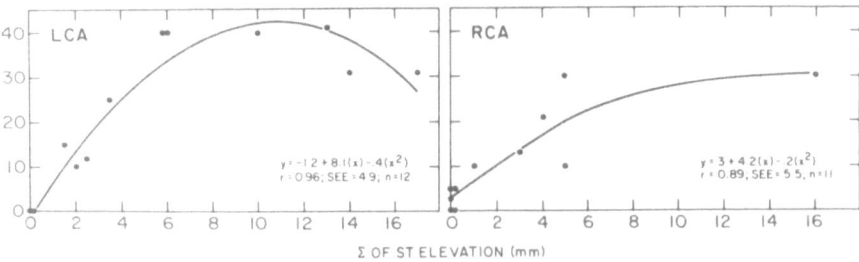

Figure 8. The relation between the sum of ST segment elevation during coronary occlusion (abscissa), and the percent hypocontractile perimeter (%HYP) (ordinate). Left panel, 12 patients with left anterior descending (LCA) dilatations; Right panel, 11 patients with right coronary artery (RCA) dilatations.

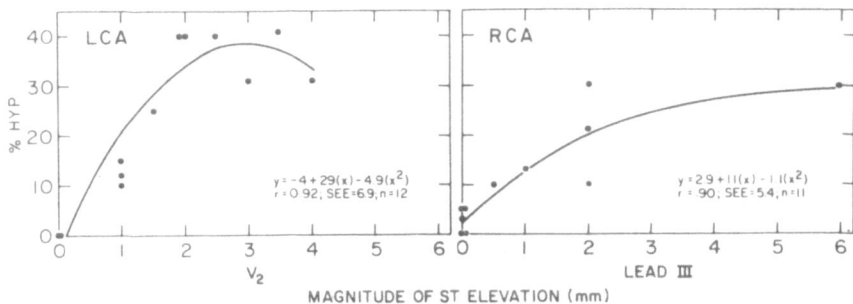

Figure 9. The relation between the magnitude of ST segment elevation during coronary occlusion in either V_2 or Lead III (abscissa), and the percent hypocontractile perimeter (%HYP) (ordinate). Left panel, lead V_2 for LAD artery dilatations; Right panel Lead III for RCA dilatations.

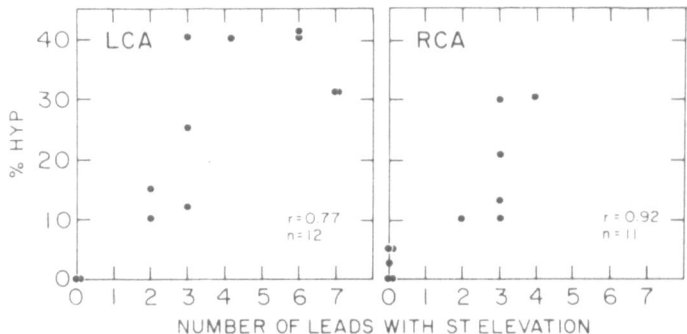

Figure 10. The relation between the total number of leads with ST segment elevation during coronary occlusion (abscissa), and the percent hypocontractile perimeter (%HYP) (ordinate).

no other stimuli to collateral flow other than fixed coronary obstruction was present.

The coronary collateral circulation is a dynamic circulation. In human subjects, with severe coronary artery disease, Bourassa et al [10], observed that changes in collateral filling occurred within two weeks of coronary bypass surgery. Patients with good collateral filling prior to surgery no longer had angiographic evidence of collateral filling after successful bypass surgery. In contrast, patients without evidence of collateral circulation prior to surgery developed angiographic evidence of collateral filling to arteries subtended by occluded grafts. A similar reduction in collateral filling was observed by Gruntzig et al who demonstrated that collateral filling disappeared immediately after successful coronary angioplasty [11].

Several investigators have evaluated the collateral circulation, in patients with coronary spasm, prone to recurrent episodes of transient severe narrowing or even total occlusion of a coronary artery. Gensini et al described a patient with coronary spasm superimposed on a severe lesion [12]. Injection of the contralateral artery at the time of spasm and total occlusion, revealed collateral filling to the diseased artery, which was not visible in the resting state. More recent work by the Japanese investigators Takeshita et al [13], and Tada et al [14], in patients with spasm and normal coronary arteries, indicated that there was evidence of collateral filling immediately after the onset of coronary spasm, which was not present angiographically on prior injections when the native coronary arteries were not in spasm.

Our observations in a larger group of patients with severe atherosclerotic heart disease, and no history of coronary spasm, suggests that this subset of patients also has the capacity to improve collateral filling after abrupt cessation of antegrade blood flow [1]. In fact, the immediate appearance of well developed collaterals in the majority of our patients during sudden total coronary occlusion was striking. Our high prevalence rate for well developed collaterals is supported by other recent investigations which have used an angioplasty model [15–17]. This high prevalence rate however, is in contrast to the prevalence rate of collateral circulation visualized during acute myocardial infarction. For example, the observations of Nohara et al [18], in the first three hours of infarction suggests that only about 40–50% of patients have good collateral filling. In addition, observations made during the Mt. Sinai Medical Center/Bellevue Reperfusion Pilot Trial indicate that only 50% of patients with total coronary occlusions have collateral circulation to the infarct-related artery [19]. One possible explanation for the difference between our prevalence rate and the lower prevalence rate observed in patients during infarction may be that our patients, in general, had more severe stenoses than the average patient presenting with an acute infarction. It is probable that in a large fraction of infarct patients, sudden coronary artery occlusion occurred on a coronary lesion that was not severe enough to stimulate collateral development [20].

Can collateral circulation limit myocardial ischemia? Early studies assessed the functional significance of the coronary collateral circulation in patients with ischemic heart disease by pathologic evaluation of postmortem hearts. Blumgart et al [21], and Baroldi et al [22], observed that a significant number of patients had sustained total coronary occlusion but had large interarterial anastomotic channels that filled the main epicardial coronary arteries retrograde. Inspite of the total obstructions, however, many of these patients had no evidence of ischemic injury. These investigators suggested that the collateral flow passing through the interarterial anastomoses protected the jeopardized zone. Several investigators applied selective coronary arteriography in-vivo and observed major inter- and intra-coronary collateral channels filling vessels retrograde [23–27]. Using these techniques, Helfant et al [24], suggested that there were no significant differences between patients with versus without collaterals with regard to the extent of ventricular aynergy or hemodynamic indices of left ventricular dysfunction. However, they did observe a trend toward less mortality during the follow-up period. In contrast, Levin et al [25], and Webster et al [26], studied patients with total occlusion of at least one coronary artery and both investigators concluded that patients with collaterals, had better ventricular function than patients who progressed to total occlusion in the absence of collaterals. More recently, the impact of collateral circulation has been assessed during the acute phase of myocardial infarction [18, 28, 29]. While several of these studies suggested that collaterals in the early hours of acute infarction was associated with relatively smaller infarcts, these studies were limited by the fact that the patients presented several hours after total occlusion of the infarct related artery, very little information was available regarding the clinical and coronary arteriographic characteristics of the patient prior to the infarction, and additional therapeutic interventions were often employed which may have also limited infarct size.

In patients with coronary spasm, Takeshita et al [13], and Tada et al [14], observed that those patients who had good collateral filling of the artery induced to spasm had only ST segment depression and not the ST segment elevation seen after sudden transmural ischemia in those patients with spasm and no collateral filling.

The data presented in the present study, comparing ventriculography during sudden coronary occlusion, with the degree of collateral filling seen during occlusion, strongly suggests that the coronary collateral circulation does limit myocardial ischemia in man. The protection afforded does not appear to be an all or none phenomenon but rather a graduated one. In general terms, grade 0 or 1 collateral filling can be viewed as conferring a negligible degree of protection. All three indices of myocardial ischemia (percent hypocontractile perimeter, sum of ST segment elevation, and onset of angina), were markedly positive in all patients with only grade 0 or 1 collateral filling. While earlier anatomic investigations demonstrated that narrow intercoronary collateral channels between 100 to 300 microns in diameter are congenitally present in normal hearts [22, 30], our data suggests that these small collateral channels are not large enough to protect myocardium in jeopardy. In contrast, grade 2 collaterals confer an intermediate degree of myocardial protection. While there was a greater variability with respect to the percent hypocontractile perimeter in patients with grade 2 collateral filling as compared to grade 0 or 3, the majority of grade 2 patients demonstrated new zones of asynergy that were intermediate in size compared to those of patients with either grade 0 or 3 collaterals. Grade 3 collaterals appear to be almost completely protective. The only patients without any new asynergy during coronary occlusion were those with grade 3 collaterals. The tendency towards greater protection with higher collateral grade applied to patients with left coronary as well as right coronary artery occlusion, and also to proximal as well as distal coronary artery occlusion.

Electrocardiographic correlation to new wall motion abnormalities. Clinical investigations reviewing the ECG changes seen during the early phase of acute coronary thrombosis or coronary spasm indicate that several ECG patterns may be observed. The most common change observed is ST segment elevation [31, 32]. Some investigators suggested that T wave peaking occurred prior to ST elevation [33], whereas others suggested that acute increases in R wave amplitude occurred along with ST elevation [32, 34, 35]. A few investigators have even observed transient Q waves within minutes of acute coronary insufficiency [36, 37].

Our study constitutes the first prospective analysis of the relation between the ECG, and an angiographic estimate of the extent of the new ischemic segment assessed within minutes of sudden coronary occlusion in a large group of human subjects with fixed, severe atherosclerotic heart disease. Using the angioplasty model described above, we assessed the ECG variables of ST segment elevation, ST segment depression, R-wave amplitude, and the corrected QT interval, and examined the acute changes in these variable relative to the extent of ischemic wall motion abnormalities. Our observations suggest that in man, there is a highly significant relation between ST segment elevation and the size of the ischemic hypocontractile zone.

Previous studies comparing ST segment changes to infarct size. In both a dog model and a pig model of sudden ischemia, several investigators suggested that the sum of ST segment elevation and the number of leads showing ST elevation correlated well with pathologic estimates of infarct size (38–40). Work in humans however, has yielded conflicting results. Two groups of investigators have observed poor correlations between the sum of ST segment elevation and infarct size estimated from creatine kinase washout curves [41, 42]. In contrast two other groups have observed good correlations between sum of ST elevation and infarct size estimated from creatine kinase washout curves [43, 44].

Our observations indicate that both the sum of ST segment elevation and the number of leads with ST segment elevation observed within the first minute of ischemia, correlate well with angiographic estimates of the size of the ischemic hypocontractile zone. This good correlation applies to patients with either left or right coronary occlusion. The curves that best describe this relation have a steep early rise followed by a plateau. This would indicate that above a certain size of hypocontractile zone other factors probably play a role in determining the ultimate extent of the ST segment elevation [40, 45]. A greater number of patients would be needed, however, to further validate the correlations we observed. Since full 12-lead ECG may not be readily available during routine coronary angioplasty, we analyzed the relation between the magnitude of ST elevation in the most sensitive lead for either anterior or inferior asynergy, and extent of hypocontractility, and found that monitoring just one lead gave a good reflection of the extent of the ischemic zone. This finding is in keeping with the observations of Capone et al [46], who showed a good correlation between the magnitude of ST segment elevation in a single precordial lead and the sum of ST segment elevation.

Previous studies on R wave amplitude and QT intervals during ischemia. Earlier investigators suggested that giant R waves was a common early sign of acute ischemia [32, 34, 35]. Using atrial pacing to induce ischemia, David et al observed an increase in R wave amplitude in lead V_5 in 15 of 17 patients [47]. Barnhill et al assessed the changes in the QRS complex using digital computer analysis in 5 patients with spontaneous variant angina, and observed significant changes in the absolute height of the QRS complex during ischemia [48]. In contrast, Myers et al [49], measured spatial R wave amplitude during exercise testing and observed no relation between changes in R wave height and evidence of ischemia based on thallium-201 imaging. Recently, Feldman et al using precordial and intracoronary unipolar electrograms during angioplasty, failed to show any acute changes in R wave height during balloon occlusion [50].

In the present study, no significant differences were observed between the R wave amplitudes during ischemia compared to baseline. In an attempt to minimize any dilutional effect of random changes in R wave height, an additional analysis was performed of R wave changes only in those leads showing ischemic ST segment elevation. This too however, did not reveal any significant differences. Several individual patients did experience a large change in their R wave height. However, analysis of two repeated baseline measurements revealed a large intrinsic variability in R wave amplitude. Therefore, given the size of our patient population, the changes observed did not reach statistical significance.

Acute ischemia may also affect the QT interval. Mandel et al [51], observed a significant shortening in the refractory period within the ischemic zone, early after coronary occlusion in a dog model. In a prospective study in humans, Cinca et al measured the QT interval within 6 hours of acute transmural infarction [52]. They observed a relative shortening in the QT interval in the lead overlying the ischemic zone in the early phase, followed by a prolongation in the QT interval after 12 hours. Doroghazi et al [53], and Taylor et al [54], suggested that QT interval prolongation was relatively common in the early phase of acute myocardial infarction.

Our study indicates that within the first minute of coronary insufficiency there is a small but significant increase in the QT_c interval assessed over all 12 leads for both left and right coronary occlusions. Since previous investigations used only one particular lead to assess changes in the QT_c interval we also analyzed the QT interval in the lead with the longest QT. Significant prolongation occurred in patients with left coronary occlusion but not with right occlusion. The implication of these QT changes in any one particular lead however, should be viewed with caution because of the relatively large intrinsic variability observed in our analysis of two repeated baseline electrocardiograms.

Limitations of the study. All patients received the vasodilators nitroglycerine and nifedipine. However, the effects of these drugs on the collateral circulation are still uncertain. Second, our study did not evaluate absolute flow through the collateral. Third, while our evaluation suggests that collaterals are protective during the first minute of coronary occlusion, their impact after several hours remains to be determined.

Clinical implications. Our observations suggest greater myocardial protection with higher collateral grades. Second, proof of the protective effect of collateral filling provides impetus for studying markers of collateral reserve and testing therapeutic modalities that may augment collateral filling. Lastly, this study shows that the ECG is a very sensitive and simple tool for assessing sudden onset of myocardial ischemia during coronary angioplasty. Of the ECG parameters analyzed, ST segment elevation best parallels the development of new asynergy during PTCA. The close association between ST segment elevation and the extent of asynergy may be useful in predicting the impact of sudden coronary dissection and occlusion on ventricular function during coronary angioplasty. These findings may be helpful in stratifying the risk for patients undergoing elective PTCA and may help the physician better assess the need for emergency revascularization after such a complication.

References

1. Rentrop KP, Cohen M, Blanke H, Phillips RA (1985) Changes in collateral channel filling immediately after controlled coronary artery occlusion by an angioplasty balloon in human subjects. *J Am Coll Cardiol* 5:587–92
2. Cohen M, Rentrop KP (1986) Limitation of myocardial ischemia by collateral circulation during sudden controlled coronary artery occlusion in human subjects: A prospective study. *Circulation* 74:469–76
3. The Principal Investigators of CASS and Their Associates (1981) The National Heart, Lung, and Blood Institute Coronary Artery Surgery Study (CASS). *Circulation* 63 (Suppl I): I–15
4. Cohen M, Scharpf SJ, Rentrop KP (1987) Prospective analysis of electrocardiographic variables as markers for extent and location of acute wall motion abnormalities observed during coronary angioplasty in human subjects. *J Am Coll Cardiol* 10:17–24
5. Rude RE, Poole K, Muller JE et al, and the Mills Study Group (1983) Electrocardiographic and clinical criteria for recognition of acute myocardial infarction based on analysis of 3,697 patients. *Am J. Cardiol* 52:936–942
6. Bazett HC (1920) An analysis of the time relationship of the electrocardiogram. *Heart* 7:353–370
7. Gensini GG (1975) *Coronary Angiography*. Mt. Kisko, NY, Futura, p 260
8. Ingels NB Jr, Mead CW, Daughters GT II, Stinson EB, Alderman EL (1978) A new method for assessment of left ventricular wall motion. *Comput Cardiol IEEE* 57–61
9. Ingels NB Jr, Daughters GT II, Stinson EB, Alderman EL (1980) Evaluaton of methods for quantitating left ventricular segmental wall motion in man using myocardial markers as a standard. *Circulation* 61:966–972
10. Bourassa MG, Solignac A, Goulet C, Lesperance J (1974) Regression and appearance of coronary collaterals in humans during life. *Circulation* 49 (Suppl II): II–127–138
11. Gruntzig A, Pyle R, Goebel N, Schlumpf M (1980) The fate of collaterals after percutaneous transluminal coronary angioplasty (abstr). *Circulation* 62 (Suppl III): III–120
12. Gensini GG (1975) *Coronary Angiography*. Mt. Kisko, NY, Futura, p 331–332
13. Takeshita A, Koiwaya Y, Nakamura M, Yamamoto K, Torii S (1982) Immediate appearance of coronary collaterals during ergonovine-induced arterial spasm. *Chest* 82:319–322
14. Tada M, Yamagishi M, Kodama K, Kuzuya T, Nanto S, Inoue M, Abe H (1983) Transient

collateral augmentation during coronary arterial spasm associated with ST-segment depression. *Circulation* 67:693–698

15. Bass TA, O'Brien JT, Conetta DA, Perryman, RA, Miller AB (1984) Dynamic appearance of collaterals during transluminal coronary angioplasty (abstr). *Circulation* 70 (Suppl II): II–36

16. Hill JA, Feldman RL, Macdonald RG, Pepine CJ (1985) Coronary artery collateral visualization during acute coronary artery occlusion *Am J Cardiol* 55:1216–1218

17. Meier B, Luethy P, Finci L, Steffenino GD, Rutishauser W (1987) Coronary wedge pressure in relation to spontaneously visible and recruitable collaterals. *Circulation* 75:906–13

18. Nohara R, Kambara H, Murakami T, Kadota K, Tamaki S, Kawai C (1983) Collateral function in early acute myocardial infarction. *Am J Cardiol* 52:955–959

19. Rentrop KP, Feit F, Blanke H, Stecy P, Schneider R, Rey M, Horowitz S, Goldman M, Karsch K, Meilman H, Cohen M, Seigel S, Sanger J, Slater J, Gorlin R, Fox A, Fagerstrom R, Calhoun WF (1984) Effects of intracoronary streptokinase and intracoronary nitroglycerin infusion on coronary angiographic patterns and mortality in patients with acute myocardial infarction. *N Eng J Med* 311:1457–1463

20. Cohen M, Sherman W, Rentrop KP, Gorlin R (1988) Determinants of collateral filling observed during sudden controlled coronary artery occlusion in human subjects: A prospective study. *J Am Coll Cardiol* (in press)

21. Blumgart HL, Schlesinger MJ, Davis D (1940) Studies on the relation of the clinical manifestations of angina pectoris, coronary thrombosis, and myocardial infarction to the pathological findings: With particular reference to the significance of the collateral circulation. *Am Heart J* 19:1–91

22. Baroldi G, Mantero O, Scomazzoni G (1956) The collaterals of the coronary arteries in normal and pathologic hearts. *Circ Res* 4:223–229

23. Gensini GG, Bruto da Costa BC (1969) The coronary collateral circulation in living man. *Am J Cardiol* 24:393–400

24. Helfant RH, Vokonas PS, Gorlin R (1971) Functional importance of the human coronary collateral circulation. *N Eng J Med* 284:1277–1281

25. Levin DC, Sos TA, Lee JG, Baltaxe HA (1973) Coronary collateral circulation and distal coronary runoff: The key factors in preserving myocardial contracility in patients with coronary artery disease. *Am J Cardiol* 119:474

26. Webster J, Moberg C, Rincon G (1974) Natural history of severe proximal cornary artery disease as documented by coronary cineangiography. *Am J Cardiol* 33:195

27. Fuster V, Frye RL, Kennedy MA, Connolly DC, Mankin HT (1979) The role of collateral circulation in the various coronary syndromes. *Circulation* 59:1137–1144

28. Rogers WJ, Hood WPJr, Mantle JA, Baxley WA, Kirklin JK, Zorn GL, Nath HP (1984) Return of left ventricular function after reperfusion in patients with myocardial infarction: Importance of subtotal stenosis or intact collaterals. *Circulation* 69:338–349

29. Blanke H, Cohen M, Karsch KR, Fagerstrom R, Rentrop KP (1985) Prevalence and significance of residual flow to the infarct zone during the acute phase of myocardial infarction. *J Am Coll Cardiol* 5:827–831

30. Fulton WFM (1964) The time factor in the enlargement of anastomoses in coronary artery disease. *Scot Med J* 9:18–23

31. Pardee HEB (1920) An electrocardiographic sign of coronary artery obstruction. *Arch Int Med* 26:244–50

32. Prinzmetal M, Toyoshima H, Ekmekci A, Nagaya T (1962) Angina pectoris: VI. The nature of ST segment elevation and other ECG changes in acute severe myocardial ischemia. *Clin Sci* 23:489–514

33. Dressler W, Roesler H (1947) High T waves in the earliest stage of myocardial infarction. *Am Heart J* 34:627–35

34. MacAlpin RN, Kattus AA, Alvara AB (1973) Angina pectoris at rest with preservation of exercise capacity: Prinzmetal's variant angina. *Circulation* 47:946–958

35. Madias JE, Krikelis EN (1981) Transient giant R waves in the early phase of acute myocardial infarction: Association with ventricular fibrillation. *Clin Cardiol* 4:339–349

36. Meller J, Conde CA, Donoso E, Dack S (1975) Transient Q waves in Prinzmetal's angina. *Am J Cardiol* 35:691–695
37. Roesler H, Dressler W (1954) Transient electrocardiographic changes identical with those of acute myocardial infarction accompanying attacks of angina pectoris. *Am Heart J* 47:520–526
38. Maroko PR, Kjekshus JK, Sobel BE, Watanabe T, Covell JW, Ross J Jr, Braunwald E (1971) Factors influencing infarct size following experimental coronary artery occlusions. *Circulation* 43:67–82
39. Muller JE, Marko PR, Braunwald E (1975) Evaluation of precordial electrocardiographic mapping as a means of assessing changes in myocardial ischemic injury. *Circulation* 52:16–27
40. Holland RP, Brooks H (1975) Precordial and epicardial surface potentials during myocardial ischemia in the pig: A theoretical and experimental analysis of the TQ and ST segments. *Circ Res* 37:471–480
41. Thompson PL, Katavatis V (1976) Acute myocardial infarction: Evaluation of precordial ST segment mapping. *Br Heart J* 38:1020–1024
42. Norris RM, Barrat-Boyes C, Heng MK, Singh BN (1976) Failure of ST segment elevation to predict severity of acute myocardial infarction. *Br Heart J* 38:85–92
43. Henning H, Hardarson T, Francis G, O'Rourke RA, Ryan W, Ross J Jr (1978) Approach to the estimation of myocardial infarct size by analysis of precordial ST-segment and R wave maps. *Am J Cardiol* 41:1–8
44. Inoue M, Hori M, Fukunami M, Fukushima M, Tada M, Abe H, Minamino T. Fukui S (1979) Evaluation of praecordial ST segment mapping as an index of infarct size in patients with acute myocardial infarction. *Br Heart J* 42:726–733
45. Holland RP, Brooks H (1977) Spatial and nonspatial influences on the QT–ST segment deflection of ischemia: Theoretical and experimental analysis in the pig. *J Clin Invest* 60:197–214
46. Capone RJ, Most AS (1979) The single precordial lead for ST segment monitoring: Comparison with the multiple lead map. *Am Heart J* 97:753–758
47. David D, Kitchen JG III, Michelson EL, Naito M, Sawin HS, Chen CC (1984) R-wave amplitude responses to rapid atrial pacing: A marker for myocardial ischemia. *Am Heart J* 107:53
48. Barnhill JE, Wikswo JP Jr., Dawson AK, Gundersen S, Robertson RMS, Roberson D, Virmani R, Smith RF (1985) Th QRS complex during transient myocardial ischemia: Studies in patients with variant angina pectoris and in a canine preparation. *Circulation* 71:901–911
49. Myers J, Ahnve S, Froelicher V, Sullivan M (1985) Spatial R wave amplitude changes during exercise: Relation with left ventricular ischemia and function. *J Am Coll Cardiol* 6:603–8
50. Feldman T, Chua KG, Childers RW (1986) R wave of the surface and intracoronary electrogram during acute coronary artery occlusion. *Am J Cardiol* 58:885–890
51. Mandel WJ, Burgess MJ, Neville J Jr, Abildskov JA (1968) Analysis of T wave abnormalities associated with myocardial infarction using a theoretical model. *Circulation* 38:178–188
52. Cinca J, Figueras J, Tenorio L, Valle V, Trenchs J, Segura R, Rius J (1982) Time course and rate dependence of Q–T interval changes during noncomplicated acute transmural myocardial infarction in human beings. *Am J Cardiol* 48:1023–1028
53. Dorghazi RM, Childers R (1978) Time-related changes in the Q–T interval in acute myocardial infarction: Possible relation to local hypocalcemia. *Am J Cardiol* 41:684–688
54. Taylor GJ, Crampton RS, Gibson RS, Stebbins PT, Waldman MTG, Beller GA (1981) Prolonged QT interval at onset of acute myocardial infarction in predicting early phase ventricular tachycardia. *Am Heart J* 102:16–24

6. Collaterals and coronary wedge pressure

B. DE BRUYNE and B. MEIER

Introduction

This chapter summarizes and discusses results obtained in various catheter-ization laboratories concerning the presence or absence of collaterals and the measurement of the distal coronary occlusion pressure (coronary wedge pressure) in the context of percutaneous transluminal coronary angioplasty and compares them to the preexisting literature on coronary collaterals and their function.

Assessment of coronary collateral circulation

Although collateral circulation is a common finding in coronary artery disease, its functional relevance has often been debated [6, 20, 21, 37]. Several reasons account for this controversy. First, experimental work has been done mainly in the dog. However, because of the existence of significant species differences [24], a great variety of collateralization of healthy human hearts and particularly of atherosclerotic human hearts, and the absence of a satisfactory laboratory model of human coronary artery disease, the results cannot necessarily be extrapolated to the human coronary circulation. Secondly, in previous studies, the relation between the degree of collateralization and the extent of myocardial necrosis [1, 4] or wall motion abnormalities [6, 20] has been assessed days or weeks following coronary closure. Since the collateral flow is likely to increase with time after coronary artery occlusion [36], it is probable that the effects of collaterals present at the time of occlusion are underestimated in these retrospective studies. Finally, the conclusions of most of the studies on human coronary collaterals are supported by angiographic evaluation of the extent of collaterals. Current angiographic equipment reveals only vessels with luminal diameter of at least 100 micrometers. Whether good angiographic visualization represents good flow in a given vessel remains an open issue. A morphological method such as angiography is probably far from ideal to demonstrate the potential efficacy of coronary collaterals in human patients.

P.W. Serruys, R. Simon & K.J. Beatt (eds), Percutaneous Transluminal Coronary Angioplasty. ISBN 0-7923-0346-6.
© *1990 Kluwer Academic Publishers, Dordrecht*

Coronary wedge pressure: Definition and determinants

A more physiological approach to collateral function is possible by studies of the hemodynamics of coronary collaterals in humans during aorto-coronary bypass surgery [17, 18, 19, 40]. Distal coronary occlusion pressure has been found to correlate with the amount of retrograde coronary blood flow. At present, it is an accepted index of collateral flow in animals [35]. With the advent of coronary angioplasty, it became possible to measure this distal coronary pressure in conscious humans [11, 12, 16, 23, 26, 29, 30, 32].

The coronary occlusion pressure has been termed coronary wedge pressure by analogy to the pulmonary wedge pressure [26]. The coronary wedge pressure is defined as the mean distal coronary pressure measured at the tip of the dilation catheter while the balloon is inflated in the stenosis at low pressure for at least 30 seconds (Fig. 1).

Phasic pressures can be obtained if the balloon is flushed with saline but even then, the fluid filled system and the small lumen of the catheter used induce damping of high frequency components. This suggests that only mean pressures should be used when comparison between different groups of patients is made [10, 26, 39].

A possible interference has to be kept in mind between the pressure used to fill the balloon (inflation pressure) and the pressure transmitted from the balloon tip. The catheters used in most of the pertinent studies are made of fairly stiff polyvinyl chloride and feature two semilunar lumina within the balloon shaft. Stepwise assessment of the coronary wedge pressure in four patients at inflation

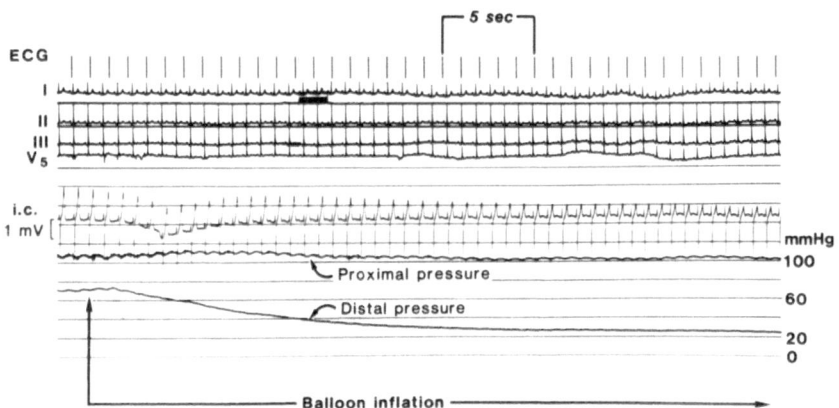

Figure 1.   Pressure tracings during balloon inflation in the left anterior descending coronary artery. The distal pressure decreases after elimination of anterograde flow and levels off after about 20 sec to a wedge pressure of 25 mmHg. ic = intra-coronary

Reprinted with permission from the American College of Cardiology, *Journal of the American College of Cardiology* (1987) 10:504–509.

pressures increasing from one to ten bars revealed no measurable changes and confirmed unbiased transmission of the coronary pressure during balloon fillings at a wide pressure range. Coronary wedge pressure used for analysis at our institution were assessed uniformly at balloon inflation pressure of about 2 bars. The coronary wedge pressure may be rendered spuriously low when the ostium of a collateral branch flowing into the artery just distal to the stenosis is occluded by the inflated balloon [38].

Since balloon inflation eliminates the contribution of antegrade flow, the coronary wedge pressure is mainly determined by the flow provided by the collaterals. There may be other significant determinants of coronary wedge pressure besides collateral flow.

Variation in mean aortic pressure can influence the level of coronary pressure. The higher the mean aortic pressure, the higher the coronary wedge pressure could be expected. Coronary wedge pressure can be corrected by using the transocclusional gradient [26, 30] or the distal coronary occlusion pressure/mean aortic pressure ratio [32]. This correction may be useful in case of marked systemic hypertension or hypotension at the moment of assessment of the coronary wedge pressure.

Coronary spasm or variation in arteriolar tone in vessels supplying both ischemic and non-ischemic myocardium could induce steal or reverse steal [8] through the collateral channels, and nitrates have been shown to decrease collateral resistance in the fibrillating heart [19].

Extravascular and intramyocardial pressures probably contribute to collateral flow and coronary wedge pressure since it has been shown in the dog that collateral flow to the distal part of an occluded vessel follows a waterfall mechanism [2, 15]. However, we found no difference in mean left ventricular end-diastolic pressure between groups with high and low coronary wedge pressure [10]. Furthermore, in previous work [26], the coronary wedge pressure was assessed at 15 and 60 sec of coronary occlusion during three consecutive balloon inflations and compared with the left ventricular end-diastolic pressure measured simultaneously with a high fidelity manometer-tipped catheter introduced through the opposite femoral artery. There was no difference in coronary wedge pressure assessed at the beginning and at the end of a 60 seconds inflation cycle, whereas the left ventricular end-diastolic pressure increased. Right atrial pressure could also influence the level of the measured pressure. These factors may be important for low coronary wedge pressures but from 20 mmHg upward, the coronary wedge pressure mainly reflects collateral flow [15].

Coronary wedge pressure and angiographic extent of collaterals

Coronary angiography demonstrates only collaterals that are already in use (spontaneously visible collaterals). PTCA provides the opportunity to uncover collaterals ready to become functional in case of occlusion of the recipient artery (recruitable collaterals). In the context of coronary angioplasty we investigated whether the coronary wedge pressure correlates with the presence of both spontaneously visible and recruitable collaterals [26].

Fifty-seven coronary arteries of 49 patients undergoing PTCA for a proximal coronary stenosis (n = 51) or occlusion (n = 6) were studied. Spontaneously visible collaterals were recorded on baseline angiograms. During the first or second balloon inflation (at about 30 sec) the following variables were assessed and recorded simultaneously: (1) coronary wedge pressure, (2) transocclusional gradient defined as the difference between the mean aortic pressure and the coronary wedge pressure; (3) electrocardiographic leads I, II, and V5 for the left anterior descending coronary artery, and leads I, II, and III for the right and the circumflex coronary artery (intracoronary ECG in 4 arteries [27]); (4) occurrence of chest pain. In addition, an ipsilateral contrast injection was performed through the guiding catheter to ascertain the completeness of balloon occlusion and to visualize recruitable ipsilateral collaterals and a contralateral contrast injection was performed through an 8F diagnostic catheter introduced via the opposite femoral artery to visualize contralateral recruitable collaterals. This injection was omitted if the attempted vessel was totally occluded, if spontaneously visible contralateral collaterals were present or if both applied. Only collaterals filling at least a segment of the recipient vessel distal to the lesion were considered (grade II and III of Rentrop's classification [31]). Spontaneously visible collaterals were defined as collaterals documented by routine coronary angiography (performed after sublingual or during intravenous nitroglycerine administration). Recruitable collaterals were defined as collaterals not visible on the routine angiogram but visible during proximal balloon occlusion of the recipient artery.

Spontaneously visible collaterals were present in 35 of the 57 arteries investigated (61%). 8 vessels (14%) had only recruitable collaterals and 14 (25%) had none. The coronary wedge pressures in the arteries with and without collaterals are depicted in Figure 2. The mean value for the arteries with collaterals was 40 ± 12 mmHg (spontaneously visible collaterals 41 ± 12 mmHg, recruitable collaterals 36 ± 12 mmHg) and that for the arteries without collaterals was 18 ± 4 mmHg (p < 0.01). A coronary wedge pressure of 30 mmHg or higher was found exclusively in arteries with collaterals. The transocclusional pressure gradient inversely reflects the coronary wedge pressure corrected for the mean systemic blood pressure. The values of the different groups were 53 ± 15 mmHg (range 25 to 100 mmHg) for arteries with collaterals (54 ± 16 mmHg, range 25 to 100 mmHg for arteries with spontaneously visible collaterals; 49 ± 8 mmHg, range 35 to 60 mm Hg) for arteries with recruitable collaterals and 75 ± 11 mmHg (range 55 to 95 mmHg) for arteries without collaterals. The mean value for arteries with spontaneously visible or recruitable collaterals were similar and each of them was significantly lower than the mean value of the arteries without collaterals. A transocclusional pressure gradient of 50 mmHg or less was found exclusively in arteries with collaterals. The mean degree of stenosis was significantly higher in arteries with collaterals ($93 \pm 8\%$, range 60 to 100%) than in arteries without collaterals ($82 \pm 16\%$, range 40 to 100%) (p < 0.005). The subgroup with spontaneously visible collaterals had a mean degree of stenosis of

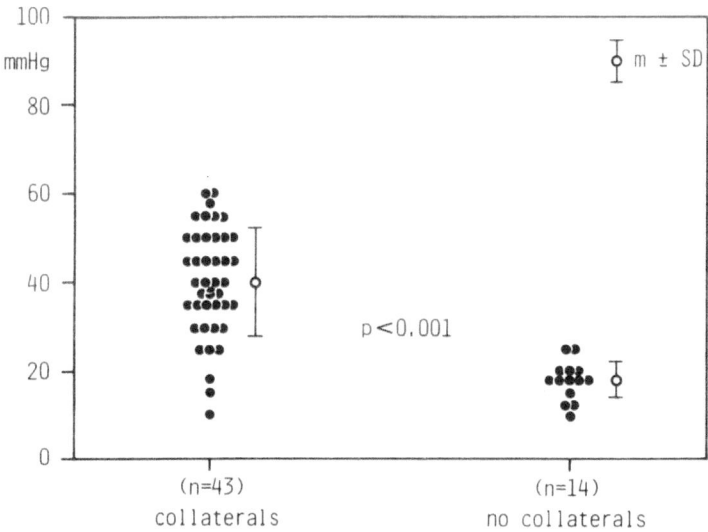

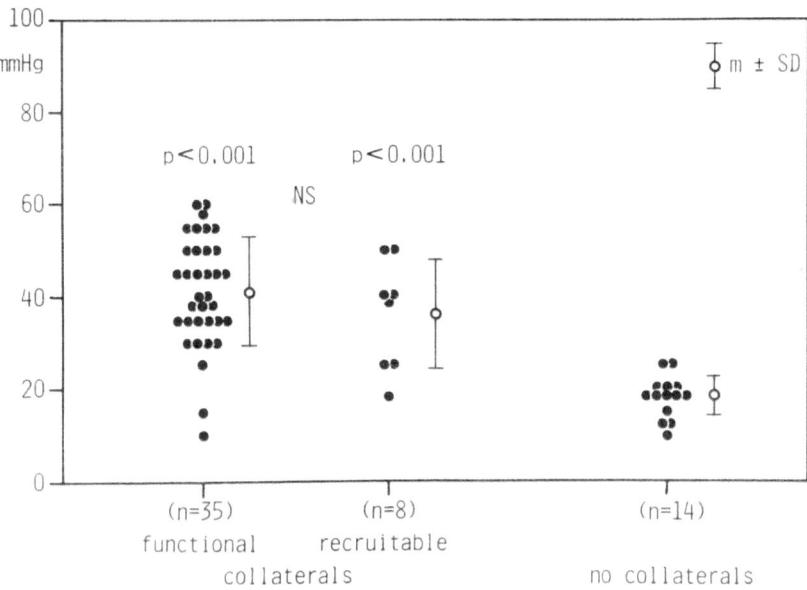

Figure 2. Coronary wedge pressures in arteries with and without collaterals (A). In panel B, the group with collaterals is divided into subgroups with functional and recruitable collaterals. The mean value of the two subgroups with collaterals were not significantly different from each other but each one was significantly higher than that of the group without collaterals. A CWP ≥ 30 mmHg was found only in arteries with collaterals.

By permission of the American Heart Association, Inc. [26].

$95 \pm 6\%$ (range 80 to 100%), significantly higher ($p < 0.001$) than that of the subgroup with recruitable collaterals ($83 \pm 10\%$, range 80 to 90%) which was quite similar to that of the group without collaterals. Electrocardiographic alteration such as ST-segment elevation, ST-segment depression, or T-wave changes occurred in 24 of 57 arteries (42%) during 30 seconds of balloon occlusion. Figure 3 shows the incidence of electrocardiographic changes in the different subgroups. The mean coronary wedge pressure was 26 ± 11 mmHg (range 10 to 60 mmHg) in arteries with electrocardiographic changes and 41 ± 11 mmHg (range 10 to 60 mmHg) in arteries without electrocardiographic changes ($p < 0.001$). Chest pain occured during a 30 seconds balloon occlusion in 27 of 57 arteries (47%) Figure 4 shows the incidence of chest pain in the different groups and subgroups. The mean coronary wedge pressure was 29 ± 16 mmHg (range 10 to 60 mmHg) in arteries producing chest pain and 39 ± 12 mmHg (range 10 to 55 mmHg) in arteries not producing chest pain ($p < 0.001$).

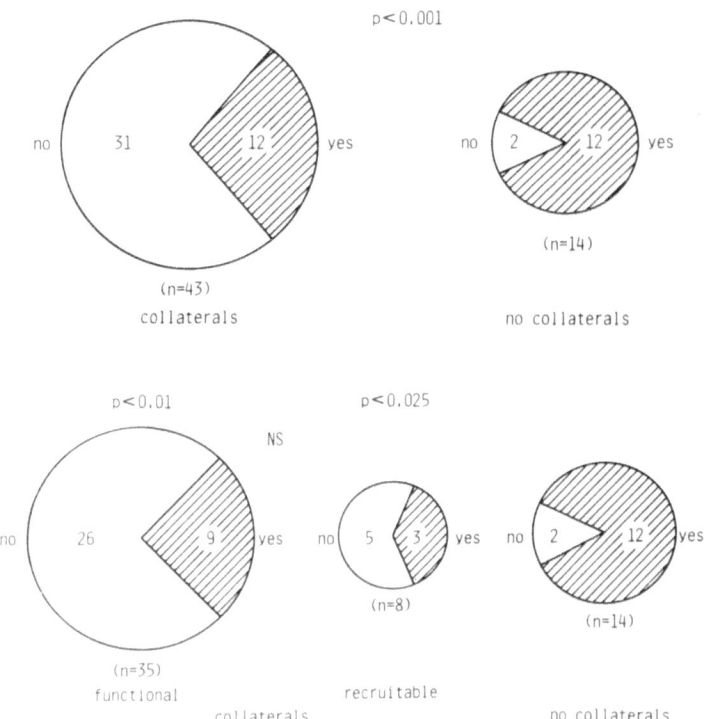

Figure 3. Ischemic electrocardiographic changes in at least one of three leads monitored during a 30 sec balloon occlusion of a coronary artery. Signs of ischemia were significantly more frequent in patients without collaterals than in patients with collaterals as a group (panel A) or divided into two subgroups with functional and recruitable collaterals (panel B).

These data indicate that the coronary wedge pressure reflects not only spontaneously visible collaterals but also recruitable collaterals not evident from diagnostic angiogram. Other studies have shown a correlation between either the systolic occlusion pressure or the mean distal occlusion pressure and the angiographically quantitated collateral circulation [12, 30]. The transocclusional pressure gradient is derived directly from the coronary wedge pressure. It provides little additional information but it is corrected for the systemic blood pressure. The transstenotic pressure gradient allows no inference on the presence of collaterals. A high transstenotic pressure gradient may well be an incentive for the development of collaterals. In parallel to their development, however, the transstenotic pressure gradient decreases. The degree of stenosis was higher in arteries with spontaneously visible collaterals than in those with recruitable or without collaterals. This is in agreement with previous studies showing that collaterals are visible only if the stenosis of the recipient vessel approaches or

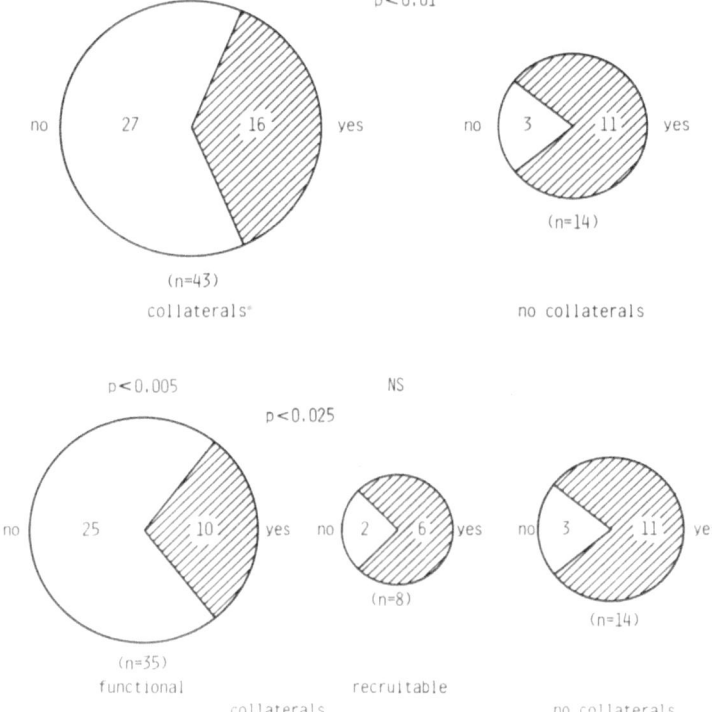

Figure 4. Chest pain during a 30 seconds balloon occlusion of a coronary artery. Chest pain occurred significantly more frequently in patients without collaterals than in those with collaterals (panel A). The subgroup of patients with recruitable collaterals, however, showed an incidence of chest pain significantly different from that of the subgroup with functional collaterals and similar to that of the group without collaterals (panel B).

reaches 100% [14]. Ischemic changes of the electrocardiogram were seen more often in patients without collaterals and chest pain was less frequently reported in patients with spontaneously visible collaterals than in those with recruitable collaterals or without collaterals. The mean coronary wedge pressure of the arteries producing such markers of ischemia was significantly lower than in arteries not producing electrocardiographic changes or chest pain. There was a cut-off value of 30 mmHg or higher for prediction of collaterals. It concurs well with coronary wedge pressure measured in arteries with and without collaterals in other studies [18, 19, 23]

Coronary wedge pressure and left ventricular function

Contradictory results have been reported regarding preservation of functional myocardium by the collaterals after coronary occlusion in man [28, 33]. To evaluate the potential protective role of the coronary collateral circulation, we studied the relation between left ventricular function in patients with occlusion of one coronary artery and the coronary collateral circulation assessed both by their angiographic estimation and by the coronary wedge pressure [10].

Among 47 patients with percutaneous transluminal coronary recanalization of a major epicardial vessel and without infarction in a region other than that supplied by the attempted vessel, 13 patients underwent recanalization during the acute phase of a myocardial infarction. The remaining 34 underwent an elective procedure for a chronic total occlusion. The date of occlusion was assumed to be the moment of the acute infarction. In patients without clinically documented acute infarction, the most marked change in anginal symptoms was considered as the occlusion date. In six patients no such acute coronary event was found and the date of occlusion remained undetermined. The coronary wedge pressure was measured at the time of recanalization as previously described. The patients were separated into two groups according to the level of coronary wedge pressure. Group 1 consisted of 31 patients with a coronary wedge pressure in the occluded artery > 30 mmHg (mean 45 ± 9, range 35 to 65 mmHg) and group 2 consisted of 16 patients whose coronary wedge pressure in the occluded artery was $\leqslant 30$ mmHg (mean 23 ± 7 mmHg, range 10 to 30 mmHg). The delay between occlusion and coronary wedge pressure measurement was not significantly different between the two groups (36 ± 42 days in group 1 vs 45 ± 90 days in group 2). Yet, the duration of anginal symptoms was significantly longer in group 1 (13 ± 11 weeks) than in group 2 (5 ± 8 weeks) ($p < 0.05$). The extent of collateral circulation was assessed on the diagnostic angiogram according to Rentrop's classification [31]. The global and regional left ventricular functions were evaluated from biplane ventriculograms. Global left ventricular ejection fraction was determined from end-systolic and end-diastolic contours with the area-length method [13]. Regional left ventricular function was assessed for each segment by computerized planimetry of the segmental area change expressed as a percent of total functions. The following relation between the occluded arteries and the myocardial segment was assumed: for the left anterior descending coronary artery, the anterolateral, apical, distal septal, and proximal septal segments; for the right coronary artery, the diaphragmatic, posterobasal, and posterior segments; for the left circumflex coronary artery, the posterior, posterolateral and posterobasal segments.

Figure 5 shows that the mean value of the left ventricular ejection fraction was significantly higher in group 1 ($63 \pm 9\%$) than in group 2 ($49 \pm 7\%$) ($p < 0.001$). This difference remained significant when only the 34 patients with elective procedures were considered ($62 \pm 10\%$ vs $48 \pm 6\%$, $p < 0.005$). The global left ventricular ejection fraction was also higher in group 1 than in group 2 when comparing patients stratified according to the vessel occluded. A significant correlation existed between the coronary wedge pressure and the global left ventricular ejection fraction ($r = 0.51$, $p < 0.001$) (Fig. 6). Furthermore, with a cut-off value of 30 mmHg, it was possible to separate the patients with a normal systolic left ventricular function (ejection fraction $> 55\%$) from those with impaired left ventricular function. There was a significant relation between the coronary wedge pressure and the angiographically determined extent of collateral circulation (Fig. 7). Yet, the latter did not significantly correlate with the global left ventricular ejection fraction (Fig. 8). Wall motion of the myocardial

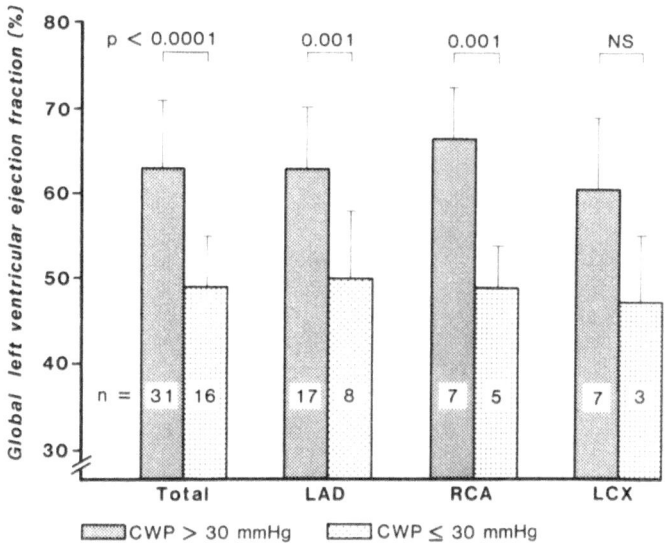

Figure 5. Mean global left ventricular ejection fraction for high (> 30 mmHg) and low ($\leqslant 30$ mmHg) coronary wedge pressure (CWP). The mean value of left ventricular ejection fraction is higher in the group with high than in the group with low coronary wedge pressure, even when comparing patients stratified to the vessel occluded.

LAD = left anterior descending coronary artery; LCx = left circumflex coronary artery; RCA = right coronary artery; NS = not significant.

By permission of the American Heart Association, Inc. [10].

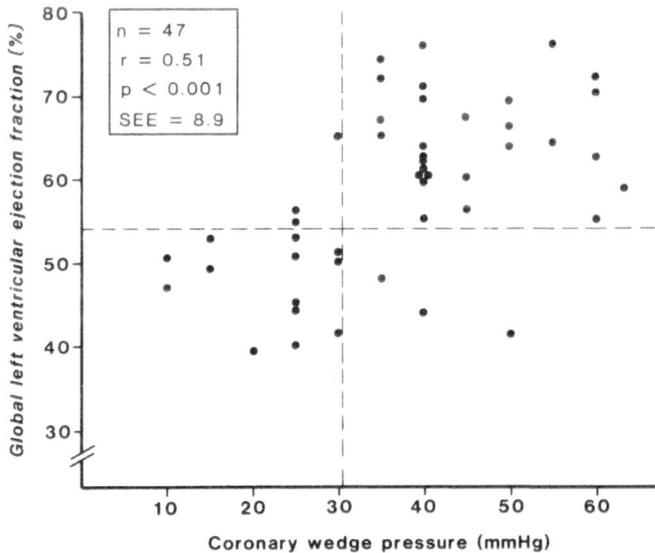

Figure 6. Relation between global left ventricular ejection fraction and coronary wedge pressure. The global left ventricular function is significantly correlated to the level of coronary wedge pressure in the occluded vessel.

By permission of the American Heart Association, Inc. [10].

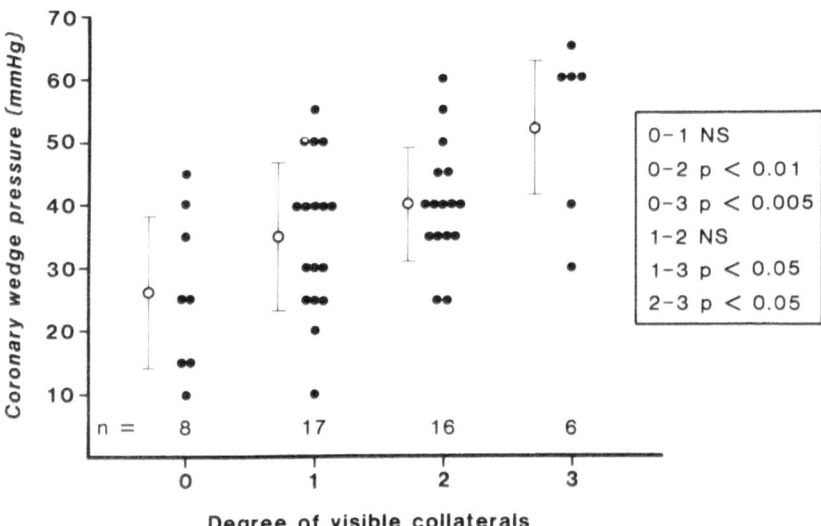

Figure 7. Relation between coronary wedge pressure and angiographic degree of collateralization. A clear relation exists between the coronary wedge pressure and the angiographically determined collaterals. NS = not significant.

By permission of the American Heart Association, Inc. [10].

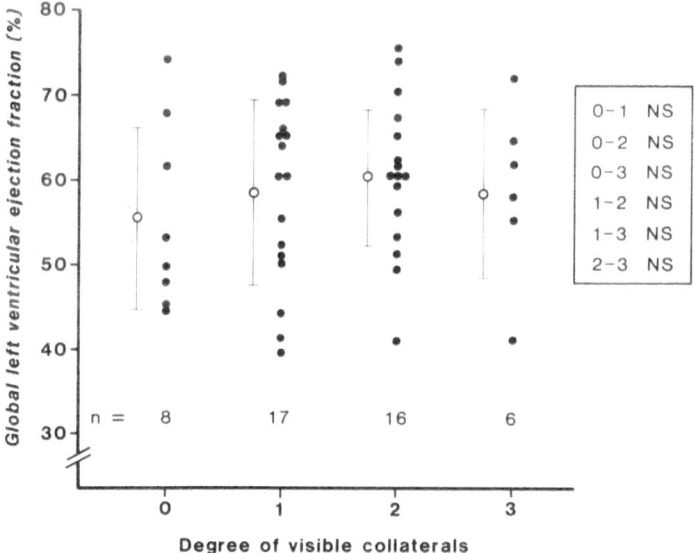

Figure 8. Global left ventricular ejection fraction for different angiographic degrees of collateralization. There is no significant relation between angiographic degrees of collateralization and global left ventricular function. NS = not significant.

By permission of the American Heart Association, Inc. [10].

area related to the occluded artery was better preserved but not normalised in group 1 with the higher coronary wedge pressure than in group 2 (Fig. 9). The difference remained significant with separate analysis of the left anterior descending and the right coronary artery. The difference was not significant in the left circumflex group, probably because of the small number of patients.

These results indicate that the higher the coronary wedge pressure measured during percutaneous transluminal coronary recanalisation, the better the systolic wall motion of the occluded artery related segment is preserved. As a consequence, global left ventricular ejection function was found to be higher in patients with high coronary wedge pressures. Not withstanding the delay between the occlusion of the vessel and assessment of the collaterals, our data support the hypothesis that a coronary wedge pressure higher than 30 mmHg preserves some but not all contractile function in the myocardial area dependent on an occluded artery. In contrast, we found no correlation between left ventricular function and the angiographically determined degree of collateral circulation. This leads us to conclude that coronary wedge pressure is a more accurate indicator of the protective role of coronary collaterals.

The introduction of coronary angiography and angioplasty at the acute stage of myocardial infarction has helped to gain a better understanding of the protective effects of collaterals on left ventricular function. It was found that among patients with successful thrombolysis those with good collaterals showed

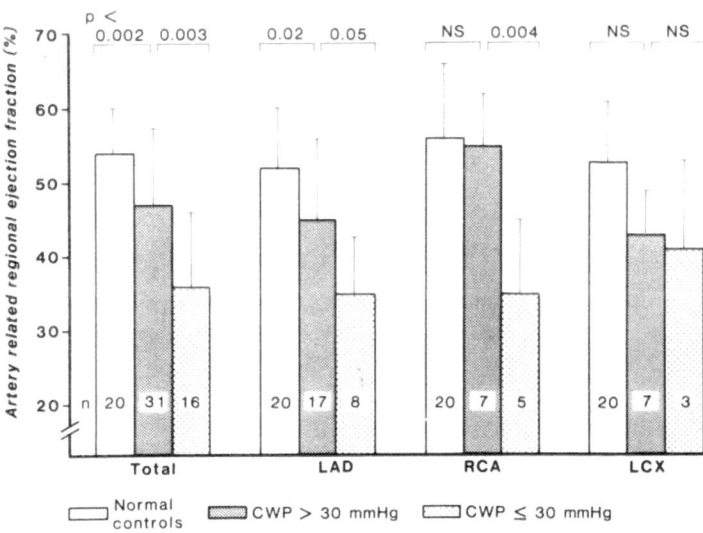

Figure 9. Occluded artery related regional left ventricular function for high (> 30 mmHg) and low (⩽ 30 mmHg) coronary wedge pressure and for normal controls. Wall motion of the myocardial area related to the occluded artery is better preserved albeit not normal in the group with high than in the group with low coronary wedge pressure. Abbreviations as in Fig. 5.

By permission of the American Heart Association, Inc. [10].

more improvement of left ventricular function (acute vs late measurements) than those without [34]. This improvement was not related to the delay between onset of symptoms and beginning of intracoronary thrombolysis suggesting that collaterals prevented complete infarction despite several hours of coronary occlusion. Two other studies emphasize the importance of residual flow attributed to subtotal occlusion or good collaterals in the first hours of acute myocardial infarction [3, 28]. Recently, Rentrop et al used left ventriculography during balloon inflation to assess collaterals both angiographically and by measuring the distal coronary occlusion pressure [9, 32]. They found that angiographically determined collateral circulation limits myocardial ischemia as assessed by the extent of new ventricular asynergy and electrocardographic changes during coronary occlusion. Furthermore, they demonstrated that ventricular function after abrupt coronary occlusion is determined by an interaction between the location of the coronary artery obstruction and the amount of collateral flow.

Coronary wedge pressure and restenosis after PTCA

Recurrence of stenosis after PTCA, constitutes one of the major limitations of the procedure [25]. Accelerated progression of native vessel disease after surgical coronary bypass grafting has been well documented [5, 7] and has been attributed to the decreased transstenotic flow induced by the graft. Postulating that native collateral flow or pressure could have a similar detrimental effect on restenosis after angioplasty, we used the coronary wedge pressure to estimate collateral flow at the time of angioplasty and observed its effect on the angiographic recurrence rate [39].

Of 170 consecutive vessels in 152 patients for which coronary wedge pressure was measured at the time of angioplasty, longterm follow-up with a control angiogram was obtained in 100 vessels with initially successful angioplasty. These 100 lesions were treated in 91 patients. Of the studied vessels, 12 had been subjected to emergency angioplasty (in patients with ongoing myocardial infarction) and 88 had been treated with elective angioplasty. Control coronary angiography at 6 to 9 months was suggested for all patients undergoing PTCA whether or not symptoms of ischemia were present but the final decision was left to the patient and the referring physician. Angiography was performed earlier if prompted by recurrent symptoms. Recurrent stenosis was defined as a luminal diameter $> 50\%$ at the site of previous angioplasty. The patients were classified into two groups according to the presence or absence of restenosis at follow-up. A cut-off value of 30 mmHg was used to define lesions with a high or low coronary wedge pressure.

The mean value of coronary wedge pressure was significantly higher for the 37 vessels with restenosis (30 ± 10 mmHg) than for the 63 vessels without restenosis (26 ± 9 mmHg) ($p < 0.01$). The presence of angiographically visible collateral flow was noted for 42% of the vessels with restenosis and 29% of the vessels without (NS). The rate of restenosis was examined for different values of coronary wedge pressure (Fig. 10). With a coronary wedge pressure < 30 mmHg, the restenosis rate was 23%; with a coronary wedge pressure $\geqslant 30$ mmHg the restenosis rate was 52% ($p < 0.001$). Thus, a coronary wedge pressure $\geqslant 30$ mmHg has a predictive value for recurrence of stenosis of 52% and a coronary wedge pressure < 30 mmHg has a predictive value for long term success of 77%. The association of a high coronary wedge pressure with an increased recurrence rate was present in both the subgroups with total occlusion (recurrence rates 69 and 20%, respectively, for coronary wedge pressures $\geqslant 30$ and < 30 mmHg, $p < 0.05$) and the subgroup with stenosis (46 and 24%, respectively, $p < 0.05$). Of the 70 vessels with an initial coronary wedge pressure measurement but without follow-up angiography, 2 had had a previous bypass surgery. The 68 remaining vessels had a mean coronary wedge pressure of 32 ± 13 mmHg and this was significantly higher than the 28 ± 10 mmHg measured for the 100 vessels with subsequent angiographic control ($p < 0.01$). It is possible that the higher coronary wedge pressure in this group afforded improved protection against symptoms and influenced the clinical decision to abstain from control angiography.

These data show that a high ($\geqslant 30$ mmHg) coronary wedge pressure is associated with a more than twofold increased incidence of restenosis at long-term follow-up. This negative influence of a high distal occlusive pressure remained significant when the subgroups of lesions with a complete occlusion

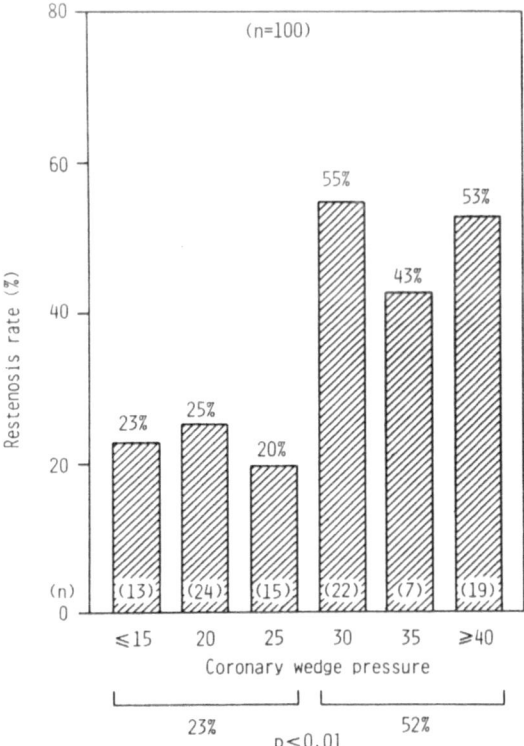

Figure 10. Restenosis rate after balloon angioplasty in relation to coronary wedge pressure in 100 vessels. The restenosis rate of lesions situated in vessels with a coronary wedge pressure < 30 mmHg is roughly half of that observed for vessels with a coronary wedge pressure ≥ 30 mmHg.

Reprinted with permission of the American College of Cardiology, *Journal of the American College of Cardiology* (1987) 10:504–509.

and those with stenosis were considered. Other authors have reported a similar detrimental effect of collateral flow on long-term angioplasty results. Dervan et al [11] observed a higher restenosis rate for chronic total occlusions than for stenosis after angioplasty, and measured a significantly higher coronary wedge pressure (35 ± 10 mmHg) in eight patients with occlusive lesions that in a group with stenosis and no visible collateral flow (mean coronary wedge pressure 20 ± 7 mmHg). Although effects on restenosis were not reported, these figures are in accordance with ours. Probst reported an increased restenosis rate associated with angiographically well developed collateral channels; a high distal pressure (systolic occlusion pressure > 45 mmHg) was significantly associated with recurrent lesions in a group of 47 patients, but neither degree of coronary obstruction nor left ventricular function before angioplasty was given [29]. It is tempting to establish a parallel between native collaterals and surgical bypass grafts. Both lead to increased distal pressure and, therefore, decrease flow through the lesion. Reduced transstenotic flow has been considered the most plausible explanation for accelerated disease progression in bypassed coronary vessels [22]. Our data support the hypothesis that decreased flow through a lesion treated by angioplasty, due to high distal pressure induced by collaterals, has a detrimental effect on long term results. To the familiar concept that collateral channels are formed as a response to a stenosis, one might add the somewhat paradoxical notion that stenosis may recur as a response to collaterals.

Conclusions

The measurement of coronary wedge pressure is a simple means to gain information about the collateralization of a coronary artery subjected to coronary angioplasty. A clear relation exists between the angiographic grade of collateralization and the coronary wedge pressure. The higher the coronary wedge pressure, the more assured the operator can be that in case of acute vessel occlusion adequate perfusion to the jeopardized myocardium will be maintained. Coronary wedge pressure reflects both spontaneously visible collaterals and recruitable collaterals not evident from diagnostic angiograms. This indicator of collateral circulation more accurately reflects the protective role of collaterals than their angiographic presence since left ventricular systolic function is significantly correlated to coronary wedge pressure but not to their angiographic assessment. Moreover, coronary wedge pressure measurements at the time of angioplasty allow some prediction about the risk for restenosis which is higher with high coronary wedge pressure.

References

1. Baroldi G, Mantero O, Scomazzoni G (1956) The collaterals of the coronary arteries in normal and pathologic hearts. *Circ Res* 4:233–229
2. Bellamy RF (1978) Diastolic coronary artery pressure-flow relations in the dog. *Circ Res* 43:92–101
3. Blanke H, Cohen M, Karsch KR, Fagerstrom R, Rentrop KP (1985) Prevalence and significance of residual flow to the infarct zone during the acute phase of myocardial infarction. *J Am Coll Cardiol* 5:827–831
4. Blumgart HL, Schlesinger MG, Davis D (1940) Studies on the relation of the clinical manifestations of angina pectoris, coronary thrombosis and myocardial infarction to the pathological findings, with particular reference to the significance of the collateral circulation. *Am Heart J* 19:1–91
5. Bourassa MG, Lespérance J, Corbara F, Saltiel J, Campeau L (1978) Progression of obstructive coronary artery disease 5 to 7 years after aortocoronary bypass surgery. *Circulation* 58 (Suppl I): I-100–106
6. Caroll RJ, Verani MS, Falsetti HL (1974) The effect of collateral circulation on segmental left ventricular contraction. *Circulation* 50:709–713
7. Cashin WL, Sanmarco ME, Nessim SA, Blankenhorn DH (1984) Accelerated progression of

atherosclerosis in coronary vessels with minimal lesions that are bypassed. *N Engl J Med* 311: 824–828

8. Chiarello M, Ribeiro LGT, Davis MA, Maroko PR (1977) 'Reverse coronary steal' induced by coronary vasoconstriction following coronary occlusion in dogs. *Circulation* 56:809–815

9. Cohen M, Rentrop KP (1986) Limitation of myocardial ischemia by collateral circulation during sudden controlled coronary artery occlusion in human subjects: a prospective study. *Circulation* 74:469–476

10. de Bruyne B, Meier B, Finci L, Urban P, Rutishauser W (1988) Potential protective effect of high coronary wedge pressure on left ventricular function after coronary occlusion. *Circulation* 78: 566–572

11. Dervan JP, Baim DS, Cherniles J, Grossman W (1983) Transluminal angioplasty of occluded coronary arteries: use of a movable guide wire system. *Circulation* 68:776–784

12. Dervan JP, McKay RG, Baim DS (1987) Assessment of the relationship between distal occluded pressure and angiographically evident collateral flow during coronary angioplasty. *Am Heart J* 114:491–497

13. Dodge HT, Sandler H, Ballen DW, Lord JD (1960) The use the biplane angiocardiography for the measurements of the left ventricular volume in man. *Am Heart J* 60:762–776

14 Elayada MA, Mathur VS, Hall RJ, Massumi GA, Garcia E, de Castro CM (1985) Collateral circulation in coronary artery disease. *Am J Cardiol* 55:58–60

15. Eng C, Kirk ES (1984) Flow into ischemic myocardium and across coronary collateral vessels is modulated by a waterfall mechanism. *Circ Res* 55:10–17

16. Feldman RL, Pepine CJ (1984) Evaluation of coronary collateral circulation in conscious humans. *Am J Cardiol* 53:1233–1238

17. Flameng W, Schwarz F, Hehrlein FW (1978) Intraoperative evaluation of the functional significance of coronary collateral vessels in patients with coronary artery disease. *Am J Cardiol* 42:187–192

18. Goldstein RE, Michaelis LL, Morrow AG, Epstein SE (1975) Coronary collateral function in patients without occlusive coronary artery disease. *Circulation* 51:118–125

19. Goldstein RE, Stinson EB, Scherer JL, Seningen RP, Grehl TM, Epstein SE (1974) Intraoperative coronary collateral function in patients with coronary occlusive disease. Nitroglycerine responsiveness and angiographic correlations. *Circulation* 64:298–308

20. Helfant RH, Vokonas PS, Gorlin R (1971) Functional importance of the human coronary collateral circulation. *N. Engl J Med* 284:1277–1281

21. Levin DC (1974) Pathways and functional significance of the coronary collateral circulation. *Circulation* 50:831–837

22. Loop FD (1984) Progression of coronary atherosclerosis. *N Engl J Med* 311: 851–853

23. MacDonald RG, Hill JA, Feldman RL (1986) ST segment response to acute coronary occlusion: coronary hemodynamic angiographic determinants of direction of ST segment shift. *Circulation* 74:973–979

24. Maxwell MP, Hearse DJ, Yellon DM (1987) Species variation in the coronary collateral circulation during regional myocardial ischemia: a critical determinant of the rate of evolution and extent of myocardial infarction. *Cardiovascular Research* 21:737–746

25. Meier B (1988) Restenosis after coronary angioplasty: Review of the literature. *Eur Heart J* 9 (Suppl C): 1–6

26. Meier B, Luethy P, Finci L, Steffenino GD, Rutishauser W (1987) Coronary wedge pressure in relation to spontaneously visible and recruitable collaterals. *Circulation* 75:906–913

27. Meier B, Rutishauser W (1985) Coronary pacing during percutaneous transluminal coronary angioplasty. *Circulation* 71:557–561

28. Nitzberg WD, Nath HP, Rogers WJ, Hood WP Jr, Withlow PL, Reeves R, Baxley WA (1985) Collateral flow in patients with acute myocardial infarction. *Am J Cardiol* 56:729–736

29. Probst P (1986) 'Collateral pressure' (occlusion pressure) during coronary angioplasty in coronary artery disease, pp. 105–114 in: Serruys PW, Meester GT (eds) *Coronary Angioplasty: A Controlled Model for Ischemia*. Dordrecht: Martinus Nijhoff (DICM 58)

30. Probst P, Zangl W, Pachinger O (1985) Relation of coronary arterial occlusion pressure during

percutaneous transluminal coronary angioplasty to the presence of collaterals. *Am J Cardiol* 55:1264–1269

31. Rentrop KP, Cohen M, Blanke H, Phillips R (1985) Changes in collateral channel filling immediately after controlled coronary artery occlusion by an angioplasty balloon in human subjects. *J Am Coll Cardiol* 5:587–592

32. Rentrop KP, Thornthon JC, Feit F, Van Buskirk M (1988) Determinants and protective potential of coronary arterial collaterals as assessed by an angioplasty model. *Am J Cardiol* 61:677–684

33. Rousseau MF, Bertrand ME, Detry JMR, Decoster PM, Lablanche JM (1982) Coronary collaterals and left ventricular function early after acute transmural myocardial infarction. *Eur Heart J* 3:223–229

34. Saito Y, Yasuno M, Ishida M, Suzuki K, Matoba Y, Emura M, Takahashi M (1985) Importance of coronary collaterals for restoration of left ventricular function after intracoronary thrombolysis. *Am J Cardiol* 55:1259–1263

35. Schaper W, Winckler B (1978) Determinants of peripheral coronary pressure in coronary artery occlusion, pp. 351–361 in: Masery A, Klassen GA, Lesch M (eds) *Primary and Secondary Angina Pectoris*. New-York: Grune and Stratton

36. Schwartz H, Leiboff RH, Bren GB, Wasserman AG, Katz RJ, Varghese PJ, Sokil AB, Ross AM (1984) Temporal evolution of the human coronary collateral circulation after myocardial infarction. *J Am Coll Cardiol* 4: 1088–1093

37. Schwarz F, Schaper J, Becker V, Kübler W, Flameng W (1982) Coronary collateral vessels: Their significance for the left ventricular histological structure. *Am J Cardiol* 49:291–295

38. Urban P, Meier B, Finci L (1987) Flow reversal in coronary collaterals. *Eur Heart J* 8:1346–1350

39. Urban P, Meier B, Finci L, de Bruyne B, Steffenino G, Rutishauser W (1987) Coronary wedge pressure: A predictor of restenosis after coronary balloon angioplasty. *J Am Coll Cardiol* 10: 504–509

40. Webb WR, Parker FB, Neville JF Jr (1973) Retrograde pressures and flows in coronary arterial disease. *Ann Thorac Surg* 15:256–262

7. Intracoronary blood flow velocity, reactive hyperemia and coronary blood flow reserve during and following PTCA

PATRICK W. SERRUYS, FELIX ZIJLSTRA, HANS H.C. REIBER,
KEVIN BEATT,* G.J. LAARMAN, JOS ROELANDT and
P.J. DE FEYTER

Introduction

Since the introduction of percutaneous transluminal coronary angioplasty (PTCA) in 1977 [1], the procedure has gained increasing importance in the treatment of coronary artery obstructions. So far, the immediate results of the procedure have been assessed by coronary angiography and the residual pressure gradient. However, the change in luminal size of an artery following the mechanical disruption of its internal wall cannot be assessed accurately from the detected angiographic contours [2, 3]. The measured residual pressure gradient may have short and long-term prognostic value, but it reflects only the hemodynamic state at rest [4, 5, 6]. Recently the assessment of coronary flow reserve has been proposed as a better method to evaluate the functional results of dilatation of a coronary artery obstruction [7, 8, 9, 10]. Papaverine is currently regarded as the vasodilator of choice for the induction of maximal hyperemia, as intracoronary administration results in an immediate, potent and short-lasting hyperemia [11, 12]. Intracoronary blood flow velocity measurements with a Doppler probe, and the radiographic assessment of myocardial perfusion with contrast media have previously been used to investigate regional coronary flow reserve [13–17]. In the present study we compared both techniques in the setting of PTCA, and compared the pharmacologically induced vasodilation after intracoronary papaverine with reactive hyperemia following transluminal occlusion.

Patients and methods

In the first study group twenty patients undergoing elective PTCA for angina pectoris were investigated (New York Heart Association functional class II to IV). Informed consent was obtained for the additional investigations. All patients

*Recipient of the Joint Fellowship from the British and Netherlands Heart Foundations.

P.W. Serruys, R. Simon & K.J. Beatt (eds), Percutaneous Transluminal Coronary Angioplasty. ISBN 0-7923-0346-6.
© *1990 Kluwer Academic Publishers, Dordrecht*

were studied without premedication, but their medical treatment (nitrates, calcium antagonists and beta-blockers) was continued on the day of the procedure. Patients with left ventricular hypertrophy, valvular heart disease, angiographic evidence of collateral circulation, anemia, polycythemia or hypertension were excluded as these conditions may influence coronary flow reserve [18–20].

Intracoronary blood flow velocity measurements

A 20 mega Hz ultrasonic crystal mounted on the tip of the angioplasty catheter was used in all patients. The Doppler crystal has a 1.0 mm diameter annulus with a 0.5 mm central hole. Two leads are soldered to the crystal and pass through the catheter between the original 0.5 mm lumen and a thin-walled tube, which serves as a new 0.4 mm lumen (Fig. 1). The leads exit near the proximal luer hub and are wired to a 2 pin plug for connection to the pulsed Doppler instrument. Blood flow velocity is measured from the catheter tip transducer using a range-gated 20 MHz pulsed Doppler instrument. The master oscillator frequency of 20 MHz is pulsed at a frequency of 62.5 kHz. Each pulse is approximately 1 ms in width and therefore contains 20 cycles of the master oscillator frequency. The frequencies chosen allow velocities of up to 100 cm/s to be recorded at distances of up to 1 cm from the catheter tip. The sampling window is individually adjusted to obtain the optimal signal, which usually results in a sampling window of 1.8 mm (range: 1.5 to 2.2).

The output of the pulsed Doppler is displayed as a frequency shift (Δf, kHz) which can be related to blood flow velocity by the Doppler equation: $\Delta f = 2F\,(V/c)\cos a$, where F is the ultrasonic frequency (20 MHz), V is the velocity within the sample volume, c is the speed of sound in blood (1500 m/s), and a is the angle between the velocity vector and the sound beam. Using an end-mounted crystal with the catheter parallel ($\pm 20°$) to the vessel axis (cos a equals $1 \pm 6\%$), the relation between the Doppler shift and velocity is approximately 3.75 cm/s

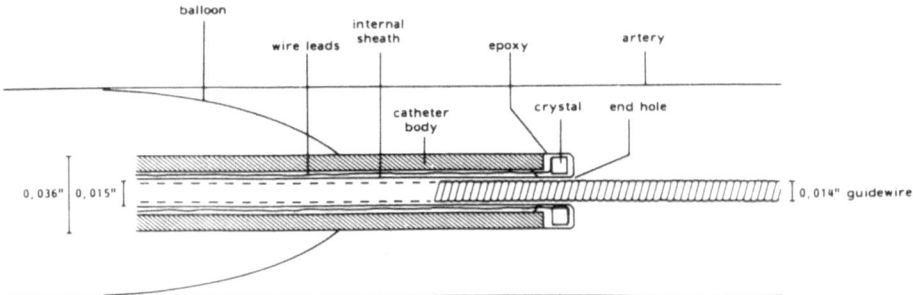

Figure 1. Schematic cross-sectional drawing of Doppler tip angioplasty catheter with inflated balloon in the artery.

per kHz [9]. Recently, Sibley et al [17] validated clinically and experimentally the ability of a similar catheter with an end-mounted piezo-electric crystal to provide accurate continuous on-line measurement of coronary blood flow velocity and vasodilator reserve. In our laboratory, we verified the accuracy of each velocity probe by correlating velocity recorded with the Doppler probe in a 9 Fr femoral sheath with the volume flow measured by a timed collection of blood from the side branch of the same sheath. Graduated flow rates (range 12 to 165 ml/min) and the corresponding velocities (range 1.2 to 8.2 kHz) were obtained by incremental balloon inflation with the balloon positioned in the sheath. This simple model allows the assessment of the flow-velocity relation at different levels. As previously demonstrated, this relation is linear with correlation coefficients generally $\geqslant 0.95$, [21, 22, 23] but underestimates true volume flow for flows over 150 ml/min [17]. Flow rates of this magnitude, or velocities exceeding 7.5 kHz, were never encountered in this study population.

Protocol

After recording the baseline intracoronary blood velocity in the proximal segment, the balloon catheter (Schneider-Shiley dilatation catheter, Shiley Inc.) with a Doppler probe at the tip was advanced across the stenosis and 3 to 7 inflations with pressures up to 12 atmospheres were used to dilate the stenosis. Resting velocities before and after each balloon inflation and those during reactive hyperemia immediately after deflation were recorded with the Doppler probe situated across the stenotic lesion and expressed in kHz.

A satisfactory functional result was considered to have been achieved if there was no further increase in peak velocity during reactive hyperemia. No additional dilatations were then performed and coronary angiography was repeated after removing the PTCA catheter. The balloon diameter size used in this study varied from 2.5 to 3.5 mm. The cross-sectional area of the catheter with the balloon deflated was 0.68 mm^2.

Quantitative analysis of the coronary artery

Coronary angiograms were performed in at least 2 orthogonal projections before and after PTCA and the same projections were repeated after the procedure (Fig. 2). The determination of coronary arterial dimensions from 35 mm cinefilm was performed with the computer-based Cardiovascular Angiographic Analysis System (CAAS) [24–26]. In essence, boundaries of the relevant coronary artery segment are detected automatically from optically magnified and video digitized regions of interest of a selected single cineframe angiogram. The absolute diameter of the stenosis (in mm) is determined using the guiding catheter as a scaling device [24]. The detected contours of the arterial and catheter segments are corrected for pincushion distortion [25]. A computer-estimation of the

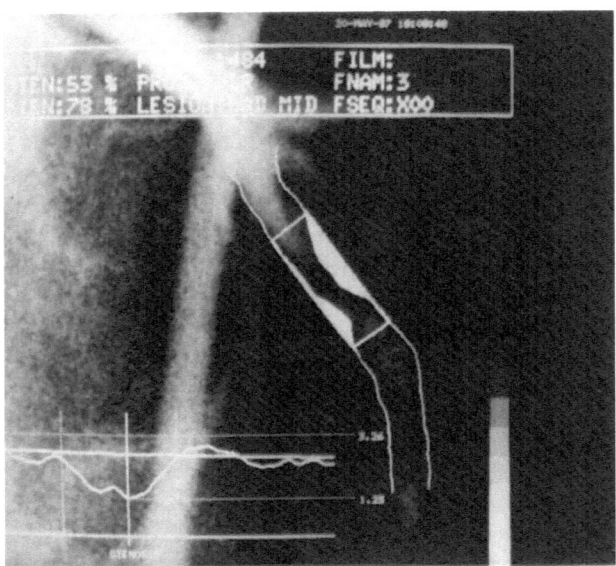

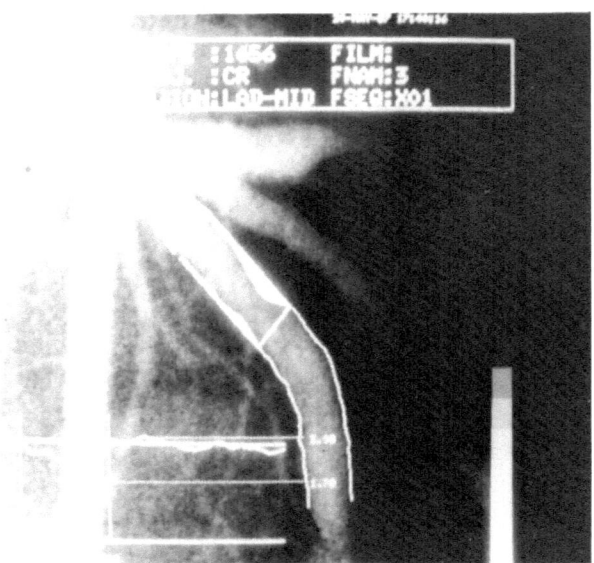

Figure 2. Angiograms of a left anterior descending coronary artery (cranial projection) before (A) and after (B) angioplasty with superimposition of the automated contours at the coronary artery segment of interest. Beneath this is shown the diameter function of the detected contours of the coronary artery. The minimal lumen diameter (vertical line) and the interpolated diameter function (horizontal line) from which the reference diameter is derived are shown.

original arterial dimension at the site of the obstruction is used to define the interpolated reference area or diameter [24–26]. The interpolated percentage area stenosis and the minimal luminal cross-sectional area (mm^2) are then calculated and averaged from at least 2, preferably orthogonal, projections.

In the second study group twenty-one patients undergoing elective PTCA for angina pectoris were studied. All patients had evidence of myocardial ischemia as indicated either by ECG changes at rest or during exercise thallium scintigraphy. Informed consent was obtained for the additional investigations. All patients were studied without premedication, but their medical treatment (nitrates, calcium antagonists and beta-blockers) was continued on the day of the procedure.

Protocol of the investigational procedure

1. Coronary cineangiography was performed in at least two, preferably ortho-gonal projections for quantitative analysis of the coronary artery stenosis, after intracoronary administration of 2 or 3 mg intracoronary isosorbide dinitrate. The intracoronary administration of isosorbide dinitrate was repeated at regular intervals (20–30 min) to ensure constant and maximal epicardial coronary vasodilation during the entire procedure [27].
2. Coronary flow reserve was measured by digital subtraction cineangiography.
3. A long guide wire (length: 315 cm; diameter: 0.014 inch) was passed through the coronary artery stenosis.
4. A balloon catheter with a Doppler probe at the tip [9] was advanced over the guide wire into the coronary artery to measure coronary blood flow velocity. The precise location of the tip of the balloon catheter with respect to the stenotic lesion – immediately proximal to the lesion and beyond any major side branches – was determined by injection of contrast medium. After recording the baseline intracoronary blood flow velocity, hyperemia was induced by injecting 12.5 mg papaverine through the guiding catheter. The ratio of peak mean intracoronary blood flow velocity to baseline was then determined as previously described by Wilson et al [13]. This measurement was obtained in 14 patients (see Table 2).
5. Thereafter the balloon was advanced across the stenosis and 3 to 7 inflations, lasting 40 to 80 s, and up to 12 atmospheres were used to dilate the stenosis until repeat cineangiography showed a good result (< 50% diameter stenosis). The mean total inflation time was 162 s/patient (range: 120–352 s). Immedia-tely following the final balloon inflation the reactive hyperemia was recorded as previously described [9].
6. After subsidence of this reactive hyperemic response, the Doppler tip was pulled back into the proximal part of the coronary artery and the ratio of peak mean intracoronary blood flow velocity after 12.5 mg papaverine i.c. to baseline velocity was again determined. This measurement was obtained in 19 patients (see Table 2).

8. After removal of the balloon catheter and the guide wire, coronary flow reserve was measured with digital subtraction cineangiography, at the same pacing rate and using the same radiographic and injection parameters as before PTCA.
9. Coronary cineangiography was repeated post-PTCA in the same projections as used at the start of the procedure, for quantitative analysis of the coronary artery stenosis.

Coronary flow reserve measurements with digital subtraction cineangiography

The coronary flow reserve measurement from 35 mm cinefilm has been implemented on the CAAS [15]. The heart was atrially paced at a rate just above the spontaneous heart rate. An ECG-triggered injection into the coronary artery was made with Iopamidol at 37°C through a Medrad Mark IV® infusion pump. This nonionic contrast agent has a viscosity of 9.4 cP at 37°, an osmolarity of 0.796 osm kg^{-1} and an iodine content of 370 mg/ml. The angiogram was repeated 30 s after a bolus injection of 12.5 mg papaverine into the coronary artery by way of the guiding catheter [11, 12]. The injection rate of the contrast medium was judged to be adequate if back flow of contrast medium into the aorta occurred. When this was not observed on the hyperemic image, baseline and hyperemic image acquisition were repeated at a higher flow rate, necessitating flow rates of up to 6 ml/s in some patients. Five or six consecutive erd-diastolic cineframes were – selected for analysis. Logarithmic nonmagnified mask-mode background subtraction was applied to the image subset to eliminate noncontrast medium densities [28]. The last end-diastolic frame prior to the administration of contrast was chosen as the mask. From the sequence of background subtracted images, a contrast arrival time image was determined using an empirically derived fixed density threshold [15]. Each pixel was labeled with the sequence number of the cardiac cycle numbered from the cycle in which the pixel intensity level first exceeded the threshold. In addition to the contrast arrival time image, a density image was computed, with the intensity of each pixel being representative of the maximal local contrast medium accumulation. The coronary flow reserve was defined as the ratio of the regional flow computed from a hyperemic image divided by the regional flow of the corresponding baseline image.

Regional flow values were quantitatively determined using the following videodensitometric principle: regional blood flow (Q) = regional vascular volume/ transit time [15]. Regional vascular volume was assessed from logarithmic mask-mode subtraction images, using the Lambert Beer relationship. Coronary flow reserve was then calculated as:

$$CFR = \frac{Qh}{Qb} = \frac{Dh}{Th} : \frac{Db}{Tb}$$

where D is the mean contrast density and T the mean appearance time at baseline (b) and hyperemia (h). Mean contrast medium appearance time and density were computed within a user-defined region of interest, which was chosen so that the epicardial coronary arteries visible on the angiogram, the coronary sinus, and the great cardiac vein were all excluded from the analysis [15]. Reproducibility data are shown in Table 1. Normal values for coronary flow reserve measured with this technique have previously been established [10, 15]. The coronary flow reserve of 12 angiographically normal coronary arteries was 5.0 ± 0.8. Therefore a flow reserve below 3.4 (2 SD below the mean) is taken to be abnormal.

Results

The first study group: Coronary blood flow velocity during PTCA as a guide line for assessment of the functional result

Clinical data (Table 2). The mean age of the 20 patients (14 men and 6 women) was 54 years (range 41–66). Eighteen patients had 1-vessel coronary narrowing and 2 patients 2-vessel narrowing. The investigated and dilated coronary artery was the left anterior descending artery in 16, the circumflex artery in 3 and the right coronary artery in 1 patient. All patients had normal systolic and diastolic wall motion and an ejection fraction of more than 55%. The mean number of balloon inflations were 4.4/patient (range 3 to 7). The PTCA was successful (diameter stenosis less than 50%) in all patients. Four patients had small localized superficial tear of the dilated coronary artery segment after the procedure.

Quantitative analysis of the coronary angiogram (Table 2). The minimal lumen cross-sectional area increased from 1.1 ± 0.8 to $2.7 \pm 1.2 \, mm^2$ (mean $\pm$ SD) (Table 2). Percent of area stenosis decreased from $83 \pm 9\%$ to $57 \pm 15\%$. Percent of diameter stenosis decreased from $60 \pm 11\%$ to $36 \pm 11\%$. The actual minimal lumen cross-sectional area before and after dilatation with the catheter across the lesion was estimated after subtraction of the area ($0.68 \, mm^2$) of the PTCA catheter.

Intracoronary Doppler shift during PTCA (Figs. 3a–d). On average, 4 dilatations were performed per patient with sequential mean inflation times of 54, 60, 63 and

Table 1. Reproducibility of the coronary flow reserve measurements.

	N	1°	2°	Difference $\pm$ SD	r	SEE
DSC	13	2.1 ± 1.2	2.1 ± 1.2	-0.02 ± 0.26	0.98	0.26
DOP	15	1.6 ± 0.3	1.6 ± 0.3	$+0.03 \pm 0.18$	0.88	0.19

1° = first determination (mean $\pm$ SD); 2° = second determination (mean $\pm$ SD); DSC = digital subtraction cineangiography, analysis of repeated image acquisition taken 5 min apart, without change in patient position, pacing rate, contrast injection parameters or X-ray gantry settings; DOP = repeated intracoronary Doppler blood flow velocity measurements 5 min apart without change in patient – or Doppler catheter position.

Table 2.   Results of quantitative coronary angiography.

				Before PTCA		
Pts	PTCA artery	Balloon size	Balloon inflation	MLCA (mm^2)	DS (%)	AS (%)
1	LAD	2.5	4	0.7	61	85
2	LC	2.5	5	0.9	56	80
3	LAD	2.5	4	0.4	66	88
4	LAD	2.5	5	1.3	53	77
5	LAD	3.0	5	0.7	66	88
6	LAD	3.0	4	0.7	55	77
7	LC	3.0	6	0.5	74	93
8	LAD	3.0	4	0.7	65	88
9	LAD	3.0	5	2.9	36	59
10	LAD	3.0	4	1.9	53	78
11	R	3.0	6	0.6	71	91
12	LAD	3.0	4	0.3	78	95
13	LAD	3.0	3	0.6	67	89
14	LAD	3.4	3	2.3	54	79
15	LAD	3.4	4	1.3	52	76
16	LAD	3.4	7	0.7	72	92
17	LC	3.4	4	3.3	48	72
18	LAD	3.4	4	1.6	47	72
19	LAD	3.4	4	0.3	74	93
20	LAD	3.4	4	0.9	63	86
Mean				1.1	60	83
±SD				±0.8	±11	±9

AS = percentage area stenosis; cor. MLCA = minimal luminal cross-sectional area taking into account the reduction in MLCA due to the catheter across the lesion. DS = percentage diameter stenosis; LAD = left anterior descending coronary artery;

68 seconds. The inflation pressure increased on average for the 4 inflations from 7.6 to 10.4, 11.4 and 12.0 atmospheres (Fig. 3). Reactive hyperemia was maximal after 27 seconds (range 21 to 33 s) after deflatioh. The time to subsidence of hyperemia was 56 seconds (range 42 to 74 s).

After each of the first 3 dilatations, both resting and hyperemic velocities increased (Table 3). On average the velocities of the last 2 dilatations did not differ statistically, suggesting that the end result was already achieved by the third dilatation (Fig. 4). However, 5 patients (1, 12, 16, 17 and 20) still had a substantial increase after the fourth dilatation and might have well benefited from additional dilatations.

The ratio of peak hyperemic velocity to resting velocity for each inflation are reported in Table 4. When calculating 'coronary flow reserve' using the peak hyperemic velocity and the resting velocity recorded before the first 2 dilatations, we observed a paradoxical decrease of the ratio from 3.9 ± 0.6 to 1.9 ± 0.2. This is

After PTCA					Before PTCA	after PTCA
MLCA (mm²)	DS (%)	AS (%)	RA (mm²)	RD (mm)	cor.MLCA (mm²)	cor.MLCA (mm²)
1.3	52	76	5.3	2.59	0.0	0.6
1.4	48	73	5.4	2.61	0.2	0.7
1.4	43	67	4.6	2.30	0.0	0.7
1.2	49	73	5.4	2.61	0.6	0.5
1.2	48	73	4.7	2.64	0.0	0.5
2.0	32	54	4.3	2.16	0.0	1.3
2.5	28	49	5.9	2.54	0.0	1.8
3.7	13	24	4.8	2.54	0.0	3.0
5.3	23	41	8.2	3.11	2.2	4.6
3.3	39	63	9.3	3.33	1.2	2.6
2.9	40	64	8.1	3.02	0.0	2.2
2.5	35	55	6.1	2.79	0.0	1.8
1.2	44	67	4.8	2.47	0.0	0.5
4.8	30	51	10.3	3.65	1.6	4.1
1.8	47	72	6.2	2.75	0.6	1.1
2.9	43	56	9.0	3.37	0.0	2.2
4.1	34	51	9.7	3.57	2.6	3.4
3.5	30	32	7.4	2.96	0.9	2.8
3.0	18	40	4.9	2.51	0.0	2.3
3.5	22	57	6.4	2.81	0.2	2.8
2.7	36	57	6.5	2.85	0.5	2.0
±1.2	±11	±15	±1.9	±0.41	±0.8	±1.2

LC = left circumflex coronary artery; MLCA = minimal luminal cross-sectional area; PTCA = percutaneous transluminal coronary angioplasty; RA = reference interpolated area; RD = reference interpolated diameter; SD = standard deviation.

due to the major increase in resting velocity whose values were very low prior before the first inflation, with the catheter across the undilated lesion. When this ratio is based on the resting velocity recorded after dilatation, the coronary flow reserve differed little from 1 inflation to the next; values ranging between 1.7 and 2.1. This absence of change was confirmed statistically by variance analysis. In other words, this ratio does not seem to be an useful functional guideline for PTCA, whereas the peak hyperemic velocity following successive balloon deflations shows a gradual and significant increase, levelling off in the most patients after the third dilatation.

Second study group: A comparison of two methods to measure coronary flow reserve in the setting of coronary angioplasty: intracoronary blood flow velocity measurements with a Doppler catheter, and digital subtraction cineangiography

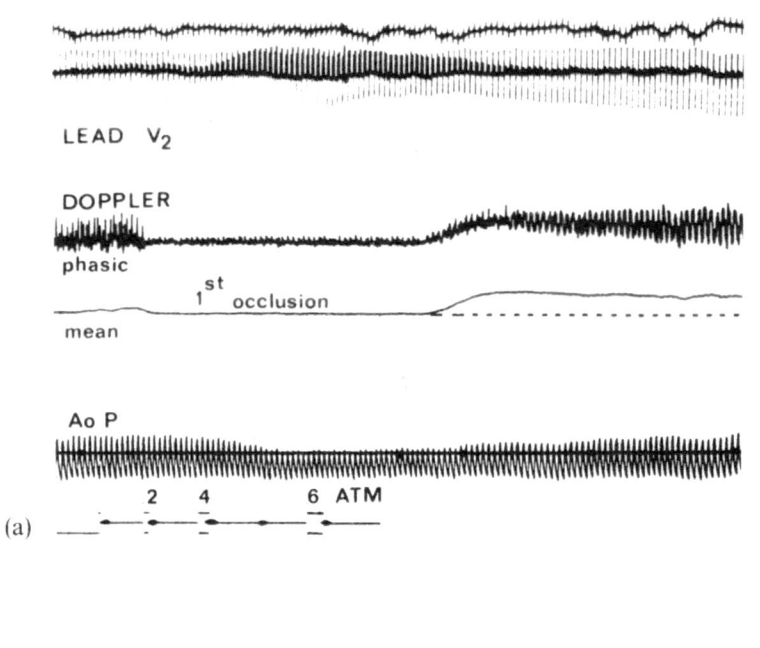

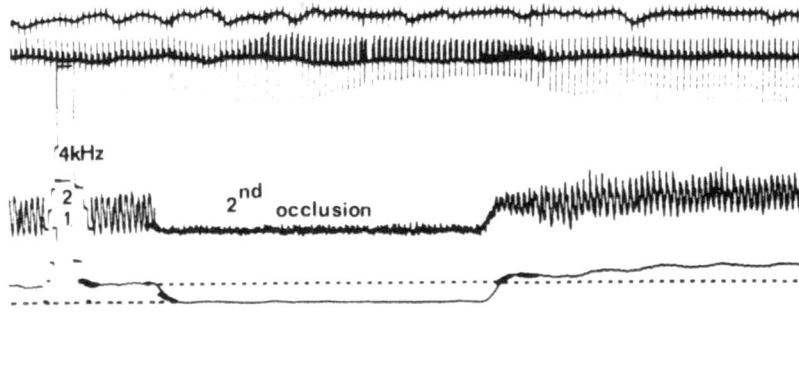

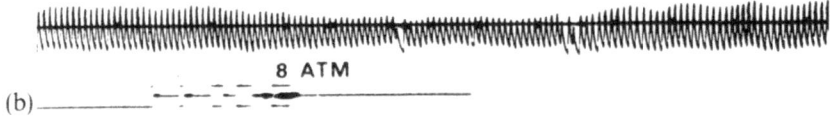

Figure 3. Examples of mean and phasic Doppler signals before, during and after balloon inflation. Reactive hyperemia occurs after balloon deflation. The precordial lead V shows ST-segment elevation.

(a) First transluminal occlusion using a balloon inflation pressure of 6 atmospheres (atm).

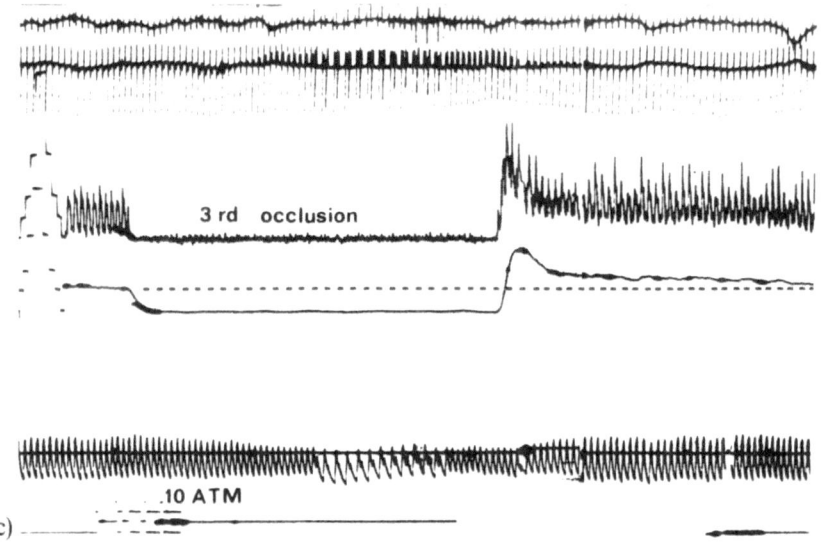

(c)

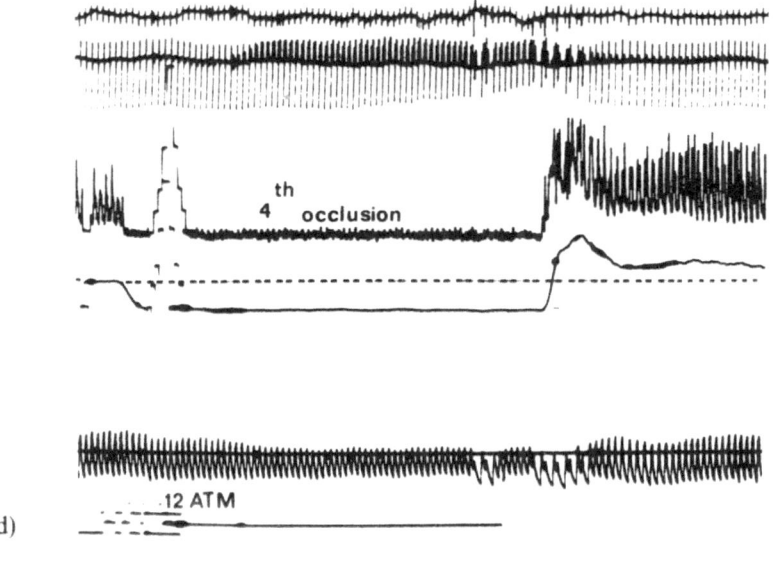

(d)

(b) Second transluminal occlusion using a balloon inflation pressure of 8 atm.
(c) Third transluminal occlusion during a balloon inflation pressure of 10 atm.
(d) Fourth transluminal occlusion using a balloon inflation pressure of 12 atm.

Table 3.   Doppler shift (kHz) during four sequential dilatations.

Pts	D1	D2	D3	D4
Vb				
Mean	0.37	0.78	1.03	1.06
±SE	±0.10	±0.19	±0.16	±0.16
		**		NS
Vh				
Mean	1.15	1.35	1.72	1.73
±SE	±0.25	±0.18	±0.26	±0.21
		*		NS
Va				
Mean	0.59	0.93	0.95	0.99
±SE	±0.12	±0.15	±0.16	±0.13
		*		NS

Data are individual and mean ± standard error (SE).
D = dilatation; Va = resting velocity after dilatation; NS = difference not significant;
Vb = resting velocity before dilatation; Vh = peak reactive hyperemia.
Variance analysis plus paired t-test: *$p < 0.05$;   **$p < 0.001$

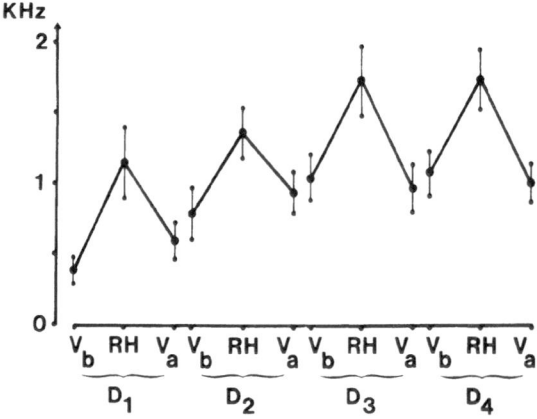

Figure 4.   Doppler shift (kHz, mean ± standard error) during 4 sequential dilatations (D). Va = resting velocity after dilatation; Vb = resting velocity before dilatation; Vh = peak reactive hyperemia.

Table 4. Ratios of peak reactive hyperemia to resting velocity after each dilatation.

Pts	Vh/Vb	Vh/Va
Dilatation 1		
Mean ($\pm$ SE)	3.93 $\pm$ 0.65	2.14 $\pm$ 0.35
Dilatation 2		
Mean ($\pm$ SE)	2.90 $\pm$ 0.63	1.70 $\pm$ 0.24
Dilatation 3		
Mean ($\pm$ SE)	1.93 $\pm$ 0.17	2.01 $\pm$ 0.14
Dilatation 4		
Mean ($\pm$ SE)	1.85 $\pm$ 0.24	1.92 $\pm$ 0.28

Data are individual and mean $\pm$ standard error (SE). Abbreviations as in Table 3.

The clinical characteristic, results of the quantitative analysis of the coronary angiogram and the coronary flow reserve measurements are shown in Table 5. The mean age of the 21 patients was 57 years (range: 37–76), 17 were male. Eighteen patients had single vessel coronary artery disease and three patients two vessel disease. The investigated and dilated coronary artery was the left anterior descending artery in 14, the circumflex artery in 3 and the right coronary artery in 4 patients. In none of the patients a sidebranch was involved at the site of the lesion. The mean left ventricular ejection fraction was 67% and ranged from 38 to 81%. Patient 9 had sustained a myocardial infarction in the anterior wall resulting in a large akinetic segment and an ejection fraction of 38%. None of the other patients had clinical evidence for a myocardial infarction and all had normal wall motion and an ejection fraction of more than 55%. In two patients (patients 4 and 11) the coronary arteriogram showed grade III/IV collateral filling of the PTCA vessel [29]. Patient 12 (see Table 5) had long standing arterial hypertension with left ventricular hypertrophy. None of the other patients had electrocardiographic, echocardiographic or angiographic evidence of left ventricular hypertrophy. The mean number of balloon inflations was 4.3/patient and ranged from 3 to 7. The dilation was successful in all patients, and none of the patients had a CPK-rise after the procedure. Seven patients had a dissection of the dilated coronary artery segment after the procedure. Five dissections were small (patients 1, 7, 10, 11 and 20), two dissections were of moderate severity (patients 17 and 18). None of the dissections had clinical repercussions. The hemodynamic data of the individual patients are shown in Table 5 and mean values ($\pm$ SD) of the heart rate and aortic pressure are given in Table 6. The cross-sectional area at the site of obstruction was $1.1 \pm 0.6 \, mm^2$ before, and $3.2 \pm 1.1 \, mm^2$ after PTCA. Percentage diameter stenosis was $58 \pm 9\%$ before, and $32 \pm 10\%$ after PTCA. Percentage area stenosis was $82 \pm 8\%$ before, and $52 \pm 14\%$ after PTCA. The interpolated reference area was $6.6 \pm 1.6 \, mm^2$ and ranged from 3.9 to 9.8 mm^2. During the measurements with the Doppler catheter just proximal to the stenosis, the tip of the catheter (1.2 mm^2) occupied $18 \pm 5\%$

Table 5. Hemodynamic data.

Pts	F/M	Age	No of DV	Vessel	B/A	OA	AS	DS
1	F	48	1	LAD	A	5.4	35	19
2	M	43	1	LAD	A	4.8	51	30
3	M	58	1	RCA	A	2.9	64	40
4	M	69	1	RCA	A	2.2	66	42
5	M	58	2	LAD	B	1.2	86	62
					A	3.3	63	39
6	M	62	1	LAD	B	0.9	86	62
					A	3.5	40	23
7	F	53	1	LAD	B	1.6	72	47
					A	3.5	51	30
8	M	56	1	LAD	B	0.7	88	64
					A	3.7	24	17
9	M	53	1	LAD	B	1.2	83	59
					A	4.5	37	21
10	M	55	1	CX	A	2.5	49	28
11	M	53	1	CX	A	2.7	69	45
12	F	57	1	LAD	B	2.9	59	35
					A	5.3	41	23
13	M	66	2	LAD	B	0.7	82	58
					A	2.9	44	25
14	M	56	1	RCA	B	0.7	87	63
15	M	67	2	CX	B	0.9	86	68
					A	1.7	69	37
16	M	60	1	LAD	B	1.3	78	53
17	M	56	1	LAD	B	0.8	86	62
					A	2.7	61	37
18	M	37	1	LAD	A	1.8	70	45
19	M	49	1	RCA	B	1.4	84	60
					A	2.5	73	48
20	F	76	1	LAD	B	1.1	75	50
					A	2.8	36	20
21	M	58	1	LAD	B	0.6	90	69
					A	2.2	64	40

Pts = patients; F = female; M = male; No of DV = number of diseased coronary arteries (diameter stenosis 50%); LAD = left anterior descending coronary artery; RCA = right coronary artery; CX = circumflex artery; B = before PTCA; A = after PTCA; OA = cross-sectional area at the site of obstruction (mm²); AS = percentage area stenosis; DS = percentage diameter stenosis; HR = Heart rate in beats/min and Ao = mean aortic pressure (mmHg) 1 = immediately preceding CFR-DSC measurements; 2 = immediately preceding the CFR-DOP and RH measurements; CFR-DSC = coronary flow reserve measured with distal subtraction cineangiography; CFR-DOP = coronary flow reserve measured with Doppler.

(range 12 to 31%) of the cross-sectional area of the coronary artery. The reactive hyperemia was measured with the balloon part of the Doppler catheter (0.65 mm²) across the stenosis. In this situation the catheter occupied 20 ± 5%, (range 12–37%) of the luminal cross-sectional area at the site of the stenosis.

Pts	HR1	Ao1	CFR DSC	HR2	Ao2	CFR DOP	RH
1	70	91	2.0	67	104	2.1	2.2
2	70	95	3.3	51	92	2.9	2.9
3	70	93	2.8	68	98	3.0	2.8
4	80	91	1.2	72	87	1.1	1.0
5	70	99	0.6	57	95	0.9	
	70	83	2.4	70	89	2.9	2.3
6	90	97	1.0	69	101	0.9	
	90	97	2.0	83	103	1.8	2.0
7	90	82	2.0	71	80	1.8	
	90	78	2.4	81	76	2.7	2.3
8	100	83	0.8	91	85	1.1	
	100	88	2.2	85	98	2.3	2.2
9	80	90	1.1	70	90	1.3	
	80	88	3.0	82	89	2.3	2.6
10	80	96	1.7	70	97	1.9	1.7
11	70	85	2.2	60	79	2.0	2.1
12	70	115	1.1	66	112	1.0	
	70	111	1.7	62	108	2.2	2.1
13	70	81	1.4	59	83	1.2	
	70	84	2.7	61	83	2.4	1.9
14	70	81	1.2	61	83	1.1	
15	70	88	1.3	58	88	1.0	
	70	76	1.8	60	79	1.7	1.5
16	80	93	1.4	73	89	1.6	
17	70	91	1.1	61	96	2.5	
	70	92	1.0	57	99	1.4	1.3
18	70	87	1.1	63	89	1.1	1.0
19	80	95	1.3	73	99	1.4	
	80	86	1.6	76	83	1.7	1.3
20	80	91	1.3	63	90	1.4	
	80	82	2.3	81	80	2.5	1.5
21	70	80	1.0	65	82	1.2	
	70	75	2.2	63	76	2.3	1.6

This implies that coronary flow reserve assessed with both techniques after PTCA was measured in the presence of an area stenosis of $52 \pm 14\%$, whereas reactive hyperemia was assessed in the presence of a residual area stenosis of $62 \pm 16\%$. In 14 patients a coronary flow reserve measurement with the angiographic technique was also obtained in a myocardial region supplied by a coronary artery which was not dilated and which had no significant stenosis (< 50% diameter stenosis). The mean coronary flow reserve of these vessels was 3.4 ± 0.8 before, and 3.3 ± 0.9 after PTCA. The relationship between coronary flow reserve measured with digital substraction cineangiography (CFR-DSC) and the cross-sectional area at the site of obstruction (OA) is shown in Fig. 5. Patients 1, 4, 7, 9, 10, 11, 12, 17, 18 and 20 had conditions associated with

Table 6.   Mean values of the heart rate and aortic pressure.

	Before PTCA		After PTCA		
	DSC-CFR	DOP-CFR	DSC-CFR	DOP-CFR	DOP-RH
HR	78 ± 10	67 ± 9	76 ± 9	69 ± 10	69 ± 10
Ao	90 ± 9	91 ± 9	88 ± 8	90 ± 10	90 ± 10

Heart rate (HR, beats/min) and mean aortic pressure (Ao, mmHg) immediately preceding the coronary flow reserve measurements with digital subtraction cineangiography (DSC-CFR) and coronary flow reserve and reactive hyperemia measurements with the Doppler catheter (DOP-CFR and DOP-RH).

a reduced coronary flow reserve, in addition to the presence of a coronary stenosis. In these patients only a weak relationship was found between these two parameters: CFR-DSC = 0.27 OA + 0.9 (r = 0.55; SEE = 0.57). In the other patients in whom the epicardial narrowing was the sole factor determining the coronary flow reserve, a good relationship was found between these two parameters: CFR-DSC = 0.51 OA + 0.7 (r = 0.88; SEE = 0.36).

The relationship between coronary flow reserve measured with Doppler (CFR-DOP) and the cross-sectional area at the site of obstruction (OA) is shown in Fig. 6. The resting Doppler-shift before PTCA was 1.4 ± 0.7 kHz and after PTCA 1.5 ± 0.7 kHz. In the patients with conditions associated with a reduced coronary flow reserve aside from the presence of a coronary stenosis the

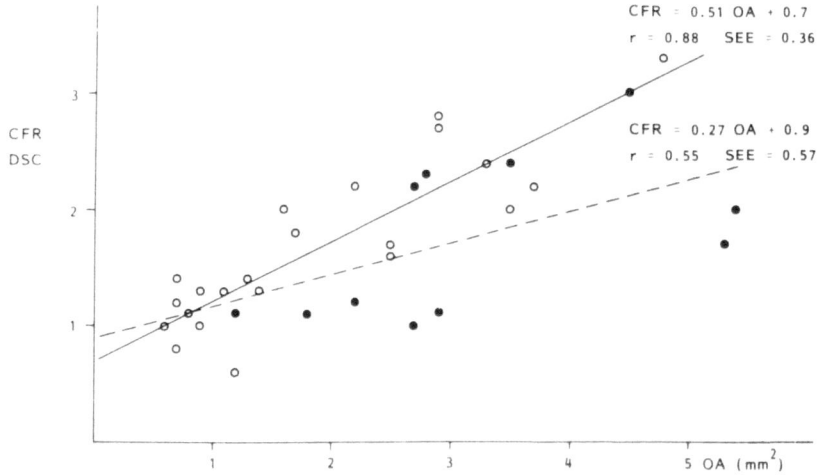

Figure 5.   Relationship between coronary flow reserve measured with digital subtraction cineangiography (CFR-DSC) and cross-sectional area at the site of obstruction (OA).

The open symbols (●) are the patients with any of the following characteristics: left ventricular hypertrophy, hypertension, previous myocardial infarction, collaterals or dissection after PTCA. The closed symbols (○) are the patients without any of the above listed characteristics.

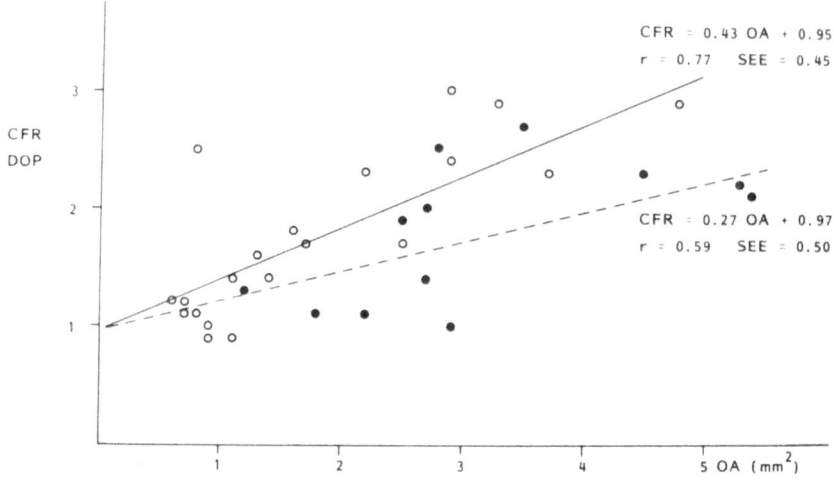

Figure 6. Relationship between coronary flow reserve measured with the Doppler probe (CFR-DO P) and cross-sectional area at the site of obstruction (OA). See for explanation of symbols Fig. 5.

relationship between these two parameters was weak: CFR-DOP = 0.27 OA + 1. 0 (r = 0.59; SEE = 0.50). In the other patients a reasonably good relationship was found between these two parameters: CFR-DOP = 0.43 OA + 1.0 (r = 0.77; SEE = 0.45).

The relationship between the coronary flow reserve measured with the angiographic technique and the coronary flow reserve measured with Doppler probe is shown in Fig. 7. There is a good relationship between the measurements made with these two techniques, irrespective of whether the flow reserve is limited solely by the severity of the coronary stenosis (CFR-DSC = 0.88 CFR-DOP + 0.12; r = 0.85; SEE = 0.38) or whether there are additional patient characteristics present such as previous infarction, hypertrophy, collaterals or dissection after PTCA (CFR-DSC = 0.96 CFR-DOP + 0.01; r = 0.87; SEE = 0.34).

The relationships between the reactive hyperemia (RH) recorded after the final balloon inflation with the angioplasty catheter still across the lesion, and coronary flow reserve measured with the angiographic technique (CFR-DSC = 0.27 + 0.95 RH; r = 0.85; SEE = 0.34) and with the Doppler catheter (CFR-DOP = 0.51 + 0.84 RH; r = 0.83; SEE = 0.32) are shown in Figs 8 and 9 respectively. As expected the mean reactive hyperemia was somewhat lower than the coronary flow reserves measured with the angiographic technique or with the Doppler probe located proximal to the dilated stenosis. Reactive hyperemia was 1.9 ± 0.6, coronary flow reserve measured with the angiographic technique 2.1 ± 0.6 and coronary flow reserve measured with the Doppler catheter 2.1 ± 0.6.

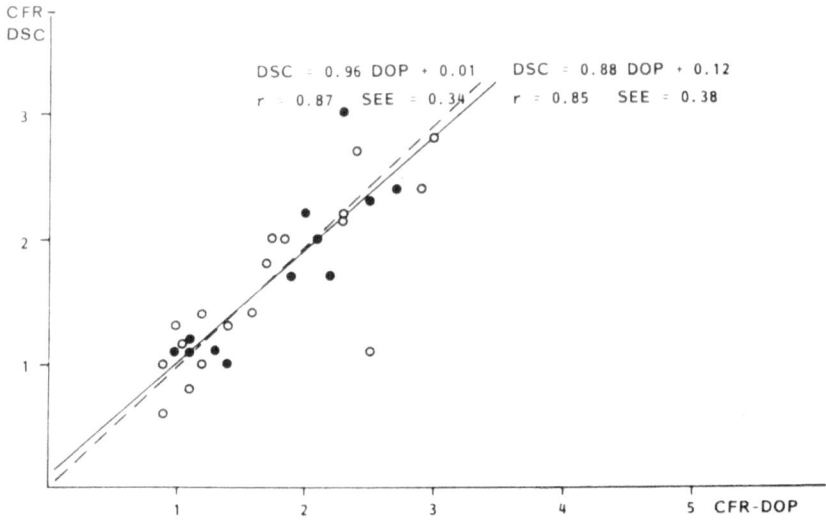

Figure 7. Relationship between coronary flow reserve measured with digital subtraction cineangio graphy (CFR-DSC) and coronary flow reserve measured with the Doppler probe (CFR-DOP). See for explanation of symbols Fig. 5.

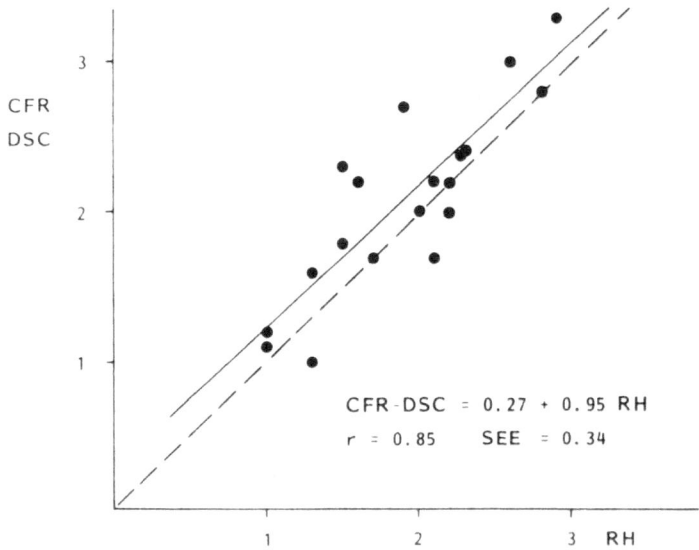

Figure 8. Relationship between coronary flow reserve measured with digital subtraction cineangio graphy (CFR-DSC) and the reactive hyperemia recorded with the Doppler probe across the dilated lesion after the final balloon inflation (RH).

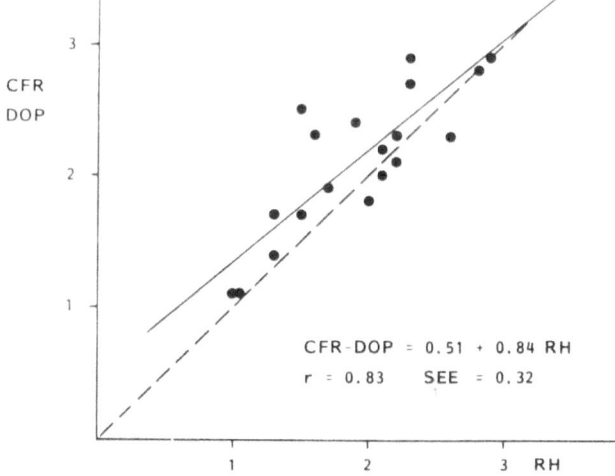

Figure 9. Relationship between coronary flow reserve measured with the Doppler probe (CFR-DOP) proximal to the dilated lesion and the reactive hyperemia recorded with the Doppler probe across the dilated lesion after the final balloon inflation (RH).

Discussion

Intracoronary blood flow velocity: An on line assessment of the functional result of the dilatation?

We measured the changes of the intracoronary blood flow velocity during PTCA by means of a Doppler tip balloon catheter. Our original purpose was to use this information as an 'on-line' assessment of the functional result of the dilatation, with the PTCA catheter still across the stenosis. The technical innovation of this catheter is the combination of a diagnostic and therapeutic tool. Although the catheter is a prototype of first generation, it provides an unique opportunity to assess the reactive hyperemia in awake human beings.

The poststenotic velocities recorded with the catheter across the lesion are low when compared with the previously published data that document values recorded proximal to the stenotic lesion [13, 18]. Recently it has been suggested [30] that the 'zero crossing' method underestimates post-stenotic velocity possibly because of disturbance of laminar flow and this may also explain the discrepancy between our results and those previously published. The routine calibration of each Doppler probe by the timed blood volume collection from the femoral sheath (cross-sectional area 6.9 mm^2) makes it unlikely that the intracoronary flow velocities recorded in this study with an end-mounted Doppler catheter are in error. The duration of the hyperemia observed in all patients was longer than that in the previously reported [10, 18, 31, 32]. However, in contrast to our results, previous results were obtained after occlusion of normal arteries and after a shorter occlusion time (20 s maximal). Marcus et al [32] have demonstrated that the duration of the hyperemic response increased progressively with increasing duration of occlusion.

Peak reactive hyperemia a useful functional guide line during the procedure

Intracoronary blood flow velocity measurements with a Doppler probe have previously been used to investigate regional coronary flow reserve, assessing the maximal reactive hyperemia induced by pharmacological vasodilation or ischemia [5–9]. However, because coronary flow reserve is a ratio between maximal and resting coronary blood flow, any increase in resting flow results in a decrease of this rato. This phenomenon was observed after the first 2 dilatations when the resting velocity preceding the inflation was used as the denominator of the ratio (peak hyperemic velocity/resting velocity). If the resting velocity after the deflation was used as denominator, the ratio remained unchanged during 4 dilatations; this alternative is therefore useless as a functional guide-line during the procedure. Because peak hyperemic velocity shows a gradual increase with successive dilatations which presumably reflects progressive enlargement of the lumen stenotis we attempted to correlate the cross-sectional area of the stenotic lesion 'corrected' for the presence of the catheter across the stenosis, with the absolute value of the peak velocity during reactive hyperemia. Despite an orderly ranking of the 2 parameters no close correlation ($r = 0.41$) could be established. Ideally cross-sectional areas measured after each stepwise enlargement of the lumen by the gradual inflation of the balloon should have been correlated with the peak hyperemic velocity after the transluminal occlusion. Unfortunately, the poor quality of the coronary angiography performed with the PTCA catheter in the guiding catheter precludes quantitative analysis.

In the setting of PTCA, the absence of precise mathematical relation between the peak hyperemic velocity measured after the last inflation and the post PTCA 'corrected' minimal lumen cross-sectional area is not so surprising. First, the changes in luminal size of an artery following the mechanical disruption of its interal wall may be difficult to assess by angiographic means [2, 3]. The irregular shape with internal tears that fill with contrast medium to a variable extent will result in some overestimation of the true functional luminal size immediately following PTCA. Second, the extent of coronary atherosclerosis may be difficult to delineate angiographically. Mc Pherson et al. [33] have documented substantial intimal atherosclerosis resulting in diffuse obstructive disease and involving the entire length of an epicardial artery, is often present, even when angiograms reveal only discrete lesions. As a consequence relative measurements of stenosis severity are an inadequate approach to assessing the severity of coronary obstructions. In addition, the calculated cross-sectional area of the stenotic lesion after the subtraction of the cross-sectional area of the catheter (mean 2.0 ± 1.2 mm^2; range 0.5–4.6 mm^2) clearly suggests that the catheter is not only impeding the flow through the stenotic lesion, even after dilatation, but might unpredictibly disturb the velocity profile in the post-stenotic segment [34]. Further miniaturization of the catheter may improve this major draw-back. For all these reasons, the measurement of the peak velocity with this prototype catheter of first generation does not permit, on-line, an accurate prediction of the morphological change of the stenotic lesion. However, during sequential dilatations the plateau observed in the peak hyperemic and resting velocity signals still provides valuable information which indicates that no further improvement in flow velocity can be expected from additional dilatations.

The purpose of the investigation in the second study group was twofold: firstly, to compare in the setting of an angioplasty procedure two different techniques of assessing regional coronary blood flow; secondly, to compare the pharmacologically induced vasodilation after intracoronary papaverine with reactive hyperemia following transluminal occlusion.

Rationale for comparison of the two techniques to measure coronary flow reserve

Extensive validation studies with the Doppler technique have been performed in which the measured changes in velocity have been compared with changes in perfusion measured with timed-venous coronary sinus collection [13, 32], labeled microspheres [35], and electromagnetic flow probes [32]. These studies indicate that under a great variety of conditions, changes in coronary blood flow velocity measured by the Doppler technique accurately reflect changes in flow [36]. Recently, small sized Doppler catheters have been developed and validated. They are able to make selective measurements of flow velocity in the major proximal coronary arteries [9, 13, 17], without causing coronary obstruction [36]. For instance, in this report the cross-sectional area of the Doppler balloon catheter was only $18 \pm 5\%$ of the cross-sectional area of the coronary artery in the segment proximal to the stenosis. However, two important limitations of the Doppler technique are: (1) it measures flow velocity rather than volume flow – which may lead to inaccurate values for flow reserve if significant change occurs in cross-sectional areas between baseline and hyperemia [18], and (2) subselective coronary cannulation increases the risk during cardiac catheterization [13, 36]. Therefore less invasive approaches to determine the regional coronary flow reserve are urgently needed.

Selective coronary angiography is the standard means for obtaining anatomical information and is the most important tool for clinical decision making used by the clinician caring for patients with coronary artery disease. Recently, several attempts have been made to measure coronary blood flow parameters during cardiac catheterization using . recent developments in radiographic technology [16]. However, radiographic contrast media cannot be used to measure coronary blood flow by the traditional methodological approaches [16]; an essential prerequisite of indicator-dilution (Stewart-Hamilton), inert substance washout (Kety-Schmidt), or firstpass distribution (Sapirstein) techniques is that the indicator substance does not affect the regional flow being measured [8]. Unfortunately, all radiographic media have substantial vascular effects [37], although nonionic media may disturb blood flow less than ionic agents [16]. Using ECG-gated power injection of a contrast agent at a rate that is presumed to be sufficiently rapid to achieve complete replacement of blood with contrast, Hodgson et al. [38] developed a mask mode subtraction technique that determines myocardial time-density curves before and during maximal hyperemia before the vascular effects of the contrast medium disturb the ratio between resting and hyperemic coronary blood flow. Since some of this techniques fundamental assumptions may not be met under clinical conditions, validation studies are of special interest [39]. In this study we found a reasonable good correlation between radiographically determined coronary flow reserve and the coronary flow velocity reserve measured with a Doppler probe, despite the fact that the two approaches have methodologically nothing in common and that their respective regions of interest (myocardium for the radiographic technique and intracoronary lumen for the Doppler technique) are basically different.

Maximal coronary blood flow after pharmacological vasodilation versus reactive hyperemia induced by coronary occlusion

In the animal laboratory it has been shown that pharmacologically induced vasodilation after intracoronary administration of papaverine is of the same magnitude as the reactive hyperemia after a 15 s occlusion of the coronary artery [40]. There is some question as to whether the same quantity of flow reserve that can be recruited pharmacologically, can be recruited during ischemia [39]. In this study, we found that reactive hyperemia in patients without hypertrophy, infarction, hypertension, collaterals or dissection was 2.1 ± 0.6 (range 1.3 to 2.9), whereas coronary flow reserves in these patients both with the Doppler probe and the radiographic technique were 2.3 ± 0.6 (range 1.6 to 3.3) after PTCA. The cross-sectional area at the site of obstruction averaged $3.05\,mm^2$ in these patients. Since the balloon catheter was still across the lesion the functional lumen averaged $2.4\,mm^2$ (see Table 2). In a previous study from this laboratory we established the relationship between cross-sectional area at the site of obstruction and the measured coronary flow reserve in a patient population with single vessel coronary disease and the absence of other factors that might reduce flow reserve such as hypertrophy, infarction, hypertension, collaterals or dissection [15]. This relationship is shown in Fig. 10. A coronary artery with an obstruction area of $2.4\,mm^2$ would be expected to have a vascular reserve of 2.2 with confidence limits extending from 1.3 to 3.0, which corresponds almost exactly to the range found in this study. Therefore, we feel that our data support the conclusion that the coronary vasodilation after an optimal dose of intracoronary papaverine [11] is equipotent to the reactive hyperemia following a transluminal occlusion of more than 40 s in patients with significant coronary artery disease.

Limitations

When comparing these three measures of the functional capacity of a coronary artery one has to bear in mind the potential sources of data scatter. Fortunately, the radiographic technique as well as the Doppler technique have a good reproducibility (see *Methods*). Coronary flow reserve and reactive hyperemia are both ratios between maximal coronary blood flow and resting flow. Resting coronary blood flow is mainly determined by aortic pressure and heart rate and coronary blood flow during maximal vasodilation is linearly related to the prevailing perfusion pressure [7, 8]. These two hemodynamic parameters change little between the measurements of flow reserve and reactive hyperemia (see Tables 1 and 3), although they certainly contribute to the scatter of the data (see Figs. 3, 4 and 5).

Several studies have shown that in selected patients a close relationship exists between quantitatively determined stenosis geometry and measured coronary flow reserve [15, 41]. However, coronary flow reserve can be influenced by many factors other than epicardial coronary stenosis, such as myocardial hypertrophy, tachycardia, hypertension, prior myocardial infarction, collaterals, dissection after PTCA [42, 43], changes in coronary vasomotor tone and changes in ventricular end-diastolic and intrathoracic pressures [7, 8]. Therefore, in order to relate the measured coronary flow reserve to quantitatively determined stenosis geometry, we have carefully divided our study population into a group of patients (A) with one or more of the above mentioned characteristics and a group of patients (B) without any of these characteristics (see Figs. 1 and 2). We tried to prevent changes in vasomotor tone which is relevant to both techniques [24] by inducing a constant maximal epicardial coronary vasodilation with repeated intracoronary administration of isosorbide dinitrate [27]. In accordance with previous reports [15, 41] we found a good correlation between cross-sectional area at the site of obstruction and measured coronary flow reserve in group B, in contrast to a poor correlation between these two parameters in group A.

Coronary flow reserve immediately after PTCA

Several authors [10, 42] have shown that the coronary flow reserve of the myocardial region supplied by the dilated vessel increases substantially after PTCA, but is not restored to normal values. The measurements obtained in the present study with two independent techniques confirm this fact. We also measured the coronary flow reserve of an adjacent myocardial region supplied by a not significantly diseased coronary artery, by the radiographic technique and found a marked difference in vasodilator response. For ethical reasons we did not obtain this measurement with the Doppler catheter as we felt that introduction of the Doppler probe into a second coronary artery might introduce additional risks to the investigational part of the procedure. Nevertheless, the results of the radiographic technique indicate that the abnormal vasodilatory response is restricted to the myocardium supplied by the dilated coronary artery. There are several potential explanations for this phenomenon.

1. Since coronary flow reserve is a ratio between resting flow and maximal coronary blood flow, any increase in resting flow results in a decrease of this ratio. Neither of the techniques we used, provided us with absolute measurements of volume flow. Therefore, we cannot make a definite conclusion regarding resting coronary volume flow after the PTCA. However, the resting Doppler shift was virtually the same before and after the PTCA procedure, $1.4 \pm 0.7 \, \text{kHz}$ and $1.5 \pm 0.7 \, \text{kHz}$ respectively. Furthermore, several authors using the thermodilution technique in the coronary sinus or the great cardiac vein have reported comparable resting volume flows before and after PTCA [44, 45, 46].

2. Metabolic, humoral or myogenic factors could potentially play a role in the limited restoration of coronary flow reserve after PTCA. However, the metabolic derangements due to the PTCA seem quickly reversible [44, 47, 48]. Although humoral factors may play a role in a specific subgroup of patients with complicated PTCA, sofar no evidence has been presented that implicates that humoral factors are important in this regard in the majority of

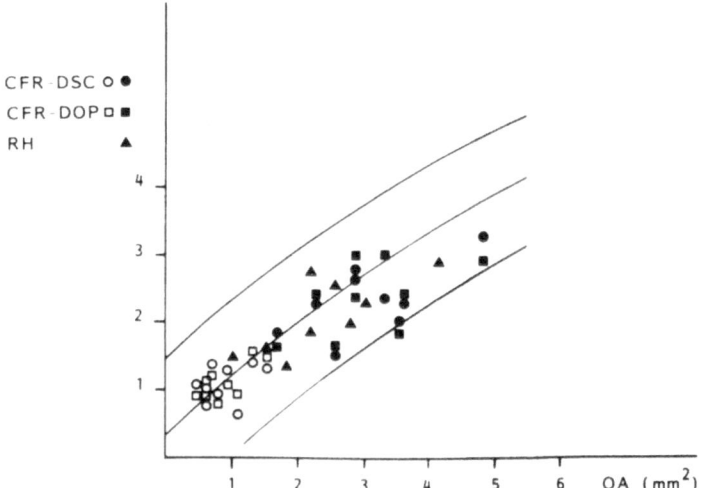

Figure 10. Relationship between flow reserve and cross-sectional area at the site of obstruction (OA) as described in a previous report of our laboratory [16]. The lines indicate the best fit curve and the 95% confidence limits. The data of the present study are superimposed.

The open symbols are the measurements obtained before PTCA. The closed symbols are the measurements obtained after PTCA.

CFR-DSC = coronary flow reserve measured with digital subtraction cineangiography, CFR-DOP = coronary flow reserve measured with the Doppler probe, RH = reactive hyperemia recorded following the final balloon inflation.

patients [49]. The chronic reduction in perfusion pressure distal to the stenotic lesion may induce alterations in the complex mechanism of autoregulation and a prolonged period of time may be needed before these abnormalities subside [50].

3. Finally, the impaired coronary flow reserve could be directly related to the residual stenosis [10]. Cross-sectional area measured immediately after PTCA generally increases about threefold due to the procedure but remains grossly abnormal [10, 51]. The relationship between cross-sectional area at the site of obstruction and coronary flow reserve as found in a previous study from our laboratory [15], is shown in Fig. 10 with the 95% confidence intervals. The data of the present study for patients fullfilling the same exclusion criteria (group B) are superimposed: coronary flow reserve measured with both techniques and the reactive hyperemia following the final balloon inflation with residual obstruction area corrected for the presence of the Doppler balloon catheter. The large majority of measurements fall within the 95% confidence limits of this relation, suggesting that the persisting reduction in cross-sectional area perse constitutes a sufficient explanation for the limited restoration of coronary flow reserve, although it does not exclude other contributing pathophysiological mechanisms.

Acknowledgements

We gratefully acknowledge to Anja van Huuksloot en Claudia Sprenger de Rover for their secretarial assistance.

References

1. Grüntzig AR, Senning A, Siegenthaler WE (1979) Nonoperative dilatation of coronary artery stenosis: percutaneous transluminal angioplasty. *N Engl J Med* 301:61–8
2. Block PC, Myler RK, Stertzer S, Fallon JT (1981) Morphology after transluminal angioplasty in human beings. *N Engl J Med* 305:382–5
3. Serruys PW, Reiber JHC, Wijns W, van den Brand M, Kooyman CJ, ten Katen HJ, Hugenholtz PG (1984) Assessment of percutaneous transluminal coronary angioplasty by quantitative coronary angiography: Diameter versus densitometric area measurements. *Am J Cardiol* 54: 482–488
4. Leimgruber PP, Roubin GS, Hollman J, Cotsonis GA, Meier B, Douglas JS, King SB, Gruentzig AR (1986) Restenosis after successful coronary angioplasty in patients with single-vessel disease. *Circulation* 73:710–717
5. Serruys PW, Wijns W, Reiber JHC, de Feyter P, van den Brand M, Piscione F, Hugenholtz PG (1985) Values and limitations of transstenotic pressure gradients measured during percutaneous coronary angioplasty. *Herz* 6:337–342
6. Redd DCB, Roubin GS, Leimgruber PP, Abi-Mansour P, Douglas JS, King SB (1987) The transstenotic pressure gradient trend as a predictor of acute complications after percutaneous transluminal coronary angioplasty. *Circulation* 76:792–801
7. Hoffman JIE (1984) Maximal coronary flow and the concept of vascular reserve. *Circulation* 70:153–159

8. Klocke FJ (1983) Measurements of coronary blood flow and degree of stenosis: current clinical implications and continuing uncertainties. *J Am Coll Cardiol* 1:31–41
9. Serruys PW, Juillière Y, Zijlstra F, Beatt KJ, de Feyter PJ, Suryapranata H, vd Brand M, Roelandt J (1988) Coronary Blood Flow velocity during PTCA: a guide-line for assessment of functional results. *Am J Cardiol* 61:253–259
10. Zijlstra F, Reiber JC, Juillière Y, Serruys PW (1988) Normalization of coronary flow reserve by percutaneous transluminal coronary angioplasty. *Am J Cardiol* 61:55–60
11. Wilson RF, White CW (1986) Intracoronary papaverine: an ideal coronary vasodilator for studies of the coronary circulation in conscious humans. *Circulation* 73:444–451
12. Zijlstra F, Serruys PW, Hugenholtz PG (1986) Papaverine: The ideal coronary vasodilator for investigating coronary flow reserve. A study of timing, magnitude, reproducibility and safety of the coronary hyperemic response after intracoronary papaverine. *Cath Cardiovasc Diagn* 12:298–303
13. Wilson RF, Laughlin DE, Ackell PH, Chilian WM, Holida MD, Hartley CJ, Armstrong ML, Marcus ML, White CW (1985) Transluminal subselective measurement of coronary artery blood flow velocity and vasodilator reserve in man. *Circulation* 72:82–92
14. Bates ER, Aueron FM, Le Grand V, Le Free MT, Mancini GBJ, Hodgson JM, Vogel RA (1985) Comparative long-term effects of coronary artery bypass graft surgery and percutaneous transluminal coronary angioplasty on regional coronary flow reserve. *Circulation* 72:833–839
15. Zijlstra F, van Ommeren J, Reiber JHC, Serruys PW (1987) Does quantitative assessment of coronary artery dimensions predict the physiological significance of a coronary stenosis? *Circulation* 75:1154–1161
16. Vogel RA (1985) The radiographic assessment of coronary blood flow parameters. *Circulation* 72:460–465
17. Sibley DH, Millar HD, Hartley CJ, Whitlow PL (1986) Subselective measurement of coronary blood flow velocity using a steerable Doppler catheter. *JACC* 8:1332–1340
18. Marcus ML (1983) Physiological effects of a coronary stenosis, pp. 242–269 in: *The Coronary Circulation in Health and Disease*. New York: McGraw-Hill
19. Marcus ML (1983) Effects of cardiac hypertrophy on the coronary circulation, pp. 285–306 in: *The Coronary Circulation in Health and Disease*. New York: McGraw-Hill
20. Marcus ML, Doty DB, Hiratzka LP, Whight CB, Eastham CL (1985) Decrease coronary reserve: a mechanism for angina pectoris in patients with aortic stenosis and normal coronary arteries. *N Engl J Med* 307:1362–1366
21. Cole JS, Hartley CJ (1977) The pulsed Doppler coronary artery catheter. Preliminary report of a new technique for measuring rapid changes in coronary artery flow velocity in man. *Circulation* 56:18–25
22. Hartley CJ, Cole JS (1974) An ultrasonic pulsed Doppler system for measuring blood flow in small vessels. *J Appl Physiol* 37:626–629
23. Wilson RF, Laughlin DE, Ackell PH, Chilean WM, Holida MD, Hartley CJ, Armstrong ML, Marcus ML, White CW (1985) Transluminal subelective measurement of coronary artery blood flow velocity and vasodilator reserve in man. *Circulation* 72:82–92
24. Reiber JHC, Serruys PW, Kooyman CJ, Wijns W, Slager CJ, Gerbrand JJ, Schuurbiers JCH, den Boer A, Hugenholtz PG (1985) Assessment of short-, medium-, and long-term variations in arterial dimensions from computer-assisted quantification of coronary cineangiograms. *Circulation* 71:280–288
25. Reiber JHC, Kooijman CJ, Slager CJ, Gerbrands JJ, Schuurbiers JHC, den Boer A, Wijns W, Serruys PW, Hugenholtz PG (1984) Coronary artery dimensions from cineangiograms; methodology and vasodilation of a computer-assisted analysis procedure. *IEEE Trans Med Imaging* MI-3:131–141
26. Reiber JHC, Kooijaman CJ, den Boer A, Serruys PW (1985) Assessment of dimensions and image quality of coronary contrast catheters from cineangiograms. *Cath Cardiovasc Diagn* 11:521–531
27. Zijlstra F, Reiber JHC, Serruys PW (1988) Does intracoronary papaverine dilate epicardial coronary arteries? Implications for the assessment of coronary flow reserve. *Cath Cardiovasc Diagn* 14:1–6

28. van der Werf T, Heethaar RM, Stegehuis H, Meyler FL (1984) The concept of apparent cardiac arrest as a prerequisite for coronary digital subtraction angiography. *J Am Coll Cardiol* 4:239–244

29. Rentrop KP, Cohen M, Blanke H, Philips RA (1985) Changes in collateral channel filling immediately after controlled coronary artery occlusion by an angioplasty balloon in human subjects. *J Am Coll Cardiol* 5:587–592

30. Kajiva F, Ogasawara Y, Tsuyioka K, Nakai M, Coto M, Wada Y, Tadaoka S, Matsuoka S, Mito K, Fuwruara T (1986) Evaluation of human coronary blood flow with an 80 channel transform methods during cardiac surgery. *Circulation* 74 (suppl III):53–60

31. Sibley D, Bulle T, Baxley W, Dean L, Whitlow P (1986) Continuous on-line assessment of coronary angioplasty with a Doppler tipped balloon dilatation catheter (abstr). *Circulation* 74 (Suppl II):459

32. Marcus M, Wright C, Doty D, Eastham C, Laughlin D, Krumm P, Fastenow C, Brody M (1981) Measurements of coronary velocity and reactive hyperemia in the coronary circulation of humans. *Circ Res* 49:877–897

33. Mc Pherson DD, Hiratzka LF, Lamberth WC, Brandt B, Hunt M, Kieso RA, Marcus ML, Kerber RF (1987) Delineation of the extent of coronary atherosclerosis by high-frequency epicardial echocardiography. *N Engl Med* 316:304–309

34. Kilpatrick D, Webber SB (1986) Intravascular blood velocity in simulated coronary artery stenoses. *Cath Cardiovasc Diagn* 12:317–313

35. Wangler RD, Peters KG, Laughlin DE, Tomanek RJ, Marcus ML (1981) A method for continuously assessing coronary velocity in the rat. *Am J Physiol* 10:H816–820

36. Marcus ML, Wilson RF, White CW (1987) Methods of measurements of myocardial blood flow in patients: a critical review. *Circulation* 76:245–253

37. Hodgson JM, Mancini GBJ, LeGrand V, Vogel RA (1985) Characterization of changes in coronary blood flow during the first six seconds after intracoronary contrast injection. *Invest Radiol* 20:246–252

38. Hodgson JM, LeGrand V, Bates ER, Mancini GBJ, Aueron FM, O'Neill WW, Simon SB, Beauman GJ, LeFree MT, Vogel RA (1985) Validation in dogs of a rapid angiographic technique to measure relative coronary blood flow during routine cardiac catheterization. *Am J Cardiol* 55:188–193

39. Klocke FJ (1987) Measurements of coronary flow reserve: Defining pathophysiology versus making decisions about patient care. *Circulation* 76:1183–1189

40. Bookstein JJ, Higgins CB (1977) Comparative efficacy of coronary vasodilatory methods. *Investigate Radiology* 12:121–127

41. Wilson RF, Marcus ML, White CW (1987) Prediction of the physiologic significance of coronary arterial lesions by quantitative lesion geometry in patients with limited coronary artery disease. *Circulation* 75:723–732

42. Hodgson JM, Riley RS, Most AS, Williams DO (1987) Assessment of coronary flow reserve using digital angiography before and after successful percutaneous transluminal coronary angioplasty. *Am J Cardiol* 60:61–65

43. Bates ER, Mc Gillem MJ, Beats TF, DeBoe SF, Mickelson JK, Mancini GBJ, Vogel RA (1987) Effect of angioplasty induced endothelial denudation compared with medial injury on regional coronary blood flow. *Circulation* 76:710–716

44. Serruys PW, Wijns W, van den Brand M, Mey S, Slager C, Schuurbiers JCH, Hugenholtz PG, Brower RW (1984) Left ventricular performance, regional blood flow, wall motion, and lactate metabolism during transluminal angioplasty. *Circulation* 70:25–36

45. Feldman RL, Conti R, Pepine CJ (1983) Regional coronary venous flow responses to transient coronary artery occlusion in human beings. *J Am Coll Cardiol* 2:1–10

46. Rothman MT, Baim DS, Simpson JB, Harrison DC (1982) Coronary hemodynamics during percutaneous transluminal coronary angioplasty. *Am J Cardiol* 49:1615–1622

47. Serruys PW, Piscione F, Wijns W, Harmsen E, van den Brand M, de Feyter P, Hugenholtz PG, de Jong JW (1986) Myocardial release of hypoxanthine and lactate during percutaneous transluminal coronary angioplasty: A quickly reversible phenomenon, but for how long? pp 75ff in:

Serruys PW, Transluminal coronary angioplasty: An investigational tool and a non-operative treatment of acute myocardial ischemia. (Doctoral Thesis, Erasmus University, Rotterdam, The Netherlands)

48. Webb SC, Rickards AF, Poole-Wilson PA (1983) Coronary sinus potassium concentration recorded during coronary angioplasty. *Br Heart J* 50:146–152

49. Peterson MB, Machay V, Block PC, Palacios I, Philbin D, Watkins WD (1986) Thromboxane release during percutaneous transluminal coronary angioplasty. *Am Heart J* 1:111–119

50. Wilson RF, Aylward PE, Leimbach WH, Talman CL, White CW (1986) Coronary flow reserve late after PTCA. – Do the early alterations persist? (abstr). *J Am Coll Cardiol* 7:212A (suppl)

51. Johnson MR, Brayden GP, Ericksen EE, Collins SM, Skaton DJ, Harrison DG, Marcus ML, White CW (1986) Changes in cross-sectional area of the coronary lumen in the six months after angioplasty: a quantitative analysis of the variable response to percutaneous transluminal angioplasty. *Circulation* 73:467–475

8. Loss of hydrogen and potassium ions after short periods of myocardial ischaemia in man

P.A. POOLE-WILSON

Introduction

Angioplasty has provided an opportunity to study the metabolic and ionic events early during ischaemia in the human heart. Almost all previous studies have used animal models in vivo or isolated cardiac muscle preparations in vitro. The findings have sometimes been conflicting. Methods for the direct measurement of intracellular ion concentrations in the human heart are not yet available. Whole tissue measurements on biopsies, even if possible and ethical, would be uninterpretable and inaccurate because of the difficulties in sampling of the myocardium and in quantitation of the extracellular space. Techniques based on magnetic resonance or using ion sensitive indicators are not yet sufficiently developed.

Measurement of arterio-venous differences

The only practical approach to the problem is to measure the arterio-venous difference. If the arterial concentration is constant net gain or loss of a metabolite or ion can be detected. If however the arterial concentration changes or the arterio-venous difference alters in magnitude without a change in direction (uptake to production for example) the interpretation of findings can be difficult without precise information on coronary blood flow. A further limitation in the use of arterio-venous differences is that regional abnormalities within the heart may not be reflected in samples of blood from the coronary sinus draining the whole heart after mixing of blood from diseased and normal myocardium. In the past arterio-venous differences have been calculated from measurements on samples of blood obtained at selected times. This gives rise to difficulties of interpretation if the blood flow is changing rapidly or if a non steady state exists. For example the assessment of lactate metabolism in the heart during an atrial pacing test depends critically on the time of sampling [1, 2]. If samples are obtained at the end of the pacing period but before pacing is stopped a non steady state exists and lactate will still be retained in the ischaemic myocardium so that

P.W. Serruys, R. Simon & K.J. Beatt (eds), Percutaneous Transluminal Coronary Angioplasty. ISBN 0-7923-0346-6.
© *1990 Kluwer Academic Publishers, Dordrecht*

the arterio-venous difference is not indicative of the state of the myocardium. If samples are obtained immediately after pacing is discontinued then again a non steady state exists and the arterio-venous difference is influenced by the rapidly changing coronary flow and the washout of lactate from ischaemic myocardium. Despite these well known problems observations on the concentration of ions and oxygen in the coronary sinus particularly if obtained by a device which provides a continuous record do provide important insights into the metabolic changes occurring in the human heart early during ischaemia.

Oxygen

The limiting substrate for the heart is oxygen. While oxygen saturation has not been reported during angioplasty results are available on the effects of vasoconstriction [3] and atrial pacing [4]. In normal persons the coronary sinus oxygen saturation is maintained constant despite increases in oxygen consumption of the heart. Oxygen saturation falls immediately heart rate is increased but within fifteen seconds the oxygen saturation has returned to the control value [4] (Fig. 1). Presumably coronary blood flow has increased (metabolic regulation of coronary flow). This mechanism cannot occur in the presence of atheromatous obstructive coronary artery disease and the oxygen saturation remains low and falls further with increasing heart rate and presumed increasing ischaemia [4]. Vasoconstriction leads to an almost immediate fall of oxygen saturation [3].

Potassium

Experiments in vivo and in vitro have demonstrated that the extracellular potassium increases rapidly during ischaemia [5–9]. The concentration can reach 10 mmol/l within 10 min. The early loss from the myocardium is reversible and is not associated with tissue necrosis [10]. Isotopic flux experiments have

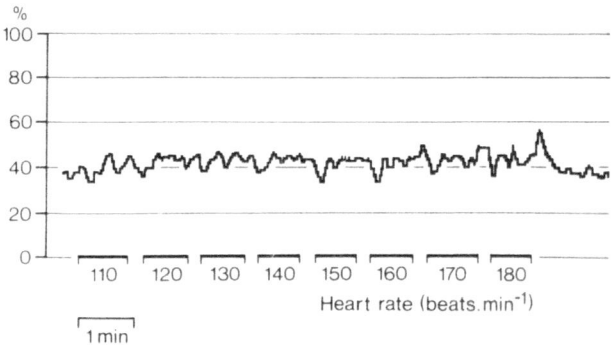

Figure 1. Coronary sinus oxygen in a normal person during atrial pacing. Note that at the higher heart rates a fall of oxygen saturation occurs as the rate is increased but recovery to normal is apparent within 15 sec (metabolic regulation of coronary flow) [4].

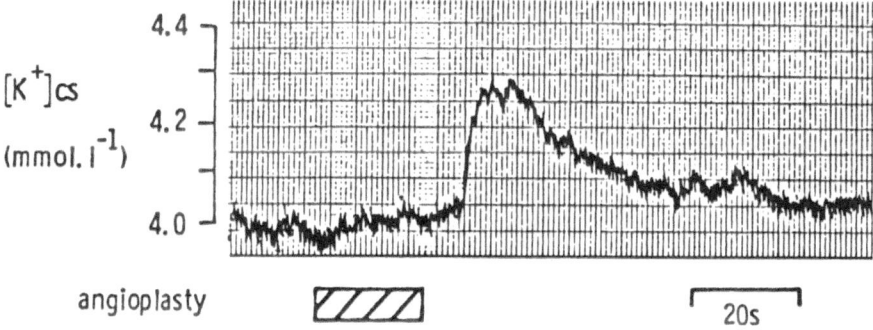

Figure 2. The potassium concentration in the great cardiac vein during angioplasty (occlusion of the left anterior descending coronary artery). A washout of potassium is evident soon after deflation of the angioplasty balloon [13–16].

demonstrated that the loss of potassium is due to a increased efflux of potassium in the presence of a largely unchanged influx.

In man the arterio-venous difference across the heart has been measured continuously during angioplasty [13–15]. The potassium concentration in the coronary sinus or great cardiac vein was recorded from a catheter tip electrode sensitive to potassium. Patients had lesions of the left anterior descending coronary artery. A typical result is shown in Fig. 2. During occlusion the potassium concentration was unchanged presumably because the flow of blood from the ischaemic muscle was substantially reduced. On deflating the angioplasty balloon a transient washout of potassium was evident. The detection of the washout was delayed about four seconds by the time for deflation of the balloon and for blood to travel from the ischaemic muscle to the electrode in the coronary sinus or great cardiac vein. The amount of potassium loss is difficult to calculate because coronary flow is unknown and is presumably changing rapidly at this time. The peak potassium concentration was highest in those patients in whom the occlusion was longest. By plotting the peak potassium concentration against the duration of the occlusion, it could be demonstrated that the loss of potassium was evident after occlusions of 15 sec duration. Shorter occlusions of less than 5 sec did not affect venous potassium concentration demonstrating that the compression of the atheromatous plaque was not the source of potassium loss. In other studies transient potassium loss was demonstrated with change of heart rate in normal persons and a further increased loss with the development of ischaemia during an atrial pacing test [16].

Hydrogen

The same techniques which were used to record potassium loss from the heart have been used to detect acidosis during angioplasty [17]. The loss of hydrogen

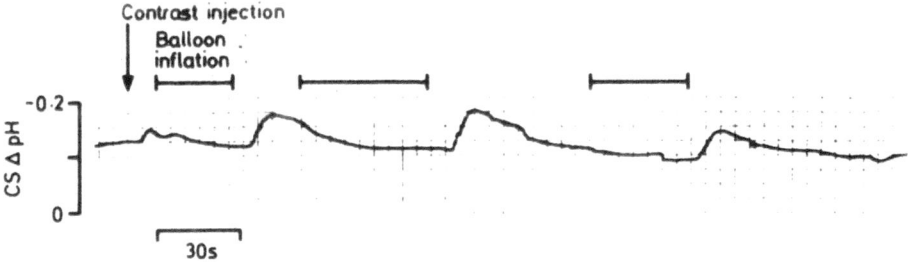

Figure 3. The hydrogen concentration in the great cardiac vein during angioplasty. The pattern is similar to the loss of potassium. Hydrogen ions are washed out from the ischaemic myocardium on reperfusion [17].

ions was similar to that of potassium ions (Fig. 3) and was evident after occlusions of between 10 and 15 sec. Thus acidosis was shown in the human myocardium early durng ischaemia. Acidosis has also been shown after atrial pacing when ischaemia has been induced [2]. An alkalosis was never observed. Under some conditions in in vitro experimental models alkalosis has been reported [18–20]. Presumably this is due to the breakdown of creatine phosphate which consumes protons. In man [17] and in dogs in vivo [21] it seems that alkalosis is not found. Those biochemical reactions generating protons (adenosine triphosphate breakdown (ATP) and glycogenolysis) predominate over the effect of creatine phosphate breakdown.

The magnitude of the acidosis in the myocardium is difficult to determine from these measurements. The change in the myocardium is likely to be greater than that recorded because of dilution of blood from the ischaemic muscle with blood from adjacent normal muscle. The acidosis is sufficient to cause approximately 50% reduction of contractile function [22] even in this short period of time.

Other effects of angioplasty

Changes on the surface electrocardiogram occur after about 30 sec of coronary occlusion and chest pain after 45 sec. The precise time depends on many variables including blood flow into the ischaemic muscle bed from collateral vessels. The monophasic action potential alters within 15 sec [23] and the earliest changes of both contraction and relaxation of the myocardium occur at the same time [24].

A unifying hypothesis

The origin of acidosis early in ischaemic muscle is explained by the breakdown of ATP an glycogenolysis. There are several other potential biochemical sources of hydrogen ions and intracellular buffering could be altered thereby affecting the pH change for a given acid load. The cause of the concurrent loss of potassium is less easily explained. The loss cannot be directly due to the acidosis since acidosis in ventricular muscle causes a gain of potassium not a loss [25]. The loss is not due to reduced function of the sodium pump since that would affect potassium influx and could not account for an increase of potassium efflux. Two explanations have recently been proposed. The first is that potassium is lost through a potassium channel which is opened by a fall of ATP concentration [26, 27]. A difficulty with that suggestion is whether ATP or a fraction in association with the cell membrane falls within 15 sec of ischaemia. Furthermore the ATP dependent potassium channel is only sensitive to rather low concentrations of ATP which may not be reached until much later during ischaemia. An alternative explanation for the loss of potassium is that potassium moves out of the myocyte in association with anions [5, 12, 28]. That the accumulation of anions and lactate does cause a loss of cell potassium due to an increase of potassium efflux has been shown in isolated tissues [12, 28].

The proposal is that as soon as tissue oxygen is consumed (2 or 3 heart beats) creatine phosphate and ATP are broken down and glycogenolysis stimulated. The sum of these reactions leads to an acidosis which is of sufficient magnitude to account for at least an appreciable part of the decline in contractile function. The accumulation of lactate in the cell causes a loss of potassium. The accumulation of this potassium in the extracellular space and the fall of pH can account for the changes of the action potential [29].

Myocardial ischaemia gives rise to many complex and interacting biochemical changes. Mechanisms other than those discussed contribute to the loss of contractile function (for example the accumulation of intracellular phosphate) and to the altered morphology of the action potential. Nevertheless this simplistic hypothesis does account for many, if not most, of the mechanical and electrophysiological changes which are seen early during ischaemia.

References

1. Remme WJ, Van den Berg R, Mantel M, Cox PH, van Hugenhuyse DCA, Krauss XH, Storm CJ, Kruyssen DACM (1986) Temporal relation of changes in regional coronary flow and myocardial lactate and nucleoside metabolism during pacing-induced angina. *Am J Cardiol* 58:1188–1194
2. Cobbe SM, Poole-Wilson Pa (1982) Continuous coronary sinus and arterial pH monitoring during pacing-induced ischaemia in coronary artery disease. *Br Heart J* 47:369–74
3. Chierchia S, Brunelli C, Simonetti, I, Lazzari M, Maseri A (1980) Sequence of events in angina at rest: primary reduction in coronary flow. *Circulation* 61:759–768
4. Crake T, Crean P, Shapiro L, Canepa-Anson RC, Poole-Wilson PA (1988) Continuous recording of coronary sinus oxygen saturation during atrial pacing in patients with coronary artery disease or with syndrome X. *Br Heart J* 59:31–38
5. Kleber AG (1984) Extracellular potassium accumulation in acute myocardial ischemia. *J. Mol Cell Cardiol* 16:389–394
6. Hirche HJ, Franz C, Bos L, Bissig R, Lang R, Schramm M (1980) Myocardial extracellular K + and H + increase and noradrenaline release as possible cause of early arrhythmias following acute coronary artery occlusion in pigs. *J Mol Cell Cardiol* 12:579–594

7. Hill JL, Gettes LS (1980) Effect of acute coronary artery occlusion on local myocardial extracellular K+ activity in swine. *Circulation* 61:768–778

8. Webb SC, Fleetwood GG, Montgomery RAP, Poole-Wilson (1984) Absence of a relationship between extracellular potassium accumulation and contractile failure in the ischemic or hypoxic rabbit heart. In: *Advances in Myocardiology*, Vol. 6 Ed. Dhalla NS, Hearse DJ pp 405–415

9. Wiegand V, Guggi M, Meesmann W, Kessler M, Greitschus F (1979) Extracellular potassium activity changes with canine myocardium after acute coronary occlusion and the influence of blockade. *Cardiovas Res* 13:297–302

10. Conrad GL, Rau EE, Shine KI (1979) Creatine kinase release, potassium-42 content, and mechanical performance in anoxic rabbit myocardium. *J Clin Invest* 64:155–161

11. Rau EE, Langer GA (1978) Dissociation of energetic state and potassium loss from anoxic myocardium. *Am J Physiol* 235:H537–H543

12. Gaspardone A, Shine KI, Seabrooke SR, Seabrooke SR, Poole-Wilson PA (1986) Potassium loss from rabbit myocardium during hypoxia: evidence for passive efflux linked to anion extrusion. *J Mol Cell Cardiol* 18:389–399

13. Webb SC, Canepa-Anson R, Rickards AF, Poole-Wilson PA (1983) High potassium concentration in a parenteral preparation of glyceryl trinitrate. Need for caution if given by intracoronary injection. *Br Heart J* 50:395–396

14. Webb SC, Rickards AF, Poole-Wilson PA (1983) Coronary sinus potassium concentration recorded during coronary angioplasty. *Brit Heart J* 50:146–148

15. Webb SC, Canepa-Anson R, Rickards AF, Poole-Wilson PA (1987) Myocardial potassium loss after coronary occlusion in humans. *J Am Coll Cardiol* 9:1230–1234

16. Webb SC, Poole-Wilson PA (1986) Potassium exchange in the human heart during atrial pacing and myocardial ischaemia. *Br Heart J* 55:554–559

17. Crake T, Crean P, Shapiro L, Rickards AF, Poole-Wilson PA (1987) Coronary sinus pH during percutaneous transluminal angioplasty: early development of acidosis during myocardial ischaemia in man. *Br Heart J* 58:110–115

18. Allen DG, Morris PG, Orchard CH, Pirolo JS (1985) A nuclear magnetic resonance study of metabolism in the ferret heart during hypoxia and inhibition of glycolysis. *J Physiol* 361:185–204

19. Gebert G, Benzing H, Strohm M (1971) Changes in the interstitial pH of dog myocardium in response to local ischemia, hypoxia, hyper- and hypo-capnia, measured continuously by means of glass micro-electrodes. *Pflugers Archiv* 339:72–81

20. Jacobus WE, Pores IH, Lucas SK, Clayton HK, Weisfeldt ML, Flaherty TJ (1984) The role of intracellular pH in the control of normal and ischaemic myocardial contractility: a 31P nuclear magnetic resonance and mass spectrometry study. In: Intracellular pH: Its function, regulation and utilisation in cellular functions. Ed. R Nuccitelli, DW Deamer Alan Liss, New York. pp 537–565

21. Cobbe SM, Parker DJ, Poole-Wilsn PA (1982) Tissue and coronary venous pH in ischaemic canine myocardium. *Clin Cardiol* 5:153–156

22. Poole-Wilson PA, Seabrooke SR (1985) Relationship between intracellular pH and contractility in guinea-pig papillary muscles. *J Physiol* 365:63P

23. Donaldson RM, Taggart P, Bennett JG, Rickards AF (1984) Study of electrophysiological ischaemic events during coronary angioplasty. *Texas H Inst J* 11:24–30

24. Serruys PW, Wijns W, van den Brand M, Meij S, Slager C, Schuurbiers JCH, Hugenholzts PG, Brower RW (1984) Left ventricular performance, regional blood flow, wall motion and lactate metabolism during transluminal angioplasty. *Circulation* 70(1):25–36

25. Poole-Wilson PA, Langer GA (1975) Effect of pH on ionic exchange and function in rat and rabbit myocardium. *Am J Physiol* 229:570–581

26. Noma A (1983) ATP – regulated K+ channels in cardiac muscle. *Nature* 305:147–148

27. Weiss J, Shine KI (1986) Effects of heart rate on extracellular [K+] accumulation during myocardial ischaemia. *Am J Phys* 250:H982–991

28. Crake T, Kirby MS, Poole-Wilsn PA (1987) Potassium efflux from the myocardium during hypoxia: role of lactate ions. *Cardiov Res* 21:886–891

29. Weiss J, Shine KI (1981) Extracellular potassium accumulation during myocardial ischemia: implications for arrhythmogenesis. *J Mol Cell Cardiol* 13:699–704

9. Myocardial release of hypoxanthine and lactate during coronary angioplasty

A quickly reversibe phenomenon, but for how long?

PATRICK W. SERRUYS, FEDERICO PISCIONE, WILLIAM WIJNS, JOHAN A.J. HEGGE, EEF HARMSEN, MARCEL VAN DEN BRAND, PIM DE FEYTER, PAUL G. HUGENHOLTZ and JAN W. DE JONG

Introduction

Until recently the assessment of alteration in myocardial metabolism in man early after an abrupt occlusion of a major coronary artery has not been feasible. Percutaneous transluminal coronary angioplasty (PTCA), however, now provides a unique opportunity to study the time course of these metabolic changes during the transient interruption of coronary flow by the balloon occlusion sequence in patients with single-vessel disease and without angiographically demonstrable collateral circulation [1, 2]. The need to detect any persisting metabolic or mechanical dysfunction becomes of even greater concern as the number of dilated vessels and the duration of balloon inflation tend to increase, thereby enhancing both the extent and the severity of ischemia. The risk exists that the damage induced by the intervention may exceed its benefit.

During and after ischemia, there is in the heart, as well as in other muscles, excessive ATP breakdown. This degradation of ATP causes an efflux of breakdown products, which are able to pass through the cell membrane into the blood before significant amounts of enzymes appear. The purine derivatives adenosine, inosine and hypoxanthine are therefore thought to be early markers for ischemia [3]. Because of high activities of adenosine deaminase an nucleoside phosphorylase and low amounts of xanthine oxidase in the heart and blood, hypoxanthine seems most promising as early marker for myocardial ischemia [4].

Recently high pressure liquid chromatography (HPLC) came into use for the determination of nucleosides and purine bases in the whole blood [5, 6], facilitating the determination of purine derivatives, in particular hypoxanthine. This new technical development prompted us to investigate the myocardial release of hypoxanthine during coronary angioplasty.

In a group of 28 patients blood flow, lactate and hypoxanthine metabolism were analyzed during reactive hyperemia after repeated occlusions of the left anterior descending coronary artery, the effects of ischemia proved quickly reversible, but were indicative of impending cellular dysfunction.

P.W. Serruys, R. Simon & K.J. Beatt (eds), Percutaneous Transluminal Coronary Angioplasty. ISBN 0-7923-0346-6.
© *1990 Kluwer Academic Publishers, Dordrecht*

Patients and methods

All patients met the following criteria: a brief history of angina pectoris (less than one year), an isolated obstructive lesion in one coronary vessel (the left anterior descending) and an accessible stenosis of less than 1 cm in length. All patients were candidates for coronary artery bypass graft surgery because of disabling angina, but were selected for angioplasty rather than surgery because of their anatomy.

Twenty-eight patients were studied: 21 men, 7 women, aged from 38 to 74 years. Of these 16 were in NYHA class II, 8 in class III, and 4 in class IV. In all the ejection fraction was greater than 50%. These twenty eight patients were selected from fifty eight patients in whom thermodilution coronary sinus blood flow was measured during angioplasty for various indications. They were chosen since they required at least four transluminal dilatations. These four dilatations were performed with a total duration of occlusion of 192 ± 40 s (mean $\pm$ SD). All patients in this study gave their informed consent and there were no complications directly related to the research procedure.

PTCA technique

Percutaneous transluminal coronary angioplasty (PTCA) was performed by the same technique in all patients. Via a 9F, 16 cm introducing sheath, a guiding catheter was directed into the stenotic area under fluoroscopic and pressure control. PTCA was performed according to the technique of Gruentzig, with the equipment of Schneider, via the femoral route. In all cases the pressure gradient across the obstructive lesion was recorded before, during and after balloon inflation. The dilatation catheters were either the 20–30 or 20–37 models. The inflation pressure ranged from 2–12 atmospheres, while individual dilatations ranged from 40 to 60 s. Attempts to dilate the lesion were repeated as long as the gradient persisted. Coronary angiography with non ionic contrast medium (metrizamide) was performed immediately before and after PTCA. Lateral, anteroposterior, oblique and hemi-axial angiographic views were obtained in virtually all patients.

Premedication consisted of aspirin, nifedipine and/or isosorbide dinitrate. All patients received either 3 mg of isosorbide dinitrate or 0.2 mg nifedipine selectively into the left main coronary artery during control coronary arteriography, but the coronary flow measurements we report were not carried out within the periods of the drug's effect on the coronary circulation. Beta-blockers were not discontinued. During the procedure, heparin and low molecular weight dextran were administered intravenously.

Lactate measurements

Blood (1.5 ml) for lactate measurements was rapidly deproteinized with an equal volume of cold 8% perchloric acid ($HClO_4$) and centrifuged. After centrifugation, the supernatant fluids were stored at $-20°C$. Lactate in the supernatant was analyzed enzymatically according to Apstein et al [7] with the AutoAnalyzer.* Standard curves were made with lithium lactate in 4% $HClO_4$.

Hypoxanthine determination

An isocratic high pressure liquid chromatographic system was used for the estimation of purine nucleosides and oxypurines in blood [6]. Use was made of a reversed-phase column. Since nucleotides derived from erythrocytes affected the separation, these compounds had to be removed. We used the method of Chatterjee et al [8], with some minor differences. We applied 1.5 ml of the deproteinized, neutralized blood sample onto a pre-washed column of Al_2O_3 (0.6 g) in a Pasteur pipette, and eluted it with 5.0 ml 10 mmol/l Tris/HCL, pH 7.4. For faster elution, a vacuum was applied to a sampling manifold. Twelve samples were treated at the same time.

A Waters M 6000 high pressure liquid chromatography** was employed with a WISP 710 B autosampler** a Model 440 UV-detector fixed at 254 hm wavelength connected to a BD 41 recorder. A 4 mm I.D. $\times$ 30 cm prepacked Bondapak/C_{18} column***, particle size 10 m was used in these studies. Chromatographic conditions were adapted from earlier work [9]: 200 µl samples were eluted from this column with 10 mmol/l $NH_4H_2PO_4/CH_3OH$ (10:1, v/v), pH 5.50. The flow rate was 60 ml/h (Fig. 1).

Blood samples were obtained at six consecutive measurement periods: before the PTCA procedure, 5–10 s after each transluminal occlusion, 5 min after termination of the PTCA procedure. Five minutes were allowed between each dilatation for recovery.

Flow measurements

A thermodilution coronary sinus blood flow catheter (Webster) was introduced into the coronary sinus by way of a right brachial vein. In 15 cases, the catheter tip was placed in the great cardiac vein. Coronary sinus blood flow (13 patients, group I) or great cardiac vein blood flow (15 patients, group II) was measured by the continuous thermodilution method before and after the PTCA procedure as well as during each transluminal occlusion. In the beginning of the investigation the location of the external thermistor, in the coronary sinus or in the great cardiac vein, was verified by injection of 3 ml contrast material. Each recording of blood flow during coronary angioplasty began before balloon inflation and was interrupted at the moment of balloon deflation.

Coronary vascular resistance (CVR) was calculated for great cardiac vein

---

*Technicon, Tarrytown, NY, USA.
**Millipore Waters, Bedford, Mass, USA.
***Kipp en Zonen, Delft, The Netherlands.

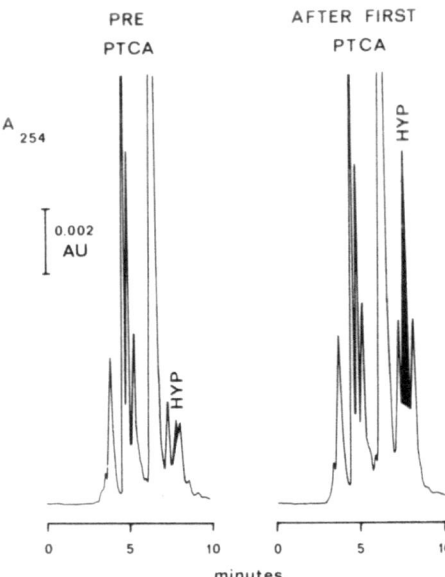

Figure 1. Isocratic high pressure liquid chromatographic separation of nucleosides and purine basis from a patient before and after a single transluminal occlusion.
Abbreviations: hyp = hypoxanthine.

(GCV) or coronary sinus (CS) [10] using the mean arterial pressure (MAP) and blood flow in the great cardiac vein (Flow (GCV)) and coronary sinus (Flow (CS)), respectively:

$$CVR\ (GCV) = MAP/Flow\ (GCV)\ (mmHg\ min/ml)$$
$$CVR\ (CS) = MAP/(Flow(CS))\ (mmHg\ min/ml).$$

Statistical analysis

Results are expressed as mean ± standard error of the mean. Comparison between pre-PTCA, post-PTCA and occlusion conditions were evaluated using analysis of variance for repeated measurements. When overall significance was found, multiple comparisons were significantly different at the 0.05 level.

Results

Coronary hemodynamic measurements

The results of the coronary hemodynamic observations are summarized in Fig. 2 and Tables 1 and 2. During initial dilatation the mean duration of balloon

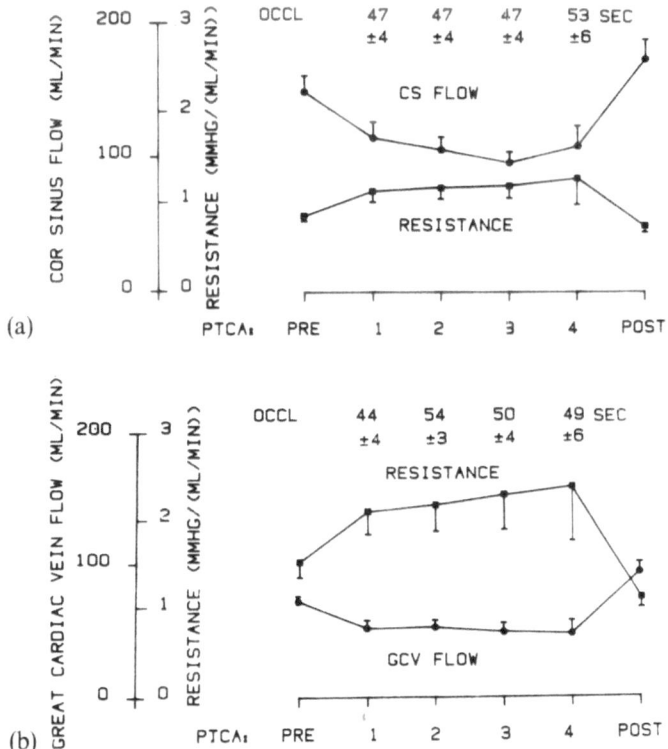

Figure 2a. (top) Changes in coronary sinus blood flow and resistance during four episodes of occlusion.
Abbreviation: CS = coronary sinus.
Figure 2b. Changes in great cardiac vein flow (ml/min) and resistance (mmHg/ml/min) during four transluminal occlusions.
Abbreviations: OCCL = occlusion time (s); GCV = great cardiac vein.

inflation was 47 ± 4 s in group I and 44 ± 4 s in group II. During the subsequent dilatations the duration of inflation was slightly increased up to 53 ± 6 s and 49 ± 6 s. Occlusion pressure did not change throughout these occlusion times of 40 to 60 s and there was a high degree of reproducibility of the occlusion pressure during these successive occlusions (Tables 1 and 2). Coronary sinus blood flow before the first dilatation was 149 ± 12 ml/min, falling to 96 ± 8 ml/min ($p < 0.005$) during the third transluminal occlusions and rising to 174 ± 15 ml/min (NS) 5 min after the last balloon deflation (Table 1). Consequently, total coronary resistance increased from 0.75 ± 0.06 to 1.2 ± 0.3 mm Hg/ml/min ($p < 0.05$) by the end of the fourth dilatation (Table 1).

The mean blood flow in the great cardiac vein in group II before the first inflation was 72 ± 4 ml/min, falling to 47 ± 10 ml/min ($p < 0.003$) during the fourth

Table 1. Coronary hemodynamics and metabolic disturbances during sequential transluminal occlusion in group I (13 patients).

	Before PTCA	First occlusion
Duration of occlusion (s)	—	47 ± 4*
Occlusion pressure (mmHg)	—	31 ± 5
CS flow (ml/min)	149 ± 12	115 ± 12[b]
Resistance (mmHg/ml/min)	0.75 ± 0.06	1.03 ± 0.12[a]
Arterial lactate (mM)	0.43 ± 0.09	0.46 ± 0.08
CS venous lactate (mM)	0.47 ± 0.10	0.81 ± 0.16[a]
Art-CS lactate (mM)	$+0.04 \pm 0.04$	-0.39 ± 0.14[a]
Arterial hypoxanthine (μM)	1.81 ± 0.5	$+2.5 \pm 1.1$
CS venous hypoxanthine (μM)	2.2 ± 0.6	4.6 ± 1.4[a]
Art-CS hypoxanthine (μM)	$+0.4 \pm 0.2$	-2.04 ± 1.3

CS = coronary sinus; Art = arterial.
*Mean $\pm$ SEM
[a]$p < 0.05$;   [b]$p < 0.005$ versus before PTCA

Table 2. Coronary hemodynamics and metabolic disturbances during sequential transluminal occlusion in group II (15 patients).

	Before PTCA	First occlusion
Duration of occlusion (s)	—	44 ± 4*
Occlusion pressure (mmHg)	—	24 ± 4
GCV flow (ml/min)	72 ± 4	51 ± 6[a]
Resistance (mmHg/ml/min)	1.42 ± 0.18	2.0 ± 0.3[a]
Arterial lactate (mM)	0.59 ± 0.12	0.67 ± 0.16
GCV lactate (mM)	0.75 ± 0.15	1.8 ± 0.4[b]
Art GCV lactate (mM)	$+0.18 \pm 0.06$	-1.1 ± 0.3[a]
Arterial hypoxanthine (μM)	3.0 ± 0.06	3.0 ± 0.7
GCV hypoxanthine (μM)	3.4 ± 0.7	5.2 ± 0.8[c]
Art-GCV hypoxanthine (μM)	$+0.3 \pm 0.3$	-2.2 ± 0.7[a]

GCV = great cardiac vein; Art = arterial.
*Mean $\pm$ SEM
[a]$p < 0.05$;   [b]$p < 0.005$;   [c]$p < 0.001$ versus before PTCA

inflation and rising slightly to 93 ± 8 ml/min ($p < 0.03$) after completion of the PTCA procedure (Table 2) while the differences in resting pre and post coronary angioplasty levels of coronary sinus blood flow did not reach a statistically significant level. Great cardiac vein coronary vascular resistance was 1.42 ± 0.18 mm Hg min/ml before balloon inflation, 2.3 ± 0.6 by the end of the fourth inflation ($p < 0.005$) and 1.02 ± 0.11 after completion of the PTCA procedure (Table 2).

Lactate and hypoxanthine metabolism

The arteriovenous lactate measurements are listed in Tables 1 and 2 and shown in Fig. 3. In group II the control measurements showed a difference of $+0.18$ mM,

Second occlusion	Third occlusion	Fourth occlusion	After PTCA
47 ± 4	47 ± 4	53 ± 6	—
28 ± 5	29 ± 3	30 ± 5	
106 ± 9[b]	96 ± 8[b]	108 ± 15[a]	174 ± 15
1.07 ± 0.13[a]	1.09 ± 0.14[a]	1.2 ± 0.3[a]	0.64 ± 0.07
0.47 ± 0.09	0.43 ± 0.06	0.42 ± 0.06	0.42 ± 0.12
0.88 ± 0.19[b]	0.75 ± 0.14[b]	0.79 ± 0.14[a]	0.46 ± 0.07
−0.41 ± 0.14[a]	−0.32 ± 0.08[b]	−0.37 ± 0.10[b]	+0.01 ± 0.07
1.9 ± 0.06	1.3 ± 0.4	1.6 ± 0.5	1.6 ± 0.5
3.0 ± 0.3	2.9 ± 0.9	2.5 ± 0.5	1.9 ± 0.3
−0.9 ± 0.5	−1.7 ± 1.0	−0.9 ± 0.6	+0.1 ± 0.4

Second occlusion	Third occlusion	Fourth occlusion	After PTCA
54 ± 3	50 ± 4	49 ± 6	—
23 ± 3	21 ± 2	25 ± 5	
52 ± 6[a]	48 ± 7[b]	47 ± 10[b]	93 ± 8[a]
2.1 ± 0.3[a]	2.2 ± 0.4[b]	2.3 ± 0.6[b]	1.02 ± 0.11
0.65 ± 0.12	0.71 ± 0.14	0.9 ± 0.3	0.58 ± 0.13
1.6 ± 0.3[c]	1.3 ± 0.3[b]	1.8 ± 0.6[a]	0.64 ± 0.12
−0.91 ± 0.18[c]	−0.60 ± 0.17[b]	−0.8 ± 0.4[b]	+0.07 ± 0.03
3.3 ± 0.6	2.9 ± 0.8	3.0 ± 1.4	3.7 ± 0.7
7.8 ± 1.4[b]	4.2 ± 1.06	4.4 ± 1.2[a]	3.8 ± 0.7
−4.52 ± 1.4[b]	−1.4 ± 0.7	−1.5 ± 0.4	+0.2 ± 0.44

which decreased to −1.1 and −0.91 mM, after the first and the second dilatations, respectively. After the third dilatation the lactate difference was −0.60 mM, which was not significantly different from the values recorded after the first and the second dilatation. As a first approximation, the amount of lactate lost from the ischemic tissue during the four consecutive occlusions seems to be more or less constant and at least did not increase with the time. As expected, the pooled A-V lactate difference obtained during PTCA in group II (great cardiac vein, −0.8 ± 0.3 mM sampling) was higher than that in group I (coronary sinus sampling, −0.35 ± 0.12 mM/l, (p < 0.01). During the four consecutive transluminal occlusions, an average rise in the great cardiac vein hypoxanthine from 3.4 ± 0.7 to 5.6 ± 1.1 M, (p < 0.01) and in coronary sinus hypoxanthine from 2.2 ± 0.6 m/l to 3.6 ± 0.8 μM, (p < 0.05) was observed, which fell off after comple-

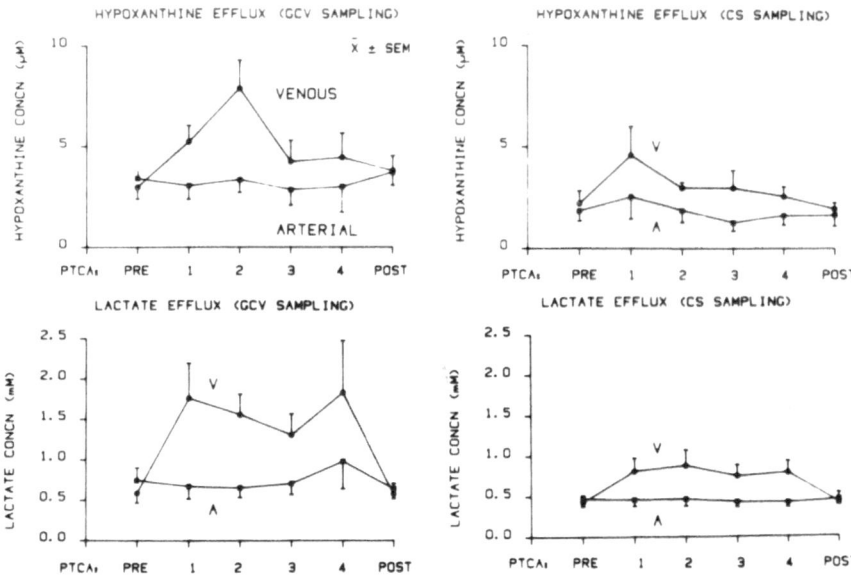

Figure 3. Changes in arterial and venous concentration of hypoxanthine and lactate during transluminal occlusion.

Abbreviations: GCV = great cardiac vein; CS = coronary sinus; PRE = pre angioplasty; POST = post angioplasty.

tion of the PTCA procedure. The arterial levels of these compounds remained constant during transluminal occlusion. The myocardial arterial-GCV difference of hypoxanthine changed from $+0.3 \pm 0.3\,\mu M$ before angioplasty at rest to $-2.4 \pm 1.2\,\mu M$ ($p < 0.001$) during sequential transluminal occlusions and was significantly larger than the changes observed in the myocardial arterial-CS difference (Table 1). Significant production of hypoxanthine, calculated either as arterial-venous difference or extraction, only took place during transluminal occlusion while hypoxanthine release was absent 5 min after completion of the PTCA procedure.

The crucial conclusion to be drawn from the observation that a few minutes after termination of the procedure no significant amount of lactate and hypoxanthine are produced is that metabolic disturbances induced by repeated ischemia are quickly reversible.

Discussion

Use of purine release as a marker for ischemia during transluminal occlusion in man

Ischemia can be defined as a situation, where coronary blood flow (and hence oxygen and substrate supply, and carbon dioxide and metabolite removal) cannot meet the tissue demand [11]. As a consequence of this O_2 deficiency, mitochondrial function is restricted [12] and the balance between ATP production and usage is disturbed, creatine phosphate (CrP) levels fall, followed by a decline in ATP [3, 13]. Creatine (Cr), ADP, phosphate and H^+ levels increase [14–16], glycolysis rate is enhanced [17, 18] and lactate levels rise. Shortly thereafter K^+, H^+ and lactate are released into the coronary venous blood. The anaerobic ATP production, however, is insufficient to meet the amount of ATP needed for contraction [15]. This is directly responsible for the decrease in local segmental wall function [19, 20] which is in turn reflected by a loss of systolic wall thickening [20] and shortening [21].

If sufficiently widespread, global hemodynamic measurements will demonstrate a decrease in contractility as reflected by a decrease in LV ejection fraction, and in the maximal velocity of the contractile element (V max) as well as an increase in regional myocardial stiffness with a reduction in LV distensibility, which manifests itself by an increase in end-diastolic pressure [1, 22]. This series of events was repeatedly observed in our patients during transluminal angioplasty.

Whether the fall in contractility is caused by a fall in ATP [15], an increase of H^+ [18, 23, 24] or a decrease in the phosphate potential $(=(ATP)/(ADP)(PI)$ [25] is known at the moment. One of the problems hampering this type of investigation relates to the compartmentalization of ATP and the interdependence of several parameters. For example, a fall in ATP or CrP would cause a decrease in phosphate potential and an increase of H^+, therefore rendering the interpretation difficult. When ATP levels decrease, cellular ADP levels increase. ATP is converted to ADP and AMP, by the action of adenylate kinase. AMP is deaminated to IMP, or dephosphorylated to adenosine, which is further catabolized to inosine and hypoxanthine (Fig. 4). These components pass the cell membrane [19, 26–28] where adenosine acts as a vasodilator [28, 29]. A slight decrease of ATP therefore results in an immediate rise in AMP-catabolites. This release can be used to monitor myocardial ATP-breakdown.

We felt therefore that measuring myocardial arterial-venous differences of blood hypoxanthine levels could give insight into the metabolic state of the heart; the method used here makes it possible to measure a number of purine metabolites in blood. In fact, since the 1960's, several studies have discussed the release of purine components during ischemia or anoxia (Table 3). A close correlation has been found between purine- and lactate release from animal and human hearts [6, 30–37]. Lactate as a marker of ischemia, however, has several disadvantages. During normoxia, lactate is preferentially taken up by the heart [38]. In fact, lactate released from a local ischemic area can be metabolized by the surrounding normoxic tissue [17]. The formation and removal of lactate is also influenced by blood fatty acid levels, acidosis and by a hyperglycemia [39], all metabolic conditions likely to be present during angioplasty. In addition, observations on the patients undergoing an atrial pacing stress test indicate that hypoxanthine is a more sensitive parameter for myocardial ischemia than adenosine, inosine, xanthine or lactate, because hypoxanthine release is more pronounced and of a longer duration than that of the other compounds [6].

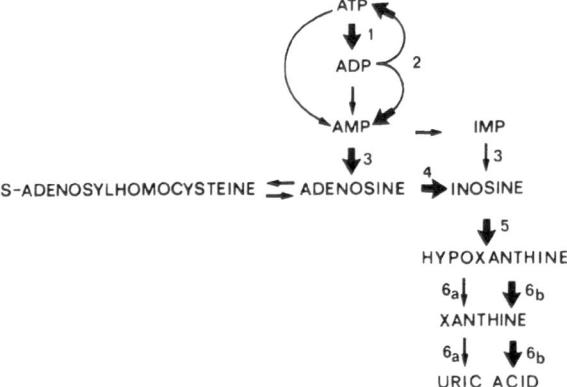

Figure 4.   Myocardial ATP catabolism. The main pathways are:
1) ATPase;   2) adenylate kinase;   3) 5′-nucleotidase;   4) adenosine deaminase;   5) nucleoside phosphorylase;   6) xanthine oxidase (a)/dehydrogenase (b).

In our patients, blood samples were obtained 5 to 10s after the start of deflation. Coronary sinus K^+ concentration has been measured continuously in patients undergoing angioplasty of significant stenoses of their left anterior descending coronary arteries [40]. The recordings obtained from these patients showed that, although coronary sinus K^+ levels did not change significantly

Table 3.   AMP-catabolites in blood as marker for myocardial ischemia in patients.

Purine	Body fluid	Clinical situation	Ref.
Adenosine	A-CS plasma	APST	30
Adenosine Inosine Hypoxanthine	A-CS plasma	CABS	30
Hypoxanthine	A-CS blood	APST	4, 6
Inosine Hypoxanthine	A-CS plasma	APST	31, 32, 33
Adenosine Inosine Hypoxanthine Xanthine	A blood	CABS	34
Hypoxanthine	A-CS blood	2 × APST	35
Adenosine Hypoxanthine	A-CS blood	APST	36
Hypoxanthine	A blood	AS	37

A = arterial; CS = coronary sinus; APST = atrial pacing stress test; CABS = coronary-aorta bypass surgery; AS = aortic surgery.

during coronary occlusion, a transient rise occurred when the occlusion was removed. After reducing pressure in the balloon, the coronary sinus K^+ levels began to rise within 8 sec. This fits exactly with the timing of peak reactive hyperemia observed by ourselves and by Rothman et al [41] and corresponds with the timing of blood withdrawal in this study. Since we could not record the great cardiac vein or coronary sinus flow during the sampling period, we did not express our results in terms of lactate or hypoxanthine efflux. The less elevated concentrations of lactate and hypoxanthine in the great cardiac vein after the third sequential occlusion do not necessarily reflect a reduction in lactate or hypoxanthine production since the reactive hyperemia measured after the third occlusion might have been significantly greater than that measured after the first and second occlusions [1, 41].

As observed by Rothman et al [41] and ourselves [1], more pronounced reactive hyperemia developed when the residual functional coronary stenosis associated with the deflated PTCA balloon was reduced by subsequent dilatation. In a previous study we demonstrated that the mean hyperemic increase in great cardiac vein flow was 55% after the first dilatation and 91% after the third dilatation [1]. Therefore and as a first approximation, the amount of lactate and hypoxanthine lost from the ischemic tissue during the first two occlusions seems to be more or less constant and at least does not increase with sequential occlusions.

Previous work [42, 43] indicates that repetitive episodes of brief ischemia do not produce a cumulative depletion of high energy phosphate compounds. The content of nucleotide pools at any point in time is determined by the rate of synthesis versus demand. The failure to demonstrate a progressive decrease in nucleotide pools during subsequent ischemic episodes following an initial ischemic episode might be explained by a decreased degradation of nucleotides during the subsequent ischemic episodes. Decreased degradation without increased synthesis is supported by the finding of the current study that the efflux of nucleotide catabolite (such as hypoxanthine) during reperfusion after the third or the fourth occlusion was less or at least not significantly different from the values obtained after the first or the second coronary occlusion.

The mechanism for the putative decrease in coronary nucleotide degradation during subsequent episodes of ischemia is unclear, but several explanations can be proposed to account for this finding. There is growing evidence for compartmentation of myocardial nucleotide pools [44, 45]. The different compartments in the cell may have different susceptibilities to depletion during myocardial ischemia. Susceptible pools may be depleted during the first ischemic episode, with more resistant pools remaining intact during subsequent ischemic episodes of the same duration. Another factor which may have contributed to the reduction in nucleotide degradation during the second and third occlusion is the greater than normal creatine phosphate content of myocardium following a brief ischemic episode [46, 47].

Whatever the mechanism, the increased creatine phosphate stores presumably present at the onset of the second and third coronary occlusion may provide high energy phosphate which serve to protect ATP pools from further depletion. A third potential explanation for decreased nucleotide degradation during the ischemic period is decreased energy consumption from decreased contractile function. However, from our previous hemodynamic studies, it seems unlikely that more rapid contractile failure may account for the preservation of nucleotide pools observed during the third and fourth occlusion. Other hemodynamic factors have to be considered.

Rentrop et al [48] have demonstrated during balloon inflation the angiographic appearance of a previously absent coronary collateral circulation. This apparent recruitment of collaterals might play a major role in the modulation of the ischemic and metabolic phenomenon related to the angioplasty procedure, although its functional significance is not yet well defined. It has been shown that the occlusion pressure measured distally to the stenosis, during balloon inflation, correlates with the existence of a collateral circulation angiographically demonstrable before or during angioplasty [49, 50]. However, Probst et al [49], Meier et al [50] and ourselves did not observe any change in the coronary occlusion pressure during serial occlusions. In fact, our results confirm their observations. The absence of any increase in coronary sinus and great cardiac vein flow during serial occlusions precludes the gradual recruitment of collateral circulation during repeated occlusions which might have explained a progressive decrease in lactate and hypoxanthine efflux.

Metabolism during reperfusion

The crucial conclusion to be drawn from our observations is that metabolic disturbances induced by repeated ischemia are quickly reversible, provided they are of short (<90 s) durations. During reperfusion, cells are reoxygenated and waste products removed. After ischemia, for a short period of time, reperfusion induces an enhanced Ca^{2+} influx, mitochondria are reactivated and ATP and CrP are again produced [51, 52]. The latter compound is transported to the myofibrils. Because of ionogenic disturbances in the cell, contraction is still decreased at this stage probably due to disturbed Ca^{2+} concentrations in the cell [53]. This can be demonstrated by an increased ventricular wall tension [54, 55], indicating an increased Ca^{2+} level, and an increased CrP even to levels higher than the normal range [56–58]. This indicates that ATP consumption by contraction is at this state below ATP production. After activation of the ionic pumps, cellular homeostasis is restored and the cell starts beating again. However ATP levels will remain subnormal for some time, and these low ATP levels cause an extra risk in as much as a critically low ATP level will be reached earlier during the next ischemic attack [59, 60]. Recently we have demonstrated that complete coronary occlusion of the left anterior descending coronary artery in man is associated with profound alterations in diastolic chamber stiffness which persist well after restoration of myocardial blood flow and of a normal systolic function [61]. Recently it has also been demonstrated that, in isolated working rat hearts, the early restoration of oxidative metabolism during reperfusion, determines functional recovery of the reperfused ischemic myocardium despite the presence of low ATP levels [62]. Thus it seems that integrity of the pathways of oxidative metabolism rather than steady state ATP levels, plays a major role in the myocardial functional recovery after acute ischemia. Even so, the decline of high energy phosphate stores heralds the beginning of 'no return'. Therefore, further work is needed to document the time course of the recovery of a normal regional diastolic function, and address the responsible derangements of subcellular metabolism as the mechanisms of the observed abnormalities are not yet fully understood. Although recovery in terms of lactate and hypoxanthine metabolism is demonstrated the question must remain to what extent transport mechanisms and enzymatic reactions have been transiently altered.

Summary

The response of myocardial lactate and hypoxanthine metabolism during percutaneous transluminal coronary angioplasty (PTCA) was studied in a series of patients undergoing this procedure. A minimum of four balloon inflations was performed per patient with an average duration per occlusion of 49 ± 11 s (mean $\pm$ SD) for a total occlusion time of 192 ± 40 s.

Thermodilution coronary venous blood flow in the proximal coronary sinus or in the great cardiac vein was measured in 28 patients. Proximal coronary blood flow, measured in 13 patients was 149 ± 12 (mean $\pm$ SEM) ml/min in the basal condition, falling to 108 ± 15 ml/min ($p < 0.05$) during the last occlusion.

Flow measured in the great cardiac vein (15 patients) decreased from control values of 72 ± 4 ml/min (mean $\pm$ SEM) to 47 ± 10 ml/min with the fourth coronary occlusion ($p < 0.005$). Arteriovenous lactate and hypoxanthine showed peak differences during the reactive hyperemia following the first two occlusions which did not increase after subsequent occlusions. Within minutes after the procedure, lactate and hypoxanthine efflux was no longer seen, demonstrating the reversibility of the metabolic disturbances after repeated ischemia.

The results of this study indicate that there is no permanent alteration in lactate or hypoxanthine metabolism after PTCA with four coronary occlusions of 40 to 60 s, with a total occlusion time of 192 ± 40 s.

References

1. Serruys PW, Wijns W, van den Brand M et al (1984) Left ventricular performance, regional blood flow, wall motion and lactate metabolism during transluminal angioplasty. *Circulation* 70:25–36
2. Serruys PW, van den Brand M, Brower RW, Hugenholtz PG (1984) Left ventricular hemodynamics, regional blood flow and lactate metabolism during balloon occlusion: Can we alter the sequence of ischemic events? In: Rutishauser W, Roskam MW (eds) *Silent myocardial ischemia.* Berlin-Heidelberg-New York-Tokyo: Springer Verlag, 37–44

3. de Jong JW (1979) Biochemistry of acutely ischemic myocardium. Schaper W (ed) *The pathophysiology of myocardial perfusion*. Amsterdam: Elsevier/North-Holland Biomedical Press, 719–750

4. Remme WJ, de Jong JW, Verdouw PD (1979) Effect of pacing-induced myocardial ischemia on hypoxanthine efflux from the human heart. *Am J Cardiol* 40:55–62

5. Hartwick RA, Krstulovic AM, Brown PR (1979) Identification and quantitation of nucleosides, bases and other UV-absorbing compounds in serum, using reversed-phase high-performance liquid chromatography. II Evaluation of human sera. *J Chromatogr* 186:659–676

6. Harmsen E, de Jong JW, Serruys PW (1981) Hypoxanthine production by ischemic heart demonstrated by high pressure liquid chromatography of blood purine nucleosides and oxypurines. *Clin Chimica Acta* 115:73–84

7. Apstein CS, Puchner E, Brachfeld N (1979) Improved automated lactate determination. *Anal Biochem* 38:20–34

8. Chatterjee SK, Bhattacharya M, Barlow JJ (1979) A simple, specific radiometric assay for 5'-nucleotidase. *Anal Biochem* 95:497–506

9. de Jong JW, Keijzer E, Uitendaal MP, Harmsen E (1980) Further purification of adenosine kinase from rat heart using affinity and ion-exchange chromatography. *Anal Biochem* 101:407–412

10. Metha J, Pepine CJ (1978) Effect of sublingual nitroglycerin on regional flow in patients with and without coronary disease. *Circulation* 58:803–807

11. Manning AS, Hearse DJ, Dennis SC, Bullock GR, Coltard DJ (1980) Myocardial ischemia: an isolated, globally perfused rat heart model for metabolic and pharmacological studies. *Eur J Cardiol* 11:1–21

12. Wilson DF, Owens CS, Erecinska M (1979) Quantitative dependence of mitochondrial oxidative Aphosphorylation on oxygen concentration. A new mathematical model. *Arch Biochem Biophys* 195:494–504

13. Danforth WH, Naegle S, Bing RJ (1960) Effects of ischemia and reoxygenation on glycolytic reactions and adenosine triphosphate in heart muscle. *Circ Res* 8:965–971

14. Garlick BP, Radda GK, Seeley PJ (1979) Studies of acidosis in the ischemic heart by phosphorus nuclear magnetic resonance. *Biochem J* 184:547–554

15. Hearse DJ (1979) Oxygen deprivation and early myocardial contractile failure. Reassessment of the possible role of adenosine triphosphate. *Am J Cardiol* 44:1115–1120

16. Hearse DJ, Crome R, Yellon DM, Wyse R (1983) Metabolic and flow correlates of myocardial ischemia. *Cardiovasc Res* 17:452–458

17. Apstein CS, Deckelbaum L, Mueller M, Hagopian L, Hood WB (1977) Graded global ischemia and reperfusion. *Circulation* 55:864–872

18. Neely JR, Liedke AJ, Whitmer TJ, Rovetto MJ (1975) Relationship between coronary flow and adenosine triphosphate production from glycolysis and oxidative metabolism. *Recent Adv Studies Cardiac Structure Metab* 8:301–321

19. de Jong JW, Goldstein S (1974) Changes in coronary venous inosine concentration and myocardial wall thickening during regional ischemia in the pig. *Circ Res* 35:111–116

20. Das SK, Serruys PW, van den Brand M, Domenicucci S, Vletter WB, Roelandt J (1983) Acute echocardiographic changes during percutaneous coronary angioplasty and their relationship to coronary blood flow. *J Cardiovasc Ultrasonogr* 2:269–271

21. Jaski BE, Serruys PW (1985) Epicardial wall motion and left ventricular function during coronary graft angioplasty in humans. *J Am Coll Cardiol* 6:695–700

22. Serruys PW, Wijns W, Grimm J, Slager C, Hess OM (1984) Effects of repeated transluminal occlusions during angioplasty on global and regional left ventricular chamber stiffness (abstr). *Circulation* 70 (Suppl II):348

23. Bing OHL, Brooks WW, Nesser JV (1973) Heart muscle viability following hypoxia: protective effect of acidosis. *Science* 180:1297–1298

24. Dhalla NS, Das PK, Sharma GP (1978) Subcellular basis of cardiac contracture failure. *J Mol Cell Cardiol* 10:363–385

25. Kannegieser GJ, Lubbe WF, Opie LH (1975) Experimental myocardial infarction with left

ventricular failure in the isolated perfused rat heart. Effects of propranolol and pacing. *J Mol Cell Cardiol* 7:135–151

26. de Boer LWV, Ingwall JS, Kloner RA, Braunwald E (1980) Prolonged derangements of canine myocardial purine metabolism after brief coronary artery occlusion not associated with anatomic evidence of necrosis. *Proc Natl Acc Sci USA* 77:5471–5475

27. de Jong JW, Harmsen E, de Tombe PP, Keijzer E (1983) Release of purine nucleosides and oxypurines from the isolated perfused rat heart. *Adv Myocardiol* 4:339–345

28. Schrader J, Haddy FJ, Gerlach E (1979) Release of adenosine, inosine and hypoxanthine from the isolated guinea pig heart during hypoxia, flow-autoregulation and reactive hyperemia. *Pfugers Arch* 369:251–257

29. Berne RM (1980) The role of adenosine in the regulation of coronary blood flow. *Circ Res* 47:807–813

30. Fox AC, Reed GE, Mellman H, Silk BB (1979) Release of nucleosides from canine- and human hearts as an index of prior ischemia. *Am J Cardiol* 43:52–57

31. Kugler G (1978) The effects of nitroglycerin on myocardial release of inosine, hypoxanthine and lactate during pacing induced angina. *Basic Res Cardiol* 73:523–533

32. Kugler G (1979) Myocardial release of lactate, inosine and hypoxanthine during atrial pacing and exercise-induced angina. *Circulation* 59:43–49

33. Kugler G (1979) Myocardial release of inosine, hypoxanthine and lactate during pacing-induced angina in humans with coronary artery disease. *Eur J Cardiol* 9:227–240

34. Brower RW, de Jong JW, Haalebos M et al (1982) Evaluation of cardioplegia in coronary artery bypass graft surgery. In: Just H, Tschirkov A, Schlosser V (eds) *Kalziumantagonisten zur Kardioplegie und Myocardprotection in der offenen Herzchirurgie.* Stuttgart: Thieme, 69–80

35. Serruys PW, de Jong JW, Harmsen E, Verdouw PD, Hugenholtz PG (1983) Effect of intracoronary nifedipine in high-energy phosphate metabolism during repeated pacing-induced angina and during experimental ischemia. In: Kaltenbach M and Neufield HN (eds) *New therapy of ischemic heart disease and hypertension.* Amsterdam: Excerpta Medica, 340–353

36. Edlund A, Berglund B, van Dorne D et al (1985) Coronary flow regulation in patients with ischemic heart disease: release of purines and prostacyclin and the effect of inhibitors of prostaglandin formation. *Circulation* 6:1113–1120

37. Schoenberg MH, Fredholm BB, Hohlbach G (1985) Changes in acid-base status, lactate concentration and purine metabolics during reconstructive aortic surgery. *Acta Chir Scand* 151:227–233

38. Drake AJ, Haines JR, Noble MIM (1980) Preferential uptake of lactate by the normal myocardium in dogs. *Cardiovasc Res* 14:65–77

39. Verdouw PW, Stam H (1980) In: Moret PR et al (eds) *Lactate. Physiologic, methodologic and pathologic approach.* Springer Verlag, Berlin: 207–223

40. Webb SC, Rickards AF, Poole-Wilson PA (1983) Coronary sinus potassium concentration recorded during coronary angioplasty. *Br Heart J* 50:146–148

41. Rothman MT, Baim DS, Simpson JB, Harrison DC (1982) Coronary hemodynamics during percutaneous transluminal coronary angioplasty. *Am J Cardiol* 49:1615–1621

42. Swain JL, Sabina RL, Hines JJ, Greenfield Jr JC, Holmes EW (1984) Repetitive episodes of brief ischemia (12 min) do not produce a cumulative depletion of high energy phosphate compounds. *Cardiovasc Res* 18:264–269

43. Verdouw PD, Remme WJ, de Jong JW, Breeman WAP (1979) Myocardial substrate utilization and hemodynamics following repeated coronary flow reduction in pigs. *Basic Res Cardiol* 74:477–493

44 Gubdjarnason S, Mathes P, Ravens KG (1970) Functional compartmentation of ATP and creatine phosphates in heart muscle. *J Mol Cell Card* 1:325–39

45. Schrader J, Gerlach E (1976) Compartmentation of cardiac adenine nucleotides and formation of adenosine. *Pflügers Archiv* 367:129–35

46. Swain JL, Sabina RL, McHale PA, Greenfield JC Jr, Holmes EW (1982) Prolonged myocardial nucleotide depletion after brief ischemia in the open-chest dog. *Am J Physiol* 242:H818–H826

47. Vial C, Font B, Goldschmidt D, Pearlman AS, Delaye J (1978) Regional myocardial energetics during brief periods of coronary occlusion and reperfusion: Comparison with S-T segment changes. *Cardiovasc Res* 12:470–476
48. Rentrop KP, Cohen M, Blanke H, Phillips RA (1985) Changes in collateral channel filling immediately after controlled coronary artery occlusion by an angioplasty balloon in human subjects. *J Am Coll Cardiol* 5:587–592
49. Probst P, Zangl W, Pachinger O (1985) Relation of coronary arterial occlusion pressure during percutaneous transluminal coronary angioplasty to presence of collaterals. *Am J Cardiol* 55:1264–1269
50. Meier B, Luethy P (1984) Coronary wedge pressure as predictor of recruitable collateral arteries. *Circulation* 70 (Suppl II): 266
51. Hearse DJ (1977) Reperfusion of the ischemic myocardium (editorial). *J Mol Cell Cardiol* 9: 605–616
52. Mittnacht S, Sherman C, Farber JL (1981) Reversal of ischemic mitochondrial dysfunction. *J Biol Chem* 256:3199–3206
53. Puri PS (1975) Contractile and biochemical effects of coronary reperfusion after extended periods of coronary occlusion. *Am J Cardiol* 36:244–251
54. Apstein CS, Deckelbaum L, Hagopian L, Hood WB (1978) Acute cardiac ischemia and reperfusion: contractility, relaxation and glycolysis. *Am J Physiol* 235:H637–H648
55. Lewis MJ, Honsmand PR, Claes VA, Brutsaert DL, Henderson AH (1980) Myocardial stiffness during hypoxia and reoxygenation contracture. *Cardiovasc Res* 14:339–344
56. Baily IA, Seymour AML, Radda GK (1981) A ^{31}P-NMR study of the effect of reflow on the ischaemic heart. *Biochim Biophys Acta* 637:1–7
57. Flaherty JT, Weisfeld ML, Buckley BH, Gardner TJ, Gott VT, Jacobus WE (1982) Mechanism of ischemic myocardial cell damage assessed by phosphorus-31 nuclear magnetic resonance. *Circulation* 65:561–576
58. Fossel ET, Morgan HE, Ingwall JS (1980) Measurements of changes in high energy phosphates in the cardiac cycle by using gated ^{31}P-nuclear magnetic resonance. *Proc Natl Acad Sci USA* 77:3654–3658
59. Braunwald E, Kloner RA (1982) The 'stunned' myocardium. *Circulation* 66:1146–1149
60. Geft IL, Fishbein MC, Ninomiya K et al (1982) Intermittent brief periods of ischemia have a cumulative effect and may cause myocardial necrosis. *Circulation* 66:1150–1153
61. Serruys PW, Wijns W, Grimm J, Slager C, Hess OM (1984) Effects of repeated transluminal occlusion during angioplasty on global and regional left ventricular chamber stiffness. *Circulation* 70 (Suppl II):348
62. Taegtmeyer H, Roberts AFC, Raine AEG (1985) Emergency metabolism in reperfused heart muscle: metabolic correlates to return of function. *J Am Coll Cardiol* 6:864–870

10. Myocardial release of hypoxanthine and urate during angioplasty

Potential mechanism for free radical generation

JAN WILLEM DE JONG, TOM HUIZER, J. ARLY NELSON,
WLODZIMIERZ CZARNECKI, JOHANNES J.R.M. BONNIER and
PATRICK W. SERRUYS

Oxygen free radicals have been implicated in ageing, oncogenesis and athero-genesis [1]. One potential source is xanthine oxidase, the oxyradical-producing form of xanthine oxidoreductase. This enzyme catabolizes the high-energy-phosphate metabolites hypoxanthine and xanthine to urate (Fig. 1). Ischemia converts the native form of the enzyme, xanthine reductase, to xanthine oxidase [2]. During reperfusion oxygen is available for the production of superoxide and hydroxyl radicals [3, 4], both of which are strongly suspected to cause tissue damage [3, 5–7]. Xanthine oxidoreductase activity is present in the myocardium of a number of species [8], but its presence in human heart is controversial. In autopsy material several authors measured high xanthine oxidoreductase activity [9, 10]. Using histochemical techniques, Jarasch and coworkers found large amounts of the enzyme in human heart endothelium [11]. On the other hand, several authors reported very low to undetectable xanthine oxidoreductase activity in human heart [12–14]. We present evidence that the heart of (a number

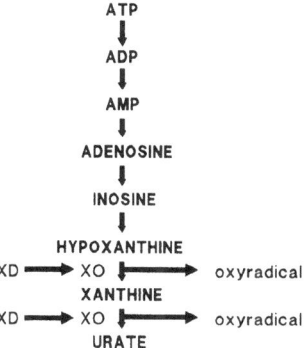

Figure 1. Catabolism of ATP, and conversion of xanthine dehydrogenase (XD) to xanthine oxidase (XO), during ischemia. XD uses NAD^+ as the electron acceptor. After conversion to XO, the enzyme uses molecular oxygen. The hydrogen peroxide produced gives rise to superoxide and hydroxyl radical formation.

P.W. Serruys, R. Simon & K.J. Beatt (eds), Percutaneous Transluminal Coronary Angioplasty. ISBN 0-7923-0346-6.
© *1990 Kluwer Academic Publishers, Dordrecht*

of) cardiac patients produces significant amounts of urate. Thus xanthine oxidoreductase may be active in the human heart in vivo.

Methods

Patients

Initial observations on apparent urate production by the human heart were done in seven patients undergoing an atrial pacing stress test at the University of Alabama, Birmingham, Ala. (group 1 [15]) and in six patients undergoing diagnostic coronary angiography in the National Institute of Cardiology, Warsaw, Poland (group 2 [16]). Arterial and coronary sinus blood was collected and immediately deproteinized with perchloric acid. Urate was determined in the extract. In addition, urate concentrations were assayed in arterial and great cardiac venous blood plasma of ten patients, catheterized for angioplasty in the Thoraxcenter, Rotterdam, The Netherlands (group 3). Subsequently, a prospective study was done in 13 patients (Catharina Hospital, Eindhoven, The Netherlands), before, during and after angioplasty. Urate and hypoxanthine were measured in arterial and coronary sinus blood plasma of these patients (group 4).

Assays

For whole blood urate levels, 2-ml samples were mixed immediately after sampling with ice-cold perchloric acid. In group 1, 6.5 ml 6% $HClO_4$ (w/v), and in group 2, 2 ml of 8% $HClO_4$ (w/v) was used to obtain the deproteinized extract. In group 1, extracts were brought to pH 5 with KOH and stored at $-20°C$ until urate quantification, according to a uricase method [17] (enzyme provided by Sigma, St. Louis, MO). In some samples urate was also quantified by high-performance liquid chromatography (HPLC). Samples from group 2 were neutralized with 6 M KOH/2 M K_2CO_3. Nucleotides (from the erythrocytes) were removed from the extract by absorption on an Al_2O_3-column. Five ml 10 mM Tris-HCl was used to elute 1.5 ml sample through a column, containing 0.6 g Al_2O_3. Eluate was stored at $-15°C$ until analysis. HPLC-determination of urate took place on a μBondapak C_{18} column (Millipore-Waters, Milford, Mass). A 100-μl sample was eluted with 1% $K_2HPO_4 - 1\%$ CH_3OH, pH 4.7, at a flow rate of 1.0 ml/min. The column was guarded by a Perisorb RP-18 pre-column (Merck, Darmstadt, GFR). The Waters-HPLC equipment consisted of: WISP 710B cooled autosampler, Model 6000A pump, Model 490 multi wavelength detector, and Model 840 computer. Peaks were identified by retention times, internal standards, and enzyme shifts. The optimal wavelength for urate detection proved to be 295 nm since absorption is maximal and disturbance by other materials is minimal. Sample preparation and assay were derived from earlier work [18].

To prepare plasma, blood was mixed in a heparinized tube with an equal volume of ice-cold 154 mM NaCl, containing 20 μM dipyridamole (Boehringer, Ingelheim, GFR) and 10 μM erythro-9-(2-hydroxy-3-nonyl)adenine (Wellcome, London, UK). These drugs were used to inhibit adenosine uptake and breakdown [19, 20]. Plasma was prepared from patients in groups 3 and 4 and kept at −80°C. Deproteinization took place with an equal volume of 8% $HClO_4$ (w/v); the supernatant fraction was neutralized with 2 M KOH/1 M K_2CO_3. HPLC-determination of urate and hypoxanthine in deproteinized, neutralized plasma took place on a μBondapak C_{18} column. A 100-μl sample was eluted with a mixture of CH_3OH (100 ml) and KH_2PO_4 (10 g/l, 1000 ml), pH 5–7, at a flow rate of 0.6 ml/min. The column was protected by an LC-18 guard-column (Supelco Inc., Bellefonte, Penn.). Detection of hypoxanthine was done at 254 nm, that of urate at 295 nm (Fig. 2), with other conditions as described above. In 27 arterial and venous plasma samples of group 4, we also assayed urate spectro-

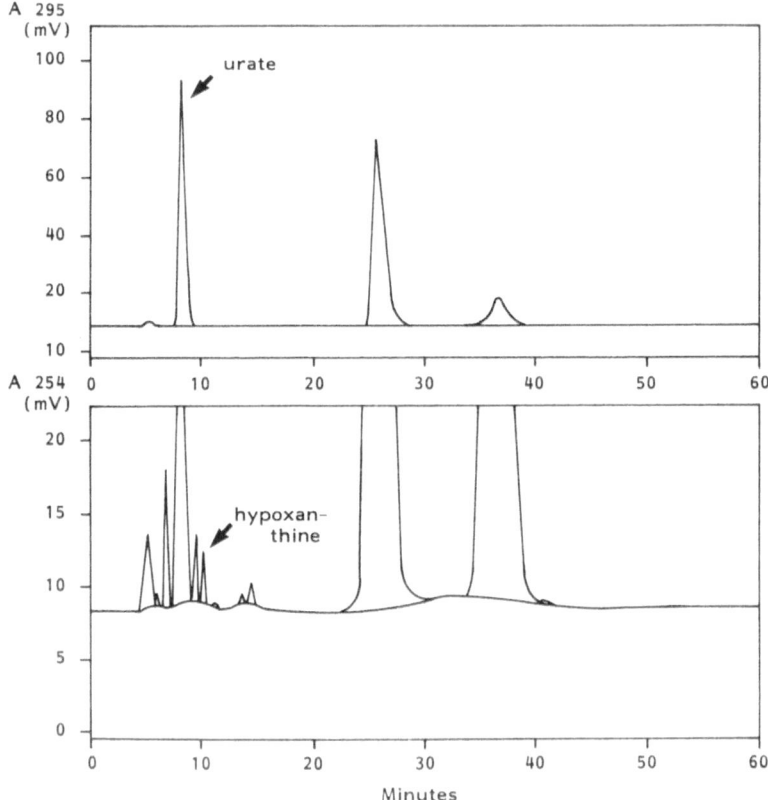

Figure 2. High-performance liquid chromatography of urate and hypoxanthine in human blood plasma. Detection took place at 295 and 254 nm, respectively. For other details, see Methods section.

photometrically with uricase [17]; enzyme was provided by Boehringer, Mannheim, GFR). The correlation coefficient between the two assay methods was 0.96. Statistical analysis was carried out with Student's t-test for paired variates, or, where appropriate, with two-way analysis of variance, considering a p-value smaller than 0.05 a significant difference.

Results

Table 1 shows that in patients with chest pain of unknown etiology, without any evidence of vessel occlusion (group 1) or with established ischemic heart disease (group 2), undergoing angiography, the urate levels in coronary sinus blood exceeded the arterial ones (p = 0.003 and p = 0.018, respectively). However, the urate levels were low in comparison to literature data [17]. We therefore also assayed the arterial and venous urate plasma concentrations in another group of patients (group 3). These catheterized patients had an isolated proximal left anterior descending artery (LAD) stenosis. All patients in this group were Canadian Cardiovascular Society grade III to IV. They were selected for percutaneous transluminal coronary angioplasty. Also in this group the arterial urate concentration was significantly lower than the coronary venous one (p = 0.028). From Fig. 3 it is clear that in all three groups, the hearts produced significant amounts of urate.

In a comparable patient population (group 4: one stenotic coronary artery, no collateral filling of the region perfused by the LAD), we measured plasma urate concentrations. They were comparable with those of group 3 (Table 2). The arterio-venous difference was relatively small and we were unable to demonstrate urate production *before* coronary angioplasty. *After* a third and fourth angioplasty attempt, urate production by the heart was statistically significant (Fig. 4; p = 0.009 and p = 0.018, respectively). Even after 15 min of recovery, urate production was still significant (p = 0.033). In this group of patients, we also measured the arterial and coronary venous plasma concentrations of hypoxanthine. This precursor of urate was produced by the heart during angioplasty (p < 0.001, Table 2). We failed to see a correlation between urate and hypoxanthine production.

Table 1.   Arterial and coronary venous urate levels.

Patient group	n	Arterial	Venous	p
		(nmol/ml)		
1	7	59 ± 20	120 ± 23	0.003
2	6	96 ± 15	145 ± 25	0.018
3	10	216 ± 17	243 ± 17	0.028

For description of patient groups, see Methods section. Extracts from arterial and coronary sinus blood were assayed in groups 1 and 2, from arterial and great cardiac venous plasma in group 3. Mean values are given ± SEM.

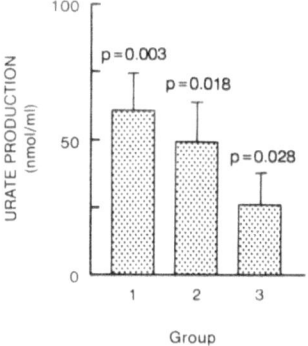

Figure 3. Significant urate production by human heart. Urate was measured in blood of catheterized patients with histories of chest pain (group 1, n = 7) and with established ischemic heart disease (group 2, n = 6). In addition, urate was assayed in plasma of patients with a proximal left anterior descending coronary artery stenosis (group 3, n = 10). Mean coronary venous-arterial differences are given with one SEM. For other details, see legend to Table 1.

Table 2. Arterial and coronary venous hypoxanthine and urate levels before, immediately after four dilations, and during recovery.

Angioplasty step	Hypoxanthine (nmol/ml)			Urate (nmol/ml)		
	Arterial	Venous	p	Arterial	Venous	p
Before	0.58 ± 0.07	0.42 ± 0.07	0.015	251 ± 18	259 ± 21	0.34
Dilation 1	0.37 ± 0.06	1.6 ± 0.4	0.013	248 ± 19	248 ± 22	0.96
Dilation 2	0.36 ± 0.07	1.3 ± 0.2	<0.001	250 ± 21	249 ± 21	0.87
Dilation 3	0.29 ± 0.06	1.18 ± 0.18	<0.001	242 ± 19	256 ± 21	0.009
Dilation 4	0.26 ± 0.06	1.10 ± 0.19	<0.001	232 ± 21	254 ± 23	0.018
Recovery	0.20 ± 0.05	0.38 ± 0.08	0.054	237 ± 20	244 ± 21	0.033

Mean values are given $\pm$ SEM (n = 11–13).

Discussion

Xanthine oxidoreductase activity is detectable in the heart of a number of species [8, 21]. In the heart of some species, e.g., pig [14, 22], it seems to be almost absent. Literature data on xanthine oxidase in human heart are conflicting. The reports vary from high [9–11] to (very) low [12–14, 23] levels. We want to emphasize that in these papers the number of samples assayed is often very small. Our data indicate that xanthine oxidoreductase could be active in the human heart in vivo. After angioplasty, the substrate (hypoxanthine) increases and the heart produces urate. A possible explanation for the discrepancies found in the studies mentioned above could be a difference in quality of the hearts examined. In the Polish study (group 2), the patients with hypokinetic myocardium or a history of subendocardial myocardial infarction produced the highest amounts of urate. Patients with

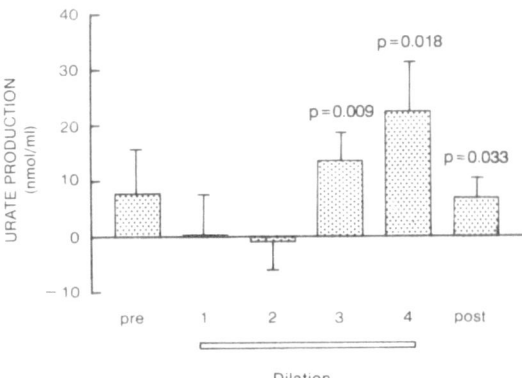

Figure 4.   Urate production by the hearts of 13 patients with single left anterior descending coronary artery stenosis, before coronary angioplasty (pre), after each balloon deflation (dilation 1 to 4) and after 15 min of recovery (post). Mean coronary sinus-arterial values are given with one SEM. Significant urate production was found immediately after the last two dilations, and during recovery.

normal myocardium or with extensive myocardial damage and abnormal left ventricular function produced much less urate. In group 1, the only two patients who experienced pain and released lactate during a pacing stress test also showed the highest urate production. The data suggest that the ischemic myocardium at risk of myocardial infarction produces urate. Eddy et al. [12] couldn't demonstrate xanthine oxidoreductase in human ventricular tissue, but supposedly their biopsies were not taken from ischemic heart. Muxfeldt and Schaper [14] found very low amounts of xanthine oxidoreductase in their two human heart samples. On the other hand, Wajner and Harkness [11] found relatively high xanthine oxidase/dehydrogenase activity in nine post-mortem specimens of human heart. Like in human heart, controversial reports exist on rabbit-heart xanthine oxidoreductase activity [8, 10, 21].

We have evidence that the relatively low urate concentrations in whole blood extracts (groups 1 and 2) are presumably due to the clean-up procedures. Nevertheless, in these studies the coronary sinus urate levels exceeded those in the artery (Table 1). When we prepared plasma (groups 3 and 4), we could use our HPLC-assay without Al_2O_3-chromatography (which removes erythrocytic nucleotides); we double-checked the values with an enzymological technique. The plasma urate levels were within the normal range. Patients with a proximal stenosis of the left anterior descending coronary artery produced again urate (group 3, Fig. 3). Only in patients with single-vessel stenosis (group 4), we were unable to see significant cardiac urate production at the beginning of the catheterization procedure. Urate production became obvious after percutaneous transluminal coronary angioplasty (Fig. 4). Presumably, this is due to cardiac ATP breakdown, with a concomitant rise in hypoxanthine as a result of myocardial ischemia due to coronary occlusion by balloon inflation (Table 2).

Hypoxanthine serves as a substrate for xanthine oxidoreductase. We conclude that the human heart seems to contain a relatively active xanthine oxidoreductase. We speculate that the enzyme generates oxyradicals after ischemia.

Acknowledgements

We greatly appreciate the technical assistance of Petra Noomen, Heleen van Loon, B.Sc., and Han Hegge, B.Sc., and the secretarial help of Ria Kanters-Stam. Dr W Rużyllo, Warsaw, provided blood of catheterized patients. In addition the nursing staff of the hospitals concerned gave valuable support.

References

1. Hearse DJ, Manning AS, Downey JM, Yellon DM (1986) Xanthine oxidase: a critical mediator of myocardial injury during ischemia and reperfusion? *Acta Physiol Scand* 548 (Suppl): 65–78.
2. McCord JM (1984) Are free radicals a major culprit? In: Hearse DJ, Yellon DM (eds) *Therapeutic Approaches to Myocardial Infarct Size Limitation*, pp. 209–218 New York: Raven Press
3. Chambers DE, Parks DA, Patterson G, Roy R, McCord JM, Yoshida S, Parmley LF, Downey JM (1985) Xanthine oxidase as a source of free radical damage in myocardial ischemia. *J Mol Cell Cardiol* 17:141–152
4. Van der Vusse GJ, Reneman RS (1985) Pharmacological intervention in acute myocardial ischemia and reperfusion. *Trends Pharmacol Sci* 6:76–79
5. England MD, Cavarocchi NC, O'Brien JF, Sollis V, Pluth JR, Orszulak TA, Kaye MP, Schaff HV (1986) Influence of antioxidants (mannitol and allopurinol) on oxygen free radical generation during and after cardiopulmonary bypass. *Circulation* 74 (Suppl 3): 134–137
6. Peterson DA, Asinger RW, Elsperger KJ, Homans DC, Eaton JW (1985) Reactive oxygen species may cause myocardial reperfusion injury. *Biochem Biophys Res Commun* 127:87–93
7. Zweier JL, Flaherty JT, Weisfeldt ML (1987) Direct measurement of free radical generation following reperfusion of ischemic myocardium. *Proc Natl Acad Sci USA* 84:1404–1407
8. Schoutsen B, De Jong JW (1987) Age-dependent increase in xanthine oxidoreductase differs in various heart cell types. *Circ Res* 61:604–607
9. Krenitsky TA, Tuttle JV, Cattau EL, Wang P (1974) A comparison of the distribution and electron acceptor specificities of xanthine oxidase and aldehyde oxidase. *Comp Biochem Physiol* 49B:687–703
10. Wajner M, Harkness RA (1988) Distribution of xanthine dehydrogenase and oxidase activities in human and rabbit tissues. *Biochem Soc Trans* 16:358–359
11. Jarasch ED, Bruder G, Heid HW (1986) Significance of xanthine oxidase in capillary endothelial cells. *Acta Physiol Scand* 548 (Suppl): 39–46
12. Eddy LJ, Stewart JR, Jones HP, Engerson TD, McCord JM, Downey JM (1987) Free radical-producing enzyme, xanthine oxidase, is undetectable in human hearts. *Am J Physiol* 253:H709–711
13. Ramboer CRH (1969) A sensitive and nonradioactive assay for serum and tissue xanthine oxidase. *J Lab Clin Med* 74:828–835
14. Muxfeldt M, Schaper W (1987) The activity of xanthine oxidase in hearts of pigs, guinea pigs, rats, and humans. *Basic Res Cardiol* 82:486–492
15. Nelson JA, McDaniel HG, Maurer BJ, Hill WA, James TN (1977) Apparent uptake of purines by the human heart (Letter to the ed). *N Eng J Med* 296:115
16. Czarnecki W (1988) Apparent inosine incorporation and concomitant haemodynamic improve-

ment in human heart. In: De Jong JW (ed) *Myocardial Energy Metabolism* pp. 257–264 Dordrecht: Martinus Nijhoff Publishers (DICM 91)

17. Scheibe B, Bernt E, Bergmeyer H-U (1974) Uric acid. In: Bergmeyer H-U (ed) *Methods of Enzymatic Analysis*, pp. 1951–1958 New York: Academic Press

18. Harmsen E, De Jong JW, Serruys PW (1981) Hypoxanthine production by ischemic heart demonstrated by high pressure liquid chromatography of blood purine nucleosides and oxypurines. *Clin Chim Acta* 115:73–84

19. Edlund A, Berglund B, Van Dorne D, Kaijser L, Nowak J, Patrono C, Sollevi A, Wennmalm A (1985) Coronary flow regulation in patients with ischemic heart disease: release of purines and prostacyclin and the effect of inhibitors of prostaglandin formation. *Circulation* 71:1113–1120

20. Ontyd J, Schrader J (1984) Measurement of adenosine, inosine and hypoxanthine in human plasma. *J Chromatogr* 307:404–409

21. Downey JM, Chambers DE, Miura T, Yellon DM, Jones D (1986) Allopurinol fails to limit infarct size in a xanthine oxidase deficient species (abstr). *Circulation* 74 (Suppl 2): 372

22. Podzuweit T, Braun W, Müller A, Schaper W (1986) Arrhythmias and infarction in the ischemic pig heart are not mediated by xanthine oxidase-derived free oxygen radicals (abstr). *Circulation* 74 (Suppl 2): 346

23. Watts RWE, Watts JEM, Seegmiller JE (1965) Xanthine oxidase activity in human tissues and its inhibition by allopurinol. *J Lab Clin Med* 66:688–697

11. Regional myocardial nitrogen-13-glutamate uptake following successful coronary angioplasty

HARALD TILLMANNS, RAINER ZIMMERMANN, WOLFRAM H. KNAPP, FRANTISEK HELUS, PETER GEORGI, BERNHARD RAUCH, FRANZ-JOSEF NEUMANN, SVEN GIRGENSOHN, WOLFGANG MAIER-BORST and WOLFGANG KÜBLER

N-13 labeled glutamate has previously been used as a positive marker of reversible myocardial ischemia in man [2, 9]. The augmented uptake of N-13 glutamate could be due to increased utilization of glutamate and its transamination products for anaerobic ATP production.

Oxidative phosphorylation is rapidly arrested in ischemic (or hypoxic) myocardium, and formation of ATP shifts to anaerobic glycolysis. Increased lactate concentrations in ischemic myocardium, however, inhibit – directly and indirectly – several enzymes of the glycolytic chain, in this way limiting glycolytic flux [3]. The observed beneficial effect of glutamate on recovery of myocardial function after transient ischemia [1] can be explained by the transamination of glutamate with pyruvate forming alanine and alpha-keto-glutarate. Alpha-ketoglutarate may subsequently serve as a fuel for the tricarboxylic acid (TCA) cycle [4, 5]. In a previous study from our laboratory performed in patients with single-vessel disease of the left anterior descending coronary artery and without previous myocardial infarction, poststenotic N-13 glutamate uptake was significantly correlated with the amount of regional [201]Th redistribution [9].

Beside conventional medical therapy and bypass surgery, percutaneous transluminal coronary angioplasty (PTCA) today is a third powerful tool in the therapeutic management of patients suffering from coronary artery disease. The present study addresses the question: Does a successful coronary angioplasty necessarily mean an instantaneous normalization of perfusion and metabolism in the poststenotic myocardial region? In order to answer this question, the behaviour of poststenotic myocardial N-13 glutamate uptake after successful coronary angioplasty was investigated; the time course of poststenotic N-13 glutamate uptake was compared to the time course of regional [201]Th activity.

Patients and methods

The present study group comprised 17 patients with single-vessel coronary artery disease (15 men and 2 women aged 53 ± 6 yr). Coronary angiography revealed at

P.W. Serruys, R. Simon & K.J. Beatt (eds), Percutaneous Transluminal Coronary Angioplasty. ISBN 0-7923-0346-6.

least 75% proximal stenoses of the left anterior descending coronary artery in all of the patients. Four of the 17 patients had a history of previous transmural myocardial infarction.

Cardiac catheterization and radionuclide studies were performed within one week before angioplasty, and radionuclide studies were repeated within 8 days after successful PTCA. Fourteen of the 17 patients were again investigated six months after angioplasty; at this time, 12 patients showed a patent left anterior descending coronary artery: These patients demonstrated a restenosis of less than 50% luminal diameter narrowing. Two patients revealed a restenosis of >75% luminal diameter narrowing and were excluded from the study. Coronary angioplasty was considered successful if residual stenosis was <25% luminal diameter narrowing, and if no pressure gradient was observed across the stenosis.

Thallium-201 serial scintigraphy was performed during graded and symptom limited exercise. Two mCi of thallium-201 were injected intravenously 1 min before the anticipated end of exercise. Five minutes after injection, the initial thallium-201 scintigram was acquired in the 30° left anterior oblique projection using a gamma camera (Searle, 1/2 in. sodium iodide crystal) equipped with a high resolution parallel-hole collimator. Redistribution imaging was performed 3 hr later in the same projection. Using a peak energy setting at 75 keV with a 30% window, encompassing the X-ray peak of ^{201}Th, imaging duration for both initial and redistribution scintigrams was the time required to collect 600000 counts. Data were collected on a minicomputer (Elsint-Dycom-80) in a 128 × 128 matrix (word mode format).

Immediately following the ^{201}Th redistribution study, N-13 glutamate scintigraphy was performed at the same exercise level as achieved during ^{201}Th scintigraphy. Five to ten mCi of N-13 glutamate was injected intravenously, and single photon imaging was performed in the 30° left anterior oblique projection using the previously described gamma camera with the addition of a high energy collimator. Peak energy setting was at 511 keV with a 15% window encompassing the annihilation radiation of N-13. Data were collected from 10 to 20 min post injection, and during this time approximately 1500000 counts were collected.

Data processing was carried out on a VAX 11/780. Regional tracer uptake was quantified by relating the poststenotic tracer uptake in the territory of the left anterior descending coronary artery (septum) to the tracer uptake in the region supplied by the non-diseased left circumflex coronary artery (posterolateral wall = 100%) using an operator independent computer algorithm [9].

Results and discussion

Before angioplasty, percent luminal diameter narrowing of the left anterior descending coronary artery amounted to 85±8%; immediately after PTCA, luminal diameter narrowing was reduced to 14±20%. Among the 14 patients reinvestigated six months after PTCA, 12 patients revealed a restenosis of less than 50% with a mean value of 25±17% luminal diameter narrowing. Likewise,

Table 1. Response of poststenotic ^{201}Th and N-13 glutamate uptake to successful percutaneous transluminal coronary angioplasty (PTCA) in patients with single-vessel coronary artery disease (LAD).

	Before PTCA	One week after PTCA	Six months after PTCA
Percent poststenotic tracer uptake			
with thallium-201	72 ± 8	78 ± 7^a	77 ± 10^b
with N-13 glutamate	94 ± 12	103 ± 11^a	94 ± 11

^{a} $p < 0.01$.
^{b} $p < 0.05$ compared to the values before PTCA.

exercise parameters – peak exercise level 117 ± 34 W after PTCA vs 92 ± 35 W before PTCA, $p < 0.05$ – were significantly improved after PTCA. The symptomatic improvement was indicated by a significant reduction of positive stress tests after PTCA (5/17 after PTCA vs 12/17 before PTCA, $p < 0.01$).

Table 1 illustrates the response of thallium-201 and N-13 glutamate uptake to angioplasty. Poststenotic ^{201}Th uptake was significantly increased after successful PTCA ($78 \pm 8\%$ vs $72 \pm 7\%$ before PTCA, $p < 0.01$) and was nearly identical after six months ($77 \pm 10\%$ after six months, $p < 0.05$ compared to the uptake before PTCA).

Surprisingly, poststenotic N-13 glutamate uptake did not decrease after successful PTCA: As compared to ^{201}Th uptake, N-13 glutamate uptake was likewise increased immediately after PTCA ($103 \pm 11\%$ vs $94 \pm 12\%$ before PTCA, $p < 0.01$). At the time of late reinvestigation six months later, however, N-13 glutamate uptake had returned to the pre-PTCA level ($94 \pm 11\%$).

Thus, repeated studies of poststenotic N-13 glutamate uptake and extraction – N-13 glutamate uptake related to estimates of regional myocardial blood flow (^{201}Th) – reveal a delayed metabolic recovery of human myocardium despite successful coronary angioplasty. This fact cannot be explained by changes in stenosis geometry, since in these patients there was no hemodynamically relevant stenosis after PTCA which otherwise theoretically could have changed the condition. The phenomenon of delayed metabolic recovery despite successful coronary angioplasty in the presence of improved exercise capacity might be explained by disturbances of the myocardial microcirculation [6, 7, 8] which disappeared within six months after successful coronary angioplasty.

References

1. Bittl JA, Shine KI (1983) Protection of ischemic rabbit myocardium by glutamic acid. *Am J Physiol* 245:H406–412
2. Knapp WH, Helus F, Ostertag H, Tillmanns H, Kübler W (1982) Uptake and turnover of L-(N-13)-glutamate in the normal human heart and in patients with coronary artery disease. *Eur J Nucl Med* 7:211–215

3. Kübler W, Spieckermann PG (1970) Regulation of glycolysis in the ischemic and anoxic myocardium. *J Mol Cell Cardiol* 1:351–358
4. Mudge GH, Mills RM, Taegtmeyer H, Gorlin R, Lesch M (1976) Alterations of myocardial amino acid metabolism in chronic ischemic heart disease. *J Clin Invest* 58:1185–1192
5. Taegtmeyer H (1978) Metabolic responses to cardiac hypoxia: increased production of succinate by rabbit papillary muscle. *Circ Res* 43:808–815
7. Tillmanns H, Leinberger H, Neumann FJ, Steinhausen M, Parekh N, Zimmermann R (1984) Early microcirculatory changes during brief ischemia – primary events in ischemic myocardial injury? *Circulation* 70:Suppl II, p 88
6. Tillmanns H, Kübler W (1984) What happens in the microcirculation? In: DJ Hearse, DM Yellon (eds), *Therapeutic Approaches to Myocardial Infarct Size Limitation*, pp 107–124, New York: Raven Press
8. Tillmanns H, Neumann FJ, Schöneck V, Zimmermann R, Dussel R, Steinhausen M (1987) Microcirculatory disturbances in stunned myocardium. *Circulation* 76 (Suppl IV): 147
9. Zimmermann R, Tillmanns H, Knapp WH, Helus F, Georgi P, Rauch B, Neumann F-J, Girgensohn S, Maier-Borst W, Kübler W (1988) Regional myocardial nitrogen-13 glutamate uptake in patients with coronary artery disease: Inverse post-stress relation to thallium-201 uptake in ischemia. *J Am Coll Cardiol* 11:549–556

12. Left atrial function in acute transient ischemia of the left ventricle

MILAN GRBIC and ULRICH SIGWART

The left atrium is a muscular contractile chamber located upstream of the left ventricle which serves as a reservoir for storing blood during left ventricular contraction, as a conduit for blood from the pulmonary veins to the left ventricle during early ventricular filling and, also, as a booster pump to complete left ventricular filling.

The role of atrial systole in maintaining optimal hemodynamic cardiac function has been studied extensively in animal models [1–3] and in humans [4–7]. A loss of atrial contraction as a result of atrial fibrillation [8] or ventricular pacing [9] reduces cardiac output by approximately 15–20%. The role of left atrial function has been demonstrated in experimental mitral regurgitation [10, 11] and in patients after myocardial infarction [12]. Braunwald and Frahn [15] have shown that the Frank-Starling mechanism may be operative in the left atrium as well in the left ventricle.

In order to assess the role of the left atrium in the presence of left ventricular failure, we have studied left atrial function during acute myocardial ischemia induced by transient occlusion of the proximal left anterior descending coronary artery in 32 patients undergoing percutaneous transluminal coronary angioplasty (PTCA).

Patients and methods

Thirty-two patients, 28 males and 4 females, aged between 34 and 63 yr (mean 52 ± 7 years) were studied. All patients were in normal sinus rhythm and none had a history of previous myocardial infarction. In each case the indication for angioplasty was a proximal stenosis of the left anterior descending coronary artery (LAD). Informed consent was obtained from each patient and the study was approved by the Hospital Ethics Committee.

All patients were premedicated with Aspirin (1 g the day before the study) and Diazepam 5 mg p.o. (1 h before the procedure). A French 7 double tipmanometer, the sensors being separated by a distance of 5 cm, was placed transseptally so that

P.W. Serruys, R. Simon & K.J. Beatt (eds), Percutaneous Transluminal Coronary Angioplasty. ISBN 0-7923-0346-6.
© *1990 Kluwer Academic Publishers, Dordrecht*

the distal sensor was located in the left ventricle and the proximal sensor in the left atrium. All pressures and their derivatives were recorded on photographic paper employing a Honeywell LS 8 photographic recorder and simultaneously stored on digital tape. The recordings were made at high paper speed before and during transluminal coronary angioplasty. In 10 patients a French 7 Pigtail catheter was advanced to the pulmonary artery for contrast injections during angioplasty. Biplane left heart cineangiography was performed at 50 frames per second during the injection of 45 ml of Iopamidol 370 into the pulmonary artery. The cineangiography was obtained before angioplasty and, after a waiting period of 20 min, during LAD balloon occlusion of 30 sec duration. The volume analysis of the left atrial and the left ventricular chambers was done according to standard methods [13, 14] employing a computer assisted analysis system (Mennen Medical). Maximum left atrial volume (LAV max(ml/m^2)) was measured just before mitral valve opening. The minimum volume (LAV min(ml/m^2)) was measured at the end of atrial contraction, and the volume before left atrial contraction (LAV-pre A(ml/m^2)) was taken just before left atrial 'a' wave. Left ventricular volumes were measured during the same cycle; we determined left ventricular volume before left atrial contraction (LVV pre A(ml/m^2)), left ventricular enddiastolic volume (LVEDV) and left ventricular endsystolic volume (LVESV). The ratio of left atrial volume change was calculated as LAV max − LAV min (ml/m^2). Left atrial contribution to left ventricular filling was determined by subtracting the left atrial stroke volume from the left ventricular stroke volume.

Pressures and derivatives were analysed on line by a computer and compared with the analog tracings. The isovolumic relaxation time (IVRT) was determined as the interval from the aortic valve closure to the mitral valve opening. In cases where no high fidelity tipmanometer was present in the aortic root, the aortic valve closure was determined from a vibration on the left atrial pressure curve which coincides exactly with the aortic pressure tracing notch (Fig. 1). The mitral valve opening corresponds to the left atrial and left ventricular pressure crossover. On pressure tracings with high gain (Fig. 3) the IVRT was measured from the lowest point of the negative dP/dt of the left ventricular pressure to the left ventricular and left atrial pressure crossover. The left atrial pressure pulse was defined as the difference between the highest and the lowest left atrial pressure.

Results

Table 1 depicts the left ventricular and left atrial pressure measurements as well as the first derivatives at rest and during the first 30 sec of LAD balloon occlusion in 32 patients. The 10 patients in whom LVEF and LA contribution to LVSVI were determined by cineangiography are included in this table.

The left ventricular peak systolic pressure decreased from 135 ± 12 to 106 ± 9 mmHg together with a simultaneous decrease of LV max dP/dt from 1634 ± 136 mmHg per second to 1137 ± 127 mmHg/sec. LVEDP rose from 12 ± 2

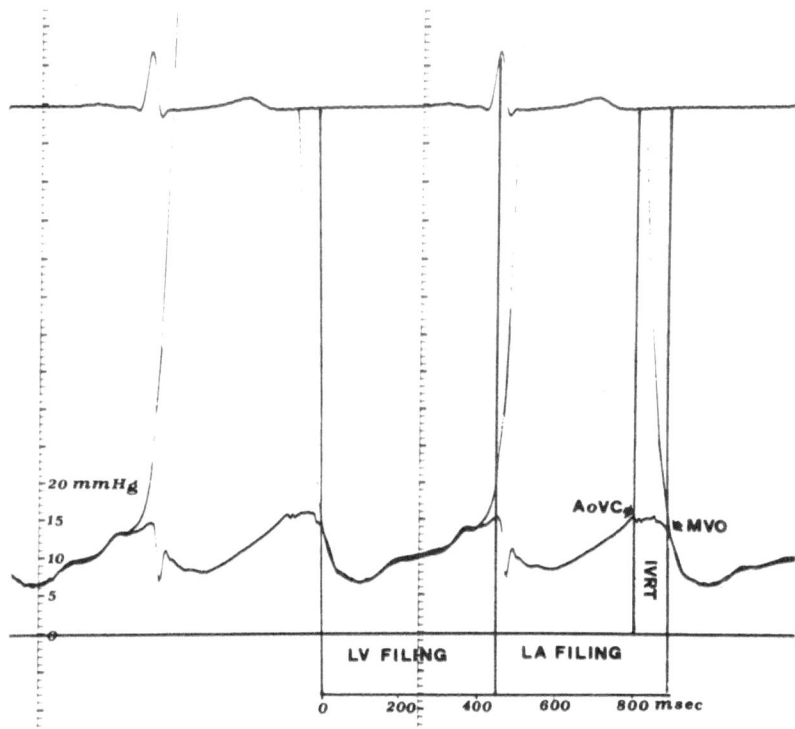

Figure 1. Left atrial and left ventricular pressures recorded at rest with high gain. Aortic valve closure (AVC) corresponds to the notch on the 'v' wave and the mitral valve opening (MVO) to the secondnotch corresponding (crossover of the LV and LA pressure curves). Isovolumic relaxation time (IVR) can easily be calculated from AoVA to MVO.

to 37 ± 3 mmHg. The left atrial mean pressure rose from 11 ± 2 to 29 ± 2 mmHg. There was a difference between LVEDP and LA mean pressure of 1.5 mmHg at rest and 7.8 mmHg after 30 sec of LAD occlusion. The LA max dP/dt increased from 177 ± 13 to 381 ± 21 mmHg/sec. The left atrial pressure amplitude (LA pulse pressure) augmented from 16 ± 3 to 26 ± 4 mmHg meaning 38% increase. Left atrial 'a' wave pressure increased from 20 ± 5 to 55 ± 6 mmHg during ischemia (Fig. 2).

The left ventricular and left atrial volumes together with other hemodynamic parameters of the 10 patients in whom cineangiography had been performed are shown in Table 2. Left enddiastolic volume index increased within the first 30 sec of LAD occlusion from 75 ± 7 ml/m^2 to 102.5 ± 10 ml/m^2 ($= 26\%$). LV-endsystolic volume rose from 30 ± 5 to 59 ± 9 ml/m^2 ($= 31\%$) during acute ischemia. Left ventricular stroke volume index diminished from 46 ± 5 to 43 ± 3 ml/m^2 while left ventricular ejection fraction decreased from 61.5 ± 7 to $42 \pm 2\%$ ($= 31\%$ reduction).

Table 1.

	Rest	7 sec.oocl.
LV PSP (mmHg)	134.75± 11.63	132.81± 11.61
LV EDP (mmHg)	12.28± 2.11	13.78± 1.95
LA mean (mmHg)	10.75± 1.68	11.71± 1.70
LV max dP/dt (mmHg/sec)	1633.66±135.93	1576.00±146.22
LA max sP/dt mmHg/sec	177.31± 13.22	194.53± 16.17
LV EF (%)	61.5 ± 6.8	
LA contribution to LVSVI (%)	25.9 ± 5.0	

LV PSP = left ventricular peak systolic pressure; LV EDP = left ventricular end-diastolic pressure; LA mean = left atrial mean pressure; LV EF = left ventricular ejection fraction in %; LA contribut. to

The left atrial volume before mitral valve opening (= LAV max) increased from 41 ± 3 to 64 ± 4 ml/m^2 (= 36%). Left atrial minimal volume (volume after left atrial contraction) increased from 18 ± 1.5 to 29 ± 3 ml/m^2 (= 37%). There was an augmentation of left atrial volume before LA contraction from 29 ± 3 to 54 ± 3 ml/m^2 (= 46%). The left atrial volume amplitude augmented from 23 ± 2 ml/m^2 to 34.5 ± 4 ml/m^2 (= 37%). The contribution of left atrial contraction to left ventricular stroke volume index increased from 26 ± 5% to 57 ± 9% at 30 sec of ischemia.

Left ventricular isovolumetric relaxation time (IVRT) was prolonged during the first 5 to 7 sec of LAD occlusion (IVRT increased from 82 ± 7 msec to 96 ± 6 msec) together with a sharp decrease of left ventricular peak negative dP/dt. IVRT started to shorten 14 ± 6 sec after LAD occlusion, reaching 57 ± 5 msec after a 30 sec occlusion. This phenomenon could be substantiated from the observation of valve movement during contrast injection.

Discussion

Myocardial ischemia is known to cause severe disturbances of myocardial function. We have observed a dramatic reduction of left ventricular peak negative dP/dt during the first seconds of acute myocardial ischemia during balloon occlusion at the time of transluminal coronary angioplasty [19]; these observations are in accordance with animal experiments [20] and have been confirmed by others [21]. Very little, however, is known about the performance of the left atrium during acute ischemia of the ventricular myocardium.

Our observations have shown an inverse relationship between left ventricular

14 sec.oocl.	21 sec.occl.	30 sec.occl.	NB
123.78 ± 10.90	115.09 ± 10.30	105.69 ± 8.85	32
22.03 ± 3.14	29.72 ± 3.52	37.16 ± 3.01	32
16.47 ± 2.02	22.25 ± 2.76	29.38 ± 2.46	32
1407.53 ± 265.38	1298.13 ± 139.38	1136.72 ± 126.65	32
253.31 ± 22.08	323.63 ± 22.76	381.28 ± 21.32	32
		41.9 ± 2	10
		57 ± 3.7	10

LVSVI = left atrial contribution to left ventricular stroke volume index
(for explanation see text).

and left atrial performance during left ventricular ischemia. While left ventricular peak systolic pressure and dP/dt max decreased by 25 and 30% respectively, left atrial mean pressure and left atrial contractility increased significantly as expressed by a 105% increment of left atrial max dP/dt. The loss of left ventricular ejection fraction of some 32% during ischemia was counterbalanced by an increased left atrial booster function resulting in a remarkable augmentation of left ventricular end-diastolic volume, thus keeping the left ventricular stroke volume almost stable despite a dramatic reduction of the ejection fraction.

These results confirm observations reported by Rahimtoola et al [16] and Matsuda et al [12] who noted an increase in atrial contraction in the intact animal when the left atrium was stretched during volume load. Other observations by Payne [17] and Braunwald [15] also suggested that the Franck Starling mechanism appears to play an important role when left atrial volume was increased with blood transfusions.

It is possible that the neurohumoral influences can play a certain role in the contractility of the left atrium, but we have not measured either of the atrial peptides or cathecholamines, so it is impossible to confirm this statement. In any case, there were no observed heart rate changes.

In animal experiments Sasayama et al [11] noted that atrial myocardial shortening was remarkably enhanced during experimental mitral regurgitation, the increase of atrial diameter leading to the appearance of a prominent atrial 'a' wave.

In our study the contraction amplitude of the left atrium increased significantly during left ventricular ischemia augmenting its contribution to left ventricular stroke volume index from 25.9 ± 5% to 57.0 ± 8.8%. Furthermore, the left atrial max dP/dt doubled during left ventricular ischemia suggesting enhanced left

Table 2. Hemodynamic values in 10 patients with angiography.

		LV PSP (mmHg) LV EDP (mmHg)	LA mean (mmHg)	LA-puls P (mmHg)	LVEDVI (ml/m²)	LVV pre 'A' (ml/m²)	LVESVI (ml/m²)
1	R	135/12	11	15	71	59	29
	I	105/36	30	23	95	73	56
2	R	119/10	9	13	69	57	24
	I	93/32	28	21	92	72	52
3	R	147/15	13	18	81	72	33
	I	108/38	31	29	115	95	69
4	R	125/9	7	12	73	62	30
	I	95/36	30	24	104	87	61
5	R	152/13	11	18	80	68	33
	I	112/39	30	28	110	95	65
6	R	131/13	11	16	82	74	40
	I	102/41	33	27	116	95	67
7	R	112/8	7	12	72	62	28
	I	95/36	30	24	97	75	45
8	R	128/12	10	17	89	78	33
	I	102/41	33	29	112	97	70
9	R	151/16	13	18	71	57	29
	I	120/39	31	25	93	73	51
10	R	133/12	10	17	69	61	25
	I	108/37	29	28	91	70	51
	R	133/12 ±13/±2.5	10.2 ±2.1	15.6 ±2.4	75.7 ±6.8	65.0 ±7.5	30.4 ±4.6
	I	104/37.5 ±8.5/±2.7	30.5 ±1.6	25.8 ±2.8	102.5 ±10.0	83.2 ±11.5	58.7 ±8.8
	p	0.001/0.001	0.001	0.001	0.001	0.05	0.001

LV PSP, LV EDP, LA mean, LV EF as in Table 1. LA-puls P = left atrial pulse pressure; LVEDVI = left ventricular end-diastolic volume index in ml/m²; LVV pre 'A' = left ventricular volume before left atrial contraction in ml/m²; LVESVI = left ventricular endsystolic volume

atrial contractility. This phenomenon is clinically known as the prominent 'atrial kick'.

The left atrial kinetics may protect the pulmonary circulation from excessive pressure increase during ischemia. After 30 seconds of occlusion, we observed left ventricular end-diastolic pressures which significantly surpassed the mean atrial pressure; this phenomenon has also been observed in other states of left

LV EF (%)	LVSVI (ml/m²)	LA max (ml/m²)	LA min (ml/m²)	LAV pre 'A' (ml/m²)	LA contribution to LVSVI (%)	LA Δ Vol (ml/m²)
61	43	41	17	30	30	24
41	39	63	26	54	72	37
65	45	39	15	27	27	24
43	40	61	30	52	55	31
59	48	42	18	27	19	24
40	46	69	31	57	57	38
59	43	39	17	29	28	22
42	44	60	32	51	43	28
59	47	41	18	30	26	23
41	45	65	25	56	47	30
51	42	43	17	28	26	26
42	49	67	30	56	53	37
61	44	41	19	30	25	22
43	42	65	31	58	64	34
63	56	45	20	31	20	25
38	42	70	33	53	52	37
59	42	45	20	35	36	25
45	42	69	30	56	62	39
78	54	36	18	26	22	18
44	40	58	24	50	65	34
61.5	46.4	41.2	17.9	29.3	25.9	23.3
±6.8	±4.9	±2.8	±1.5	±2.6	±5.0	±2.3
41.9	42.9	64.7	29.2	54.3	57.0	34.5
±2.0	±3.1	±4.1	±3.1	±2.7	±8.8	±3.7
0.05	NS	0.001	0.001	0.001	0.001	0.001

index in ml/m²; LVSVI = left ventricular stroke volume index in ml/m²; LA max = left atrial maximum volume in ml/m²; LA min = left atrial minimum volume in ml/m²; LAV pre 'A' = left atrial volume before left atrial contraction; LA Δ vol = changing of left atrial volumes.

ventricular failure. The left atrial booster pump action appears to become an important factor in forcefully filling the left ventricular chamber which is stiffened under ischemic conditions. During atrial contraction only a minor amount of blood is rejected into the pulmonary venous circulation. Since in our model the left atrium was not affected by ischemic events, the even more generous contraction may prevent important backflow into the pulmonary venous system

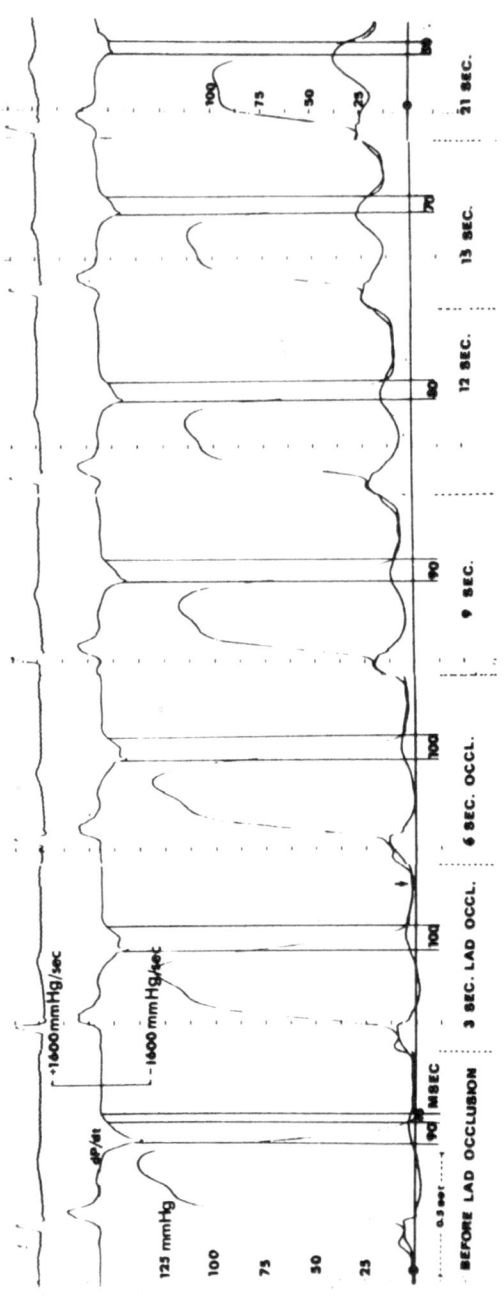

Figure 2. Left atrial pressure recorded at rest and during LAD occlusion with left atrial first derivative. During acute ischemia there is LA pressure rise (prominent 'a' wave) with LA max dP/dt rise and shortening of the isovolumic relaxation time.

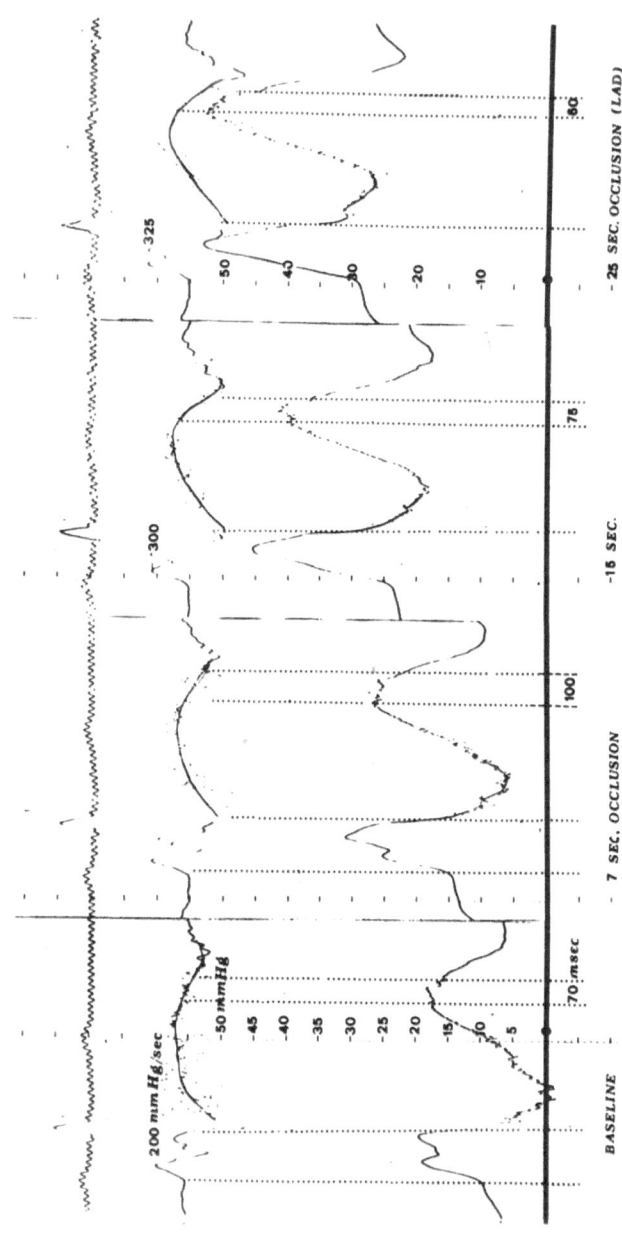

Figure 3. Simultaneously recorded LA and LV pressures with LV first derivative at rest and during LAD occlusion. The earliest phenomenon is shortening and deformation of the negative dP/dt signal with the lowest point of the LV diastolic pressure shifting into mid-diastole (arrow) together with prolongation of isovolumic relaxation time.

as observed in ventricular hypertrophy with diminished ventricular end-atrial compliance [18].

Another disease process affecting both the atria and the ventricles may explain the lack of correlation between mean left atrial pressure and mean left atrial volume in patients with valvular heart disease [13]. In our study we noted an excellent correlation between left atrial pressure, left atrial pulse pressure and left atrial volume; these parameters simultaneously increased during acute ischemia, since the left atrial myocardium happened to react physiologically to the increased load.

The observation of shortening of the isovolumic relaxation period during advanced ischemia is a by-product of our study and is in disaccordance with previous statements [22, 23]. Prolongation of the isovolumic relaxation period is a transient phenomenon during the early phase of ischemia. Left ventricular global relaxation is severely impaired during transient coronary occlusion as depicted in Fig. 3; the lowest diastolic pressure point invariably moves to the right towards mid-diastole. As left atrial pressure increases, the mitral valve opens earlier; this upward shift of the left atrial pressure curve causes the abbreviation of isovolumic relaxation.

From these observations, we can conclude that in acute ischemia an inverse correlation exists between left ventricular ejection fraction and left atrial active contribution to left ventricular filling. When left atrial pressure rises with ischemia of the left ventricle, the left atrial volume increases as well together with augmentation of left atrial pulse amplitude. The left atrial function appears to be enhanced in acute ischemia of the left ventricle suggesting an involvement of the Franck-Starling mechanism. It appears unlikely, however, that this mechanism is exclusively responsible for the recruitment of left atrial reserve; hormonal factors might play some role as well. The enhanced left atrial function and contractility may in part prevent excessive pulmonary pressure through particular kinetic phenomena. Lastly, the increased left atrial pressure reduces the time interval from aortic valve closure to mitral valve opening.

References

1. Linden RJ, Mitchell JH (1960) Relation between left ventricular diastolic pressure and myocardial segment length and observations on the contribution of atrial systole. *Circ Res* 8:1092
2. Wallace AG, Mitchell JH, Skinner NS, Sarnoff SJ (1963) Hemodynamic variables affecting the relation between mean left atrial and left ventricular end-diastolic pressures. *Circ Res* 13:261
3. Naito M, Dreyfus LS, David D, Michelson EL, Mardelli J, Kmetzo JJ (1983) Reevaluation of the role of atrial systole to cardiac hemodynamics: evidence for pulmonary venous regurgitation during abnormal atrio-ventricular sequencing. *Am Heart J* 105:295
4. Morris JJ, Entman M, North WC (1965) The changes in cardiac output with reversion of atrial fibrillation to sinus rhythm. *Circulation* 31:670
5. Killip T, Baer RA (1966) Hemodynamic effects after reversion from atrial fibrillation to sinus rhythm by precordial shock. *J Clin Invest* 45:658
6. Reale A (1965) Acute effects of countershock conversion of atrial fibrillation upon right and left heart hemodynamics. *Circulation* 32:214

7. Samet P (1973) Hemodynamic sequelae of cardiac arrhythmias. *Circulation* 47:399
8. Kaplan MA, Gray RE, Isera LT (1968) Metabolic and hemodynamic responses to exercise during atrial fibrillation and sinus rhythm. *Am J Cardiol* 22:543
9. Curtis JJ, Maloney JD, Barnhorst DA, Pluth JR, Hartzler GO, Wallace RB (1977) A critical look at temporary ventricular pacing following cardiac surgery. *Surgery* 82:888
10. Yoran C, Yellin EL, Becker RM, Gabbay S, Frater RWM, Sonnenblick EH (1979) Dynamic aspect of acute mitrala regurgitation: effects of ventricular volume, pressure and contractility on the effective regurgitation orifice area. *Circulation* 60:170
11. Sasayama S, Tarcahashi M, Osakada G, Hirose K, Hamashima H, Nishimura E, Kawai C (1979) Dynamic geometry of the left atrium and left ventricle in acute mitral regurgitation. *Circulation* 60:177
12. Matsuda Y, Toma Y, Ogawa H, Matsuzaki M, Katayama K, Fujii T, Yoshinos F, Moritani K, Kumade T, Kusukawa R (1983) Importance of left atrial function in patients with myocardial infarction. *Circulation* 7:566
13. Sauter HJ, Dodge HT, Johnston RR, Graham TP (1964) The relationship of left atrial pressure and volume in patient with heart disease *Am Heart J* 67:635
14. Dodge HT, Sandler H, Ballen DW, Lord JR Jr (1960) The use of biplane angiography for the measurement of left ventricular volume in man. *Am Heart J* 60:762
15. Braunwald E, Frahm CJ (1961) Studies on Starling's law of the heart. IV: Observations on the hemodynamic functions of the left atrium in man. *Circulation* 24:663
16. Rahimtoola HR, Ehsani A, Sinno MZ, Loeb HS, Rosen KM, Gunnar RM (1975) Left atrial transport function in myocardial infarction. Importance of its booster pump function. *Am J Med* 59:686
17. Payne RM, Stone HL, Engelken EJ (1971) Atrial function during volume loading. *J Appl Physiol* 31:326
18. Grant C, Bunnell IL, Green DG (1964) The reservoir function of the left atrium during ventricular systole. An angiographic study of atrial stroke volume and work. *Am J Med* 37:36
19. Sigwart U, Grbic M, Essinger A, Fischer A, Morin D, Sadeghi H (1982) Myocardial function in man during acute coronary balloon occlusion. *Circulation* 66:II86
20. Kumada T, Karliner JS, Pouleur H (1979) Effect of coronary occlusion on early ventricular diastolic events in conscious dogs. *Am J Physiol* 237 (5):H542–549
21. Wijns W, Serruys PW, Slager CJ, Grimm J, Krayenbuhl HP, Hugenholz PG, Hess OM (1986) Effect of coronary occlusion during percutaneous transluminal angioplasty in humans on left ventricular chamber stiffness and regional diastolic pressure-radius relations. *J Am Cardiol* 7:455–463
22. Hirota Y (1980) A clinical study of left ventricular relaxation. *Circulation* 62:756
23. Papapietro SE, Coghlan HC, Zissermann D, Russel RO Jr, Racley CE, Rogers WJ (1979) Impaired maximal rate of left ventricular relaxation in patients with coronary disease and left ventricular dysfunction. *Circulation* 59:514

13. Left ventricular filling during acute ischemia

M. GRBIC and U. SIGWART

Introduction

Left ventricular filling in the absence of aortic regurgitaion or ventricular septal defect starts with the onset of mitral valve opening and ends with mitral valve closure. The diastolic flow pattern across the mitral valve is dependent on the interrelationship of left ventricular active relaxation, chamber compliance and stiffness, the atrial contraction and blood return from the pulmonary circulation. Normally, left ventricular filling is tripartite. Immediately after mitral valve opening a rapid filling phase starts and lasts about 200 msec, followed by slow filling or diastasis, the duration of which is dependent on the heart rate and finishes with left atrial contraction.

It has become common knowledge that the filling mechanism of the left ventricle changes with myocardial impairment. Frequently the left ventricular filling pressure is being used to quantify this impairment and it is known to increase during angina pectoris. We have become interested in left ventricular filling behaviour during intermittent coronary balloon occlusion at the time of transluminal coronary angioplasty.

Methods

In 30 patients with coronary heart disease we have studied left ventricular filling during acute induced ischemia. All patients had a proximal left anterior descending artery stenosis. A double tip micromanometer (Millar PC 771) was introduced by the transeptal route with the distal sensor located in the left ventricle and the proximal transducer in the left atrium. The simultaneous LV and LA pressure tracings were recorded together with their derivatives on photographic paper and on digital tape. All recordings were obtained at rest and completed in 10 pts with left heart angiography (injection of 45 ml of contrast medium (iopamiro 370) into the pulmonary artery). The same procedure was repeated during acute ischemia when the balloon was inflated in the proximal

P.W. Serruys, R. Simon & K.J. Beatt (eds), Percutaneous Transluminal Coronary Angioplasty. ISBN 0-7923-0346-6.
© *1990 Kluwer Academic Publishers, Dordrecht*

LAD. The left heart angiography was performed 30 s after the onset of LAD occlusion. In 5 pts LV angiography was performed before and at 5–10 s of LAD occlusion.

The following observations relate three distinct features of left ventricular filling (left ventricular relaxation, left ventricular chamber stiffness and left atrial contraction) to intermittent myocardial ischemia during coronary balloon occlusion.

Results

Left ventricular relaxation

The relaxation of the heart represents a change in the material properties of the myocardium and means the return to its initial length and tension. This is a complex, energy dependent process [1]. Hirota Y. [2] considers the relaxation of the heart as a major determinant of the early diastolic filling as atrial blood rushes into the ventricle during the terminal stage of relaxation. The exact quantification process of the relaxation is difficult. The peak negative dP/dt is influenced by heart rate, systolic pressure, endsystolic volume and other factors. The time constant T of the left ventricular pressure fall during isovolumic relaxation seemed relatively independent of other determinants of cardiac performance and has been proposed as an index of LV relaxation. The conflicting results are criticized by Brutsaert [3] since they constitute a mere mathematic approximation of the pressure decay, which is a complex function (monoexponential, biexponential or asymptote?) of time, sometimes influenced in the opposite way even by minor alterations of many factors.

Fully aware of the fact that none of the as yet described indices provides a unique description of the relaxation process we have used the direct determination of the duration of isovolumic relaxation. On the simultaneously recorded high fidelity traces of the LV, LA and aortic pressure, the isovolumic LV relaxation time, defined as the interval from the aortic valve closure to the mitral valve opening, was calculated from the aortic closure notch to the crossover of the LV-LA pressure tracings. Also, we could calculate 'total relaxation time' from the aortic closure notch to the lowest point of protodiastolic pressure (Fig. 1).

Left ventricular isovolumic relaxation time is 75 ± 10 msec befor balloon occlusion and peak negative dP/dt is 1750 ± 250 mmHg/s 2 to 3 s after LAD balloon occlusion the negative dP/dt decrease and after 5 s following coronary occlusion a deformation of the ascending limb of negative dP/dt can be observed. 6 s after LAD occlusion isovolumic relaxation is prolonged to 97 ± 10 msec and peak negative dP/dt decreases to 1320 ± 210 mmHg/s. After 9 s of LAD occlusion the isovolumic relaxation starts to shorten again; between 15–25 s of LAD occlusion it dropped to 55 ± 8 msec (Fig. 2).

In 2 patients biplan left ventricular angiography was performed after 5 s of occlusion. It showed delayed shortening of the LV antero-apico-septal wall

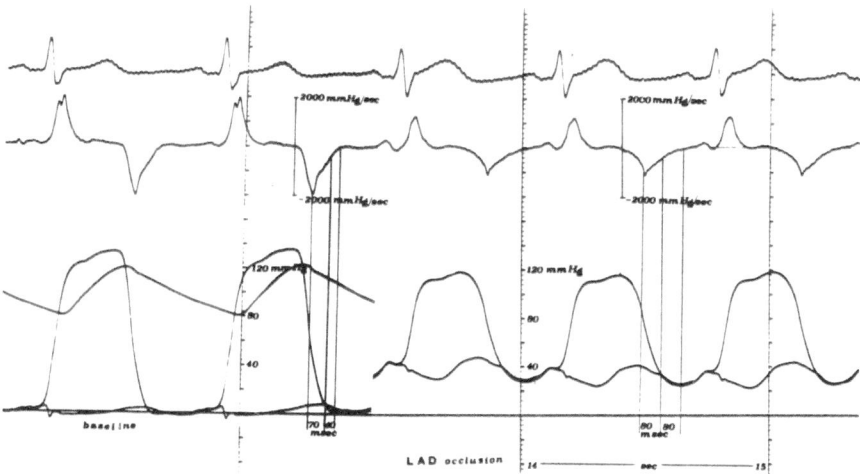

Figure 1. Simultaneous recording of left ventricular and left atrial pressures with first derivative (dP/dt) of left ventricular pressure at rest and 14 s after left anterior descending artery occlusion with left ventricular isovolumic relaxation time and 'total relaxation time' (measured to the lowest point of left ventricular diastolic pressure). Note a hammock-like pattern of LV diastolic pressure curve during acute ischemia and prolongation of LV 'total relaxation time'.

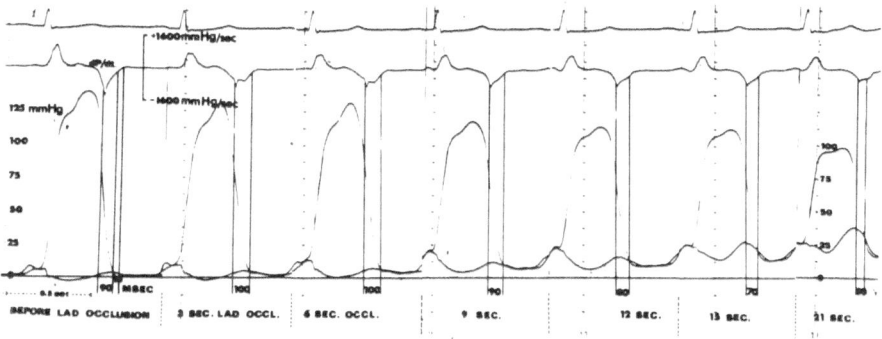

Figure 2. Left ventricular and left atrial pressures at rest and during ischemia. The LV isovolumic relaxation time prolonged only during the first 9 s of ischemia. The peak negative dP/dt deformation with notch was present during the first 6 s of ischemia and corresponded to the assynchronous LV wall motion of the antero-septal region.

coinciding with the appearance of a notched and deformed negative dP/dt (Fig. 2) as an expression of asynchronous relaxation.

The total duration of LV relaxation starts to lengthen already 3 s after LAD occlusion; 5–6 s after occlusion the lowest diastolic point moves into the middle of diastole deforming a diastolic curve into a hammock like pattern (Figs 1–3). The

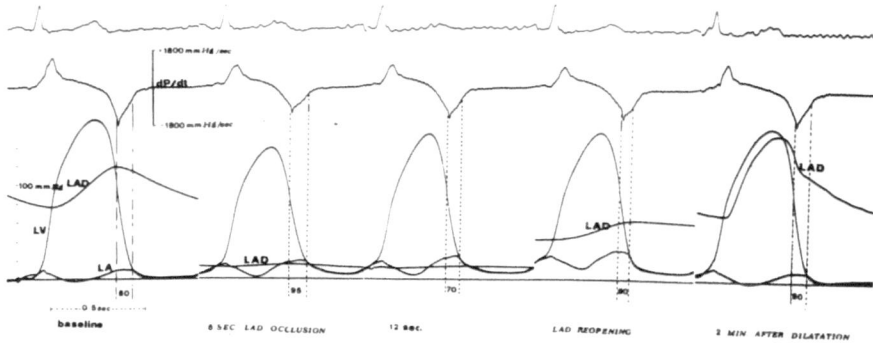

Figure 3. Six seconds after LAD artery occlusion LV diastolic curve changes into hammock-like pattern which normalises only 2 min after balloon deflation.

diastolic abnormality persists until the end of LAD occlusion. Also during left heart angiography we found markedly reduced rapid filling and left ventricular filling primarily by atrial contraction.

Left ventricular stiffness

Left ventricular chamber stiffness is determined by the level of operating pressure and the diastolic pressure-volume relation. But any analysis ought to take into account the diastolic interactions and interdependencies of the factors which influence LV diastolic pressure-volume relations: distensibility of the chamber, chamber volume and wall thickness, composition of the wall, process of relaxation, viscous properties, pericardium, atrial contraction, pleural pressure, coronary vascular volume and pressure, etc [4]. From animal and human studies, we know that left ventricular chamber stiffness increases with ischemia. Acute intermittent myocardial ischemia in our model was equally associated with a typical shift of the pressure-volume relationship. Since only segmental ischemia is achieved with selective LAD occlusion we focused our interest on regional wall motion abnormalities that may be responsible for the overall change in chamber stiffness.

Within the first 5 s of LAD occlusion we observed an asynchrony of the antero-apico-septal wall of the left ventricle with late systolic shortening occuring during the isovolumic relaxation; this coincides with a notch on the ascending limb of the negative dP/dt signal (Fig. 2). The LV filling pressure did not yet rise at that moment, but the diastolic pressure curve took the form of a hammock. After 15 s of occlusion the LV end-diastolic-pressure rose from 15 ± 2 mmHg to 22 ± 3 mmHg and after 25–30 s of LAD occlusion it rose to 27 ± 5 mmHg; together with the diastolic hammock deformation this indicates an important diastolic compliance failure. At 30 s of ischemia left heart angiography showed an

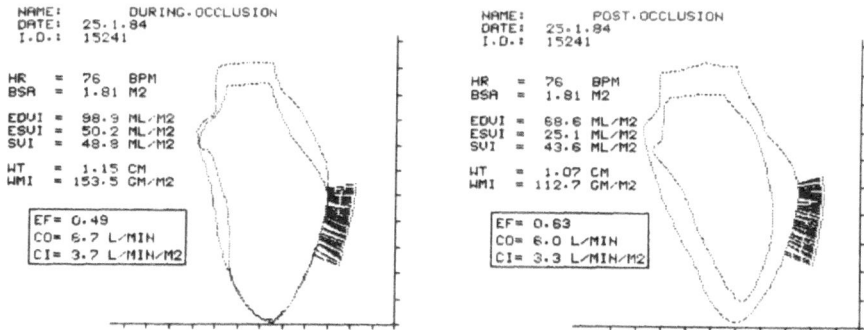

Figure 4. Left ventricular end-diastolic and end-systolic volume augmented during acute ischemia with drop of LV ejection fraction but very little decrease of LV stroke volume index.

akinesia or slight dyskinesia of the antero-septal wall with small increase of end-diastolic volume, but marked augmentation of endsystolic volume. The left ventricular ejection fraction decreased from $69 \pm 5\%$ to $41 \pm 7\%$ (Fig. 4).

The antero-apico-septal wall of the left ventricle showed a slight inward movement ('late contraction') just during the rapid filling period of the LV at the time of 30 s of LAD occlusion. This late wall contraction may contribute to the impedance of the left ventricular filling.

Left atrial contraction

It is accepted that atrial systole improves left ventricular performance by means of increasing the left ventricular preload and the end-diastolic fiber length [6]. We were interested in studying the role of the left atrium during acute intermittent left ventricular segmented ischemia.

Left atrial pressure rose within the first 7 s of LAD occlusion from 13 ± 5 to 18 ± 6 mmHg; the 'a' and 'v' waves augmented from 20 ± 3 to 30 ± 4 mmHg. After 15 s of occlusion 'a' and 'v' waves rose to 37 ± 3 and after 25 s respectively to 50 ± 5 mmHg (Fig. 5). At the same time the max dP/dt of the left atrial pressure rose from 220 ± 40 to 350 ± 20 mmHg/s (Fig. 5). This increase of left atrial max dP/dt suggested an augmented contraction of the left atrium during an acute ischemia. Left heart angiography showed left atrial volume increase from 42 ± 3 to 65 ± 4 ml/m^2 and LA minimal volume increase from 18 ± 2 to 29 ± 3 ml/m^2. The ratio of contribution of LA contraction to LV stroke volume increased from $26 \pm 5\%$ to $57 \pm 8\%$. At the same time the left ventricular ejection fraction dropped from $69 + 5\%$ to $41 + 7\%$.

30 s after the onset of LAD occlusion the left atrial mean pressure has risen to 31 ± 6 mmHg. The large increment in the height of the 'v'-wave (50 ± 8 mmHg) accounts for the reduction in isovolumic relaxation time in advanced ischemia. This 'v'-wave is not the result of papillary muscle dysfunction and mitral incompetence as we were able to confirm by left ventricular contrast injections.

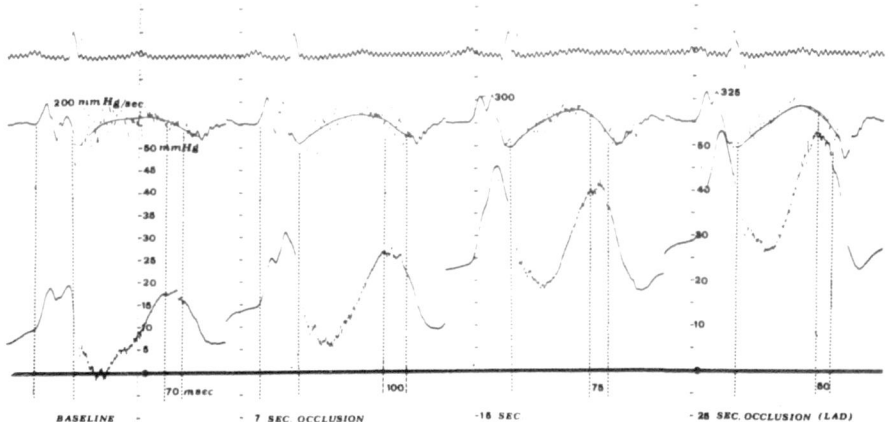

Figure 5. Left atrial pressure with it's first derivative at rest and during ischemia.

Discussion and conclusions

Left ventricular filling is a complex process dependent on a number of interrelated mechanisms that may become disorganized in disease. The ventricle has to fill appropriately to be able to eject blood adequately. Disturbances of the filling process may thus interfere with overall cardiac function. Immediately after mitral valve opening left ventricular filling is rapid, reaching a peak rate of 500 cc/s, thus exceeding ejection flow. This rapid diastolic filling lasts about 200 msec and is followed by a phase of slower volume increase, (diastasis) the duration of which is dependent on heart rate; filling finishes with the active left atrial contraction. This is the pattern that we observe during left heart angiography before a LAD occlusion.

5–6 s after LAD occlusion left ventricular geometry and filling begin to change. The isovolumic relaxation lengthens, the negative dP/dt becomes notched on its ascending limb which coincides with asynchrony of the left ventricular antero-septal wall motion. The left ventricular diastolic pressure curve change and the lower diastolic point move into the middle of diastole. Rapid filling is reduced by the diastolic late relaxation and rigidity of the antero-septal wall. When left ventricular rapid filling occurs the antero-septal wall is still contracting, thus impeding normal filling.

After 25–30 s of LAD occlusion the pattern of left ventricular filling deteriorates even more. Left ventricular antero-septal wall becomes stiff, the left ventricular volume increases, the left ventricular pressure volume curve is shifted upward and to the right, left ventricular filling pressure increases. The end-systolic volume increases with the ejection fraction reduced consequently.

Diminished rapid diastolic filling in patients with coronary artery disease have been demonstrated by Bonow [7] et al with radionuclide angiography. They found a prolonged time to peak filling rates in patients with ischemic heart disease and in patients with previous myocardial infarction. The peak filling rate correlated significantly with ejection fraction. We also found this correlation in our patients due to regional wall ischemia during LAD occlusion.

As active rapid filling of the left ventricle is impaired during acute ischemia the atrial contraction contributes significantly to terminal filling. Matsuda [8] et al have studied the left atrial volume-pressure relationship in the normal and in patients with remote myocardial infarction; they found the contribution of active atrial emptying to left ventricular stroke volume significantly higher in patients with myocardial infarction than in normal subjects. Clinically, Braunwald et al [9] suspected that Frank-Starling's law was operative in the human left atrium. Sasayama et al [10] demonstrated in an experimental study that the atrial diameter increased after the onset of acute mitral regurgitation and that atrial shortening was remarkably enhanced with a prominent 'a'-wave. This may simply be a manifestation of the Frank-Starling mechanism in atrial heart muscle. We observed augmentation of left atrial volume during acute ischemia with enhanced contraction volume emptying. The left atrial ejection fraction increased as left ventricular ejection fraction decreased: left atrial ejection fraction showed a significant inverse correlation with left ventricular ejection fraction. Furthermore, the contractility of the left atrium seems to be enhanced since the left atrial max dP/dt increased significantly. It seems that the contribution of the left atrium to left ventricular filling is significantly more important during left ventricular ischemia (LA EF 26 ± 5 to $57 \pm 8\%$).

The left atrial pressure rises and left ventricular systolic pressure reduction during ischemia of more than 25 s duration causes a shortening of the real isovolumic relaxation time. We observed a prolongation of the isovolumic relaxation only during the first 9 s of LAD occlusion. The shortening of the isovolumic relaxation time after 25–30 s was confirmed at left heart angiography. There was no delayed mitral valve opening as suggested by others.

It is now evident that the isovolumic pressure fall is not monoexponential during the first 20 s of coronary occlusion [11]. The time constant of the isovolumic pressure fall is of limited value both in animals [11] and humans [12]; it only reflects the inhomogenous behaviour of ischemic myocardium.

Theoretically it would be important to measure the total myocardial relaxation time in acute ischemia. Cardiac muscle relaxation means the return to its initial length and tension. This is controlled by 3 interacting determinants: load, inactivation and non-uniform distribution of load and inactivation in space and in time [11]. The precise measurement of the total relaxation is complex. On high fidelity pressure tracings it can possible be estimated as time from aortic valve closure to the lowest point of left ventricular diastolic pressure. During LAD occlusion this time doubled and the lowest point of the diastolic pressure moved into mid-diastole (hammock). Kumada et al [11] observed the same phenomenom during coronary occlusion in dogs. In man we noted 25 to 30 s after LAD occlusion inward movement of ischemic wall during left ventricular filling and outward movement during ejection. Using coronary occlusion during percutaneous transluminal angioplasty as a model of myocardial ischemia in man we may conclude that:

1. left ventricular filling is impaired before ejection changes occur
2. asynchronous relaxation is the first ischemic manifestation followed by prolongation of the duration of global relaxation
3. the left atrium compensates in part for the failure of the left ventricle to relax.

References

1. Strobeck JE, Bahler AS, Sonnenblick EH (1975) Isotonic relaxation in cardiac muscle. *Am J Physiol* 229:646
2. Hirota Y (1980) A clinical study of left ventricular relaxation. *Circulation* 62:756–63
3. Brutsaert DL, Rademakers FE; Syr SV(1984) Triple control of relaxation: implications in cardiac disease. *Circulation* 69:190–96
4. Gaasch WH, Levine HJ, Alexander JK (1976) Left ventricular compliance: mechanism and clinical implications. *Am J Cardiol* 38:645–53
5. Glantz SA, Parmley WW (1978) Factors which affect the diastolic pressure volume curve. *Circ Res* 42:171–80
6. Linden RJ, Mitchel JH (1960) Relation between left ventricular diastolic pressure and myocardial segment length and observations on the contribution of atrial systole. *Circ Res* 8:1092
7. Bonow RO, Bacharach SL, Green MV, Kent KM, Rosing DR, Lipson LC, Leon MB, Epstein SE (1981) Impaired left ventricular diastolic filling in patients with coronary artery disease: assessment with radionuclide angiography. *Circ* 64:315–23
8. Matsuda Y, Toma Y, Ogawa H, Matsuzazi M, Katayama K, Fujii T, Yoshino F, Moritani K, Kumada T, Kusukawa R (1983) Importance of left atrial function in patients with myocardial infarction. *Circ* 67:566–71
9. Braunwald E, Frahm CJ (1961) Studies on Starling's law of the heart. IV. Observations on the hemodynamic functions of the left atrium in man. *Circ* 24:633
10. Sasayama S, Takahashi M, Osakada G, Hirose K, Hamashima H, Nishiruma E, Kawai C (1979) Dynamic geometry of left atrium and left ventricle in acute mitral regurgitation. *Circ* 60:177–86
11. Kumada T, Karliner JS, Pouleur H, Gallagher KP, Shirato K, Ross J (1979) Effect of coronary occlusion on early ventricular diastolic events in conscious dogs. *Am J Physiol* 237(5):H542–49
12. Rousseau MF, Keriter C, Detry JMR, Brasseur L, Pouleur H (1980) Impaired left ventricular relaxation in coronary artery disease: effect of intracoronary Nifedipine. *Circ* 62:764–72

14. Left ventricular function during acute coronary artery balloon occlusion in humans

MICHEL E. BERTRAND, JEAN M. LABLANCHE, JEAN L. FOURRIER, ANTOINE GOMMEAUX and ISRAEL MIRSKY

Introduction

The acute changes in left ventricular function after coronary artery ligation have been described in numerous animal studies [1–6]. However, it is difficult to extrapolate these results to humans who have different coronary and collateral circulations [7] and where atherosclerotic coronary disease may influence the response.

The detection of ischemia-induced wall motion changes in humans has been limited to observations recorded after atrial pacing [8–10], exercise [11] or during the early stage of acute myocardial infarction [12–14]. These studies however, were conducted 2 to 10 days after the beginning of the symptoms and have not considered the immediate consequences of coronary occlusion.

Percutaneous transluminal coronary angioplasty offers the unique opportunity to study the sequential changes of left ventricular function during the transient occlusion of the vessel. As a consequence, several reports have been published concerning the modifications of myocardial relaxation [15] or coronary blood flow during percutaneous transluminal coronary angioplasty [16, 17]. Furthermore, the detection by two dimensional echocardiography of acute wall motion changes during coronary angioplasty, has been reported in recent studies [18, 19]. However, few studies have included the simultaneous recording of left ventricular pressure and left ventricular cineangiograms. Sigwart et al [20] described the abnormalities of relaxation and segmental wall motion. Serruys et al [21] reported the time course of changes during the transient interruption of coronary flow by the balloon occlusion and Wijns et al [22] recently reported the effect of acute occlusion on left ventricular chamber stiffness.

The aim of this study was to examine the possible changes in left ventricular diastolic and systolic function induced by coronary balloon occlusion in patients with single left anterior descending coronary artery disease but without angiographic evidence of collateral circulation. If dysfunction occurs, is left ventricular function restored to normal levels following coronary angioplasty?

P.W. Serruys, R. Simon & K.J. Beatt (eds), Percutaneous Transluminal Coronary Angioplasty. ISBN 0-7923-0346-6.
© *1990 Kluwer Academic Publishers, Dordrecht*

Methods

Patients. This study included 16 patients (15 males and one female) who underwent percutaneous transluminal coronary angioplasty of a proximal left anterior descending coronary artery narrowing. All patients experienced angina pain on effort and had no history of a previous myocardial infarction. All had single significant (>75%) vessel disease and normal left ventricular segmental wall motion. The diagnostic angiography showed no collateral circulation filling the distal left anterior descending artery.

Informed consent was given by all patients, and the day before the procedure, the patients received nifedipine 30 mg and aspirin 1 g. No drugs were given on the day of the procedure except heparin IV (10.000 IU–IV).

Study protocol. An 8F pigtail Millar micromanometer was introduced into the left ventricle from the left femoral route. The guiding catheter for the angioplasty was introduced from a right femoral approach. Left ventricular and aortic pressures were simultaneously recorded. A first left ventricular cineangiogram was performed in the 30° RAO projection and was obtained by injection of 0.5 ml/kg of sodium and meglumine amidotrizoate (Radioselectan). Left ventricular pressures and a frame-marker signal were recorded during cineangiography. Fifteen minutes later, the narrowing of the left anterior descending artery was crossed and dilated with a 3 mm balloon in 13 patients and a 3.5 mm balloon in 3 patients. Left ventricular and aortic pressures were recorded and a second left ventricular cineangiogram was performed during the first coronary balloon inflation. To examine the possible time-related abnormalities, patients were divided into two groups. Data were collected at 30 seconds after coronary occlusion in eight patients (group A). In a second group, balloon inflation was continued for 50 sec and left ventricular cineangiography and pressure measurements were obtained at that time (group B). All patients had ST segment elevation during the coronary occlusion and all had successful coronary angioplasty. In the group B patients, a third left venticular cineangiogram was performed and left ventricular and aortic pressures recorded fifteen minutes after completion of the procedure.

Data analysis. Left ventricular and aortic pressures were measured with a computer system (Syscomoran), Frame-by-frame left ventricular volumes and corresponding pressures were obtained simultaneously from early to end diastole. Left ventricular contours were detected with the aid of a 6502 microcomputer and left ventricular volumes were calculated according to the area length method and the formula of Kennedy et al [23]. Segmental wall motion was obtained by the radial method [24] using a center located at 69% of a line joining the upper edge of the aorta to the left ventricular apex in end systole. Nine radii were obtained in end diastole (ED) and end systole (ES) and for each, the segmental wall shortening (SWS) was calculated as SWS = 100.

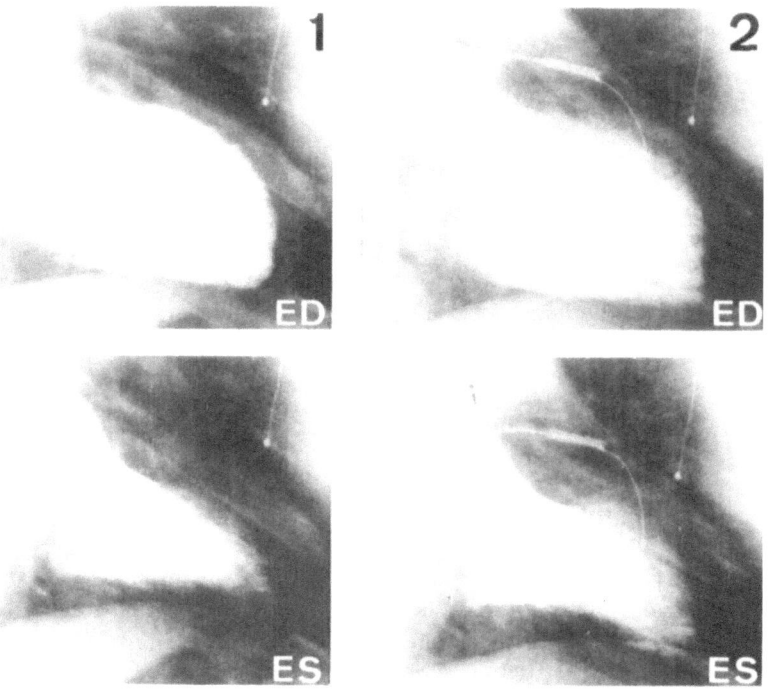

Figure 1. Left ventricular cineangiograms before and during coronary occlusion in end diastole (upper panel) and end systole (lower panel).

(ED − ES)/ED. Segments 1, 2, 3, 4 were related to the anterior wall. Segments 6, 7, 8, and 9 corresponded to the inferior wall and segment 5 was related to the apex.

Assessment of chamber and myocardial stiffness constants

Since chamber stiffness (dP/dV) depends on several factors including chamber size (V), myocardial stiffness (E), cavity volume/wall volume ratio (V/Vw) and external constraints, appropriate normalizations must be employed if comparisons between ventricles are to be made.

In Appendix 1, a rationale is provided for these appropriate normalizations in order to develop simple and clinically useful indices of chamber and myocardial stiffness. It is shown in Appendix 1 that normalization to wall volume Vw yields an index of chamber stiffness whereas normalization to cavity volume V, provides an index of myocardial stiffness.

Specifically, by curve-fitting the diastolic pressure-volume points from minimum pressure to end diastole in the forms

$$P = Ae^{\alpha(V/Vw)}; \qquad P = B\,V^{\beta};$$

we obtain

$$dP/(dV/Vw) = \alpha A e^{\alpha(V/Vw)} = \alpha P$$

and

$$dP/(dV/V) = \beta B V^{\beta} = \beta P.$$

Therefore, α (the slope of the $dP/(dV/Vw)$ vs P relation) and β (the slope of the $dP/(dV/V)$ vs P relation) may be employed as indices of chamber and myocardial stiffness respectively.

In Appendix 2, alternative methods are presented for the quantitation of global myocardial stiffness (E) and regional myocardial stiffness (Er) with the results

$$E = KDm(d\sigma/dDm) = k\sigma$$

and

$$Er = -dP/(dh/h) = \delta P$$

where K is a geometric factor, h is the left ventricular wall thickness and k, β, δ are indices of myocardial stiffness. It should be emphasized here that comparisons of chamber stiffness must be made at common levels of pressure and myocardial stiffness must be compared at common stress levels

Assessment of time constants of relaxation

The left ventricular pressure tracings were digitized from the point of peak negative dP/dt to the time at which pressure decreased to 5 mmHg above end diastolic pressure. The pressure-time data (P–t) were then curve-fitted in the forms

$$P = Ce^{-t/\tau w}; \qquad P = a + be^{-\gamma t}$$

where τ_W is the time constant as evaluated by the Weiss method (25) and $\tau_M = (1/\gamma) \log [eb/(a+b-ae)]$ is the time constant evaluated on the basis of a 3-constant curve-fit ([26] and Appendix 3).

Statistical analysis

All data were expressed as mean $\pm$ standard deviation. Paired t-tests were employed for patients in group A who were studied before and after 30 sec of coronary balloon occlusion. An analysis of variance was conducted in group B patients where 3 sequential measurements were made and the results obtained by the Bonferroni correction [27].

Results

No complications related to the angioplasty procedure were noted in any of the patients. Tables 1–4 summarize the hemodynamic data and diastolic function parameters for the patients of groups A, B.

Left ventricular pressures. Left ventricular and diastolic pressures (Tables 1, 3) were significantly increased ($p < 0.01$) at 30 sec of occlusion (group A) and in patients studied at 50 sec of occlusion (group B). The magnitudes of these increases were similar in both groups. However, little or no change was observed in peak left ventricular pressures.

Segmental wall motion. The visual analysis of the left ventricular cineangiogram clearly demonstrated a marked dyskinesia of the anterior and apical wall in all cases. Figures 2 and 3 show the important modifications occurring during total occlusion of the left anterior descending coronary artery: occlusion for only 30 sec resulted in a marked decrease of the anterior and anteroapical wall shortening with the appearance of a systolic outward displacement.

Table 1. Hemodynamic data in group A patients.

Case		LVEDP (mmHg)	LVEDVI (ml/m²)	LVESVI (ml/m²)	SVI (ml/m²)	EF (%)	Vw (ml)
1	Pre	21	83	24	58	70	211
	30 sec	27	91	47	44	48	
2	Pre	19	100	25	75	75	162
	30 sec	34	94	56	38	40	
3	Pre	25	93	24	69	74	287
	30 sec	32	99	56	33	33	
4	Pre	18	111	32	79	71	189
	30 sec	32	100	49	51	51	
5	Pre	34	93	23	70	75	173
	30 sec	46	116	78	38	32	
6	Pre	14	140	34	106	76	239
	30 sec	20	115	42	73	63	
7	Pre	6	72	13	58	81	111
	30 sec	34	93	50	43	45	
8	Pre	7	98	33	65	66	243
	30 sec	44	112	57	55	49	
Mean ± SD							
	Pre	18 ± 9	98 ± 20	26 ± 7	72 ± 15	73 ± 4	202 ± 55
	30 sec	33 ± 8*	102 ± 10	54 ± 11**	46 ± 12**	45 ± 10**	

*p < 0.01; **p < 0.001.
EF = ejection fraction; LVEDP = left ventricular end diastolic pressure; LVEDVI = left ventricular end diastolic volume index; LVESVI = left ventricular end systolic volume index; SVI = stroke index; Vw = left ventricular wall volume.

Table 2. Diastolic function parameters in group A patients.

Case		Myocardial stiffness constants			Chamber stiffness constant	Time constants of relaxation (msec)	
		k	δ	β	α	τ_W	τ_M
1	Pre	8.46	2.83	1.33	2.19	46.1	46.9
	30 sec	6.91	5.09	2.08	2.48	70.0	68.8
2	Pre	4.88	4.43	1.92	2.07	52.9	53.4
	30 sec	4.90	4.68	1.99	1.37	65.1	64.7
3	Pre	7.18	5.30	1.99	3.96	36.9	37.5
	30 sec	6.75	5.55	2.30	4.02	57.4	56.7
4	Pre	4.93	2.36	1.16	1.18	52.5	50.5
	30 sec	4.51	3.76	1.70	1.57	66.0	63.6
5	Pre	5.41	2.51	1.14	1.52	62.5	59.9
	30 sec	3.27	2.00	0.95	0.87	81.8	75.2
6	Pre	4.66	2.56	1.10	1.54	40.3	45.4
	30 sec	12.22	10.63	4.44	6.88	42.0	42.7
7[†]	Pre	6.05	2.62	3.06	1.62	43.6	49.0
	30 sec	6.17	3.43	2.05	1.73	92.7	88.8
8[†]	Pre	—	—	—	—	—	—
	30 sec	—	—	—	—	—	—
Mean ± SD							
	Pre	5.92	3.33	1.44	2.08	48.4	48.9
		±1.55	±1.23	±0.41	±1.00	± 9.4	± 7.6
	30 sec	6.43	5.29	2.24	2.87	63.7**	62.0*
		±3.16	±2.90	±1.17	±2.26	±13.3	±11.2

* $p < 0.025$; ** $p < 0.01$; † omitted from analysis.

β, δ, k = myocardial stiffness constants obtained from pressure-volume, pressure-thickness and stress-diameter relationships respectively; α = chamber stiffness constant obtained from pressure – V/Vw relation; τ_W, τ_M = time constants of relaxation obtained from 2 and 3-constant curve-fits respectively.

Left ventricular volumes and ejection fraction

Complete occlusion of the left anterior descending coronary artery resulted in a significant increase ($p < 0.001$) in end systolic volume index (ESVI) from 26 ± 7 to 54 ± 11 ml/m at 30 sec in group A (Table 1) and from 28 ± 10 to 56 ± 18 ml/m^2 in group B (Table 3). Left ventricular end diastolic volume index (EDVI) was slightly but insignificantly increased at 30 and 50 sec of occlusion. In both groups, a dramatic and significant decrease of stroke index and ejection fraction was noted ($p < 0.001$). Thus occlusion of left anterior descending coronary artery for 30 to 50 sec resulted in a marked depression of left ventricular systolic function.

Table 3. Hemodynamic data in group B patients.

Case		LVEDP (mmHg)	LVEDVI (ml/m²)	LVESVI (ml/m²)	SVI (ml/m²)	EF (%)	Vw (ml)
1	Pre	18	98	26	72	73	234
	50 sec	22	105	55	50	48	
	Post	19	111	20	91	82	
2	Pre	33	90	37	53	58	184
	50 sec	43	103	67	36	34	
	Post	27	93	37	56	60	
3	Pre	15	82	14	68	82	170
	50 sec	22	88	39	48	55	
	Post	19	85	13	72	84	
4	Pre	32	130	47	83	63	278
	50 sec	41	143	97	46	31	
	Post	24	130	63	67	51	
5	Pre	24	92	28	64	68	209
	50 sec	31	103	48	55	52	
	Post	26	115	27	88	76	
6†	Pre	18	92	20	70	77	205
	50 sec	36	102	50	52	50	
	Post	19	88	22	66	74	
7	Pre	20	100	25	75	75	204
	50 sec	36	109	46	63	57	
	Post	28	98	18	80	81	
8†	Pre	14	90	28	62	69	200
	50 sec	39	90	53	37	41	
	Post	8	79	23	56	71	
Mean ± SD							
	Pre	22 ± 7	97 ± 14	28 ± 10	68 ± 9	70 ± 7	211 ± 33
	50 sec	34 ± 7*	105 ± 16	56 ± 18**	48 ± 9**	46 ± 9**	
	Post	21 ± 6	99 ± 17	29 ± 15	72 ± 13	72 ± 11	

* $p < 0.01$; ** $p < 0.001$ (Pre vs 50 sec).
Abbreviations as in Table 1.

Time constants of relaxation (τ_W, τ_M)

The changes in time constants of relaxation are shown in Tables 2, 4. The occlusion of the left anterior descending coronary artery for 30 sec resulted in important and significant increases in τ_W from 48.5 ± 9.4 to 63.7 ± 13.3 ($p < 0.01$) and in τ_M from 48.9 ± 7.6 to 62.0 ± 11.2 ($p < 0.025$). The patients studied 50 sec after the onset of occlusion, also showed significant increases in these indices. The time constant τ_W increased from 43.4 ± 5.4 to 57.7 ± 10.5 ($p < 0.005$) and τ_M increased from 46.1 ± 7.5 to 59.2 ± 13.2 ($p < 0.03$). Both time constants returned to pre-occlusion levels 15 min after the procedure.

Table 4. Diastolic function parameters for group B patients.

Case		k	δ	β	α	τ_W	τ_M
		Myocardial stiffness constants			Chamber stiffness constant	Time constants of relaxation (msec)	
1	Pre	5.37	2.91	1.21	1.89	36.2	36.0
	50 sec	5.24	4.27	1.76	2.71	47.4	47.2
	Post	4.57	3.33	1.49	1.75	34.5	35.0
2	Pre	4.70	3.52	1.67	2.13	41.1	44.0
	50 sec	2.18	1.45	0.72	0.76	57.6	55.6
	Post	4.96	4.10	1.69	2.45	38.3	39.7
3	Pre	7.49	4.63	1.88	3.09	39.9	41.4
	50 sec	5.62	4.21	1.76	2.40	42.5	40.3
	Post	4.72	3.47	2.26	2.60	40.3	41.0
4	Pre	4.60	2.72	1.16	1.73	46.4	52.7
	50 sec	5.75	3.76	1.77	2.13	60.4	57.1
	Post	6.98	6.94	2.99	3.78	49.8	50.0
5	Pre	4.26	3.59	1.50	2.19	39.2	39.3
	50 sec	6.28	4.60	1.82	2.32	57.6	77.0
	Post	3.80	1.77	0.82	1.19	41.6	39.7
6[†]	Pre	3.63	3.18	1.26	1.92	46.1	46.2
	50 sec	8.59	5.85	2.69	3.36	54.7	54.2
	Post	—	—	—	—	39.9	42.0
7	Pre	2.46	1.35	0.52	0.92	53.2	58.3
	50 sec	3.83	2.53	1.05	1.52	76.9	77.3
	Post	2.35	1.55	0.59	1.00	54.1	58.5
8	Pre	6.36	6.60	2.70	4.02	45.4	50.9
	50 sec	4.42	2.86	1.28	1.77	64.4	65.1
	Post	3.82	3.67	1.30	2.54	41.1	44.1
Mean ± SD							
	Pre	5.03	3.62	1.52	2.28	43.4	46.1
		±1.60	±1.65	±0.68	±1.00	±5.4	±7.5
	50 sec	4.76	3.38	1.45	1.94	57.7*	59.2**
		±1.41	±1.14	±0.44	±0.66	±10.5	±13.2
	Post	4.46	3.55	1.59	2.19	42.5	43.8
		±1.41	±1.78	±0.83	±0.96	±6.4	±7.3

*$p < 0.005$, **$p < 0.03$ (pre vs 50 sec); † omitted from the statistical analysis of chamber and myocardial stiffness constant.
Abbreviations as in Table 2.

Chamber stiffness constant (α)

Since chamber stiffness must be compared at common levels of pressure, two patients from each group were excluded from the statistical analyses.

No significant alterations were observed in the chamber stiffness constant

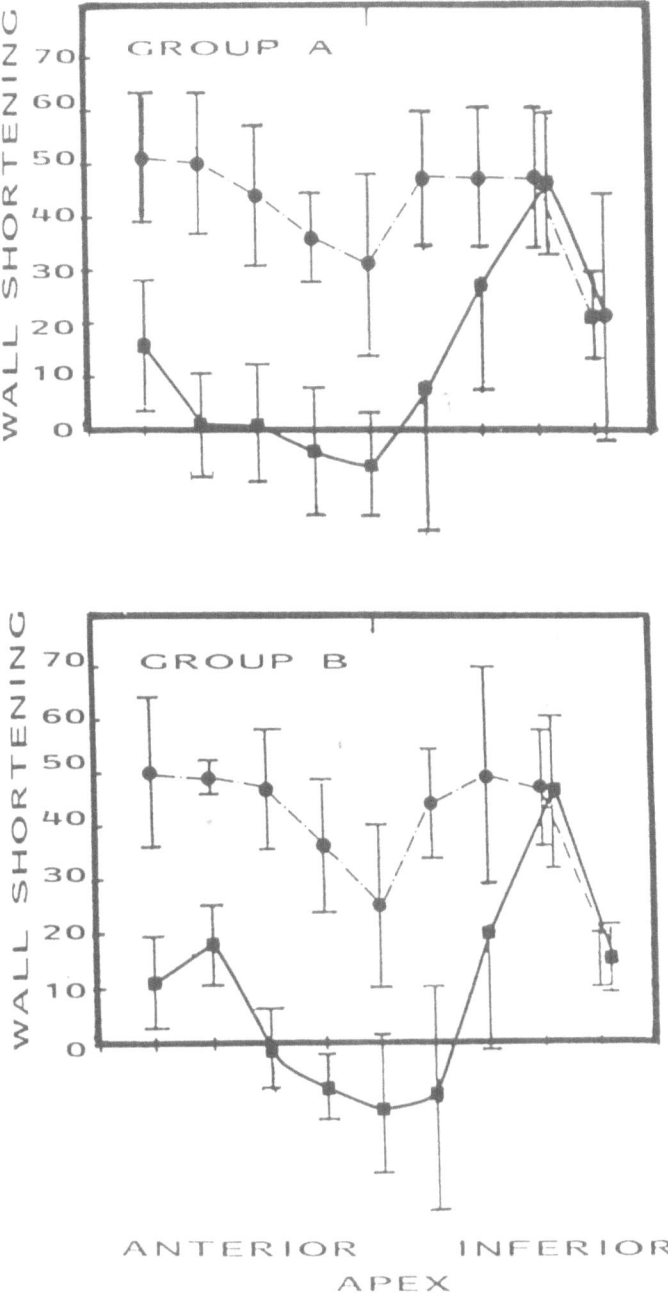

Figure 2. Radial wall motion in group A (upper panel) and in group B (low panel). Dashed lines: before occlusion. Continuous lines: During coronary occlusion.

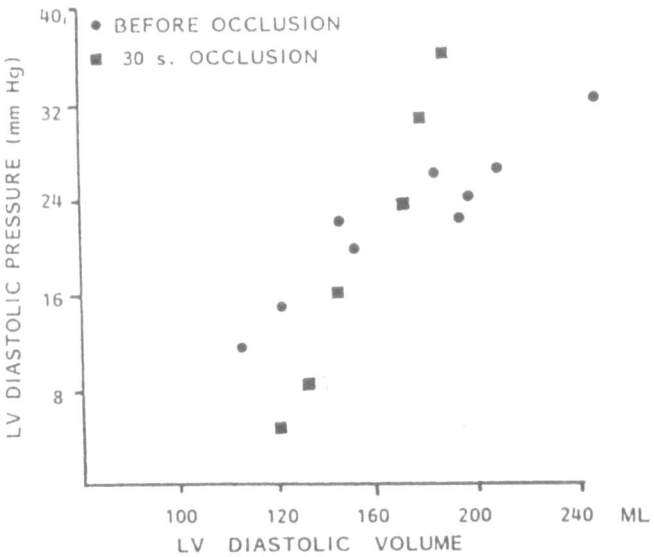

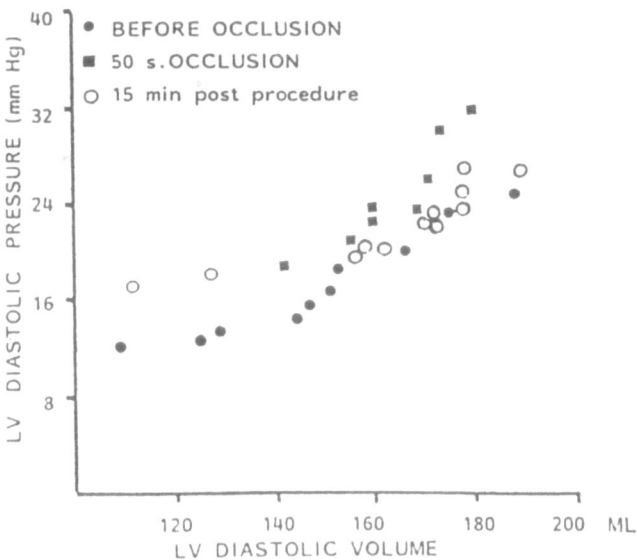

Figure 3.   Diastolic pressure-volume relations in a typical patient from each group. (A) Pressure-volume relation in a group A patient before (●) and 30 sec (■) of occlusion. (B) Pressure-volume relations in a group B patient before (●) occlusion, 50 sec of occlusion (■) and 15 min after completion of the angioplasty procedure (○). Note the upward shifts in these relationships following coronary occlusion. In group B the pressure-volume relations return to pre-occlusion levels, 15 min after the procedure.

following coronary occlusion at 30 and 50 sec although there was a tendency for an increase in the group A patients. In group A, the constant α increased from 2.08 ± 1.00 to 2.87 ± 2.26 after 30 sec and in group B after 50 sec there was no charge (pre: 2.8 ± 1.00; 50 sec: 1.94 ± 0.66). Fifteen minutes after the procedure in group B patients α remained within the pre-occlusion levels (2.19 ± 0.96).

Myocardial stiffness constants k, β, δ

The myocardial stiffness constants were evaluated by three different methods and each yielded the same qualitative results for each group. Again there were no significant alterations following coronary occlusion for 30 and 50 sec, however, the increases were more pronounced in group A (30 sec) than in group B (50 sec). Pre-occlusion levels were maintained 15 min following the procedure. The values for these constants are as follows:

		k	δ	β
Group A				
	pre	5.92 ± 1.55	3.33 ± 1.23	1.44 ± 0.41
	30 sec	6.43 ± 3.16	5.29 ± 2.90	2.24 ± 1.17
Group B				
	pre	5.03 ± 1.60	3.62 ± 1.65	1.52 ± 0.68
	50 sec	4.76 ± 1.41	3.38 ± 1.14	1.45 ± 0.44
	post	4.46 ± 1.41	3.55 ± 1.78	1.59 ± 0.83

Discussion

Left ventricular systolic and diastolic function are markedly affected shortly after occlusion of the left anterior descending coronary artery. Stroke volume and ejection fraction decreased, left ventricular end diastolic pressure increased and left ventricular relaxation was delayed. There was a tendency for both chamber and myocardial stiffness to increase indicating a reduction in left ventricular compliance, however, these changes were not statistically significant and the changes appeared to be more pronounced in the group A patients. Generally, these results were similar to those in previous animal studies [1–4], however, in coronary artery occlusion experiments, the pressure-segment length relationship has repeatedly been shown to move to the right. The present study involved patients with single vessel disease and significant narrowing of the proximal left anterior descending artery. Thus, interruption of coronary flow induced by transient balloon inflation during percutaneous transluminal coronary angioplasty, is a situation that completely mimics the experimental coronary artery ligation performed during animal studies.

The results of the present study agree in part qualitatively with those described by Serruys et al [21] and Wijns et al [22] namely (a) there were upward shifts in the diastolic pressure-volume relations immediately following the angioplasty procedure and (b) systolic function and the time constants of relaxation returned to near pre-occlusion levels 12–15 min after completion of the procedure. On the other hand, these investigators [22] showed that abnormalities in the chamber stiffness persisted 12 min after the procedure, a result not observed in the present study.

There may be several reasons for this disagreement. In their studies [22], pressure and angiographic measurements were obtained 20 sec during the second dilation and 50 sec during the fourth dilation. The interval between two sequential angiograms was at least 10 min, and one cannot exclude the possible influence of contrast medium in these consecutive examinations. Moreover, immediate collateral circulation may occur after a first coronary occlusion. In the present study, all measurements at 30 and 50 sec were done during the first balloon inflation. Another possible explanation for these differences may reside in the different methods employed for the assessment of chamber stiffness. Global stiffness was analyzed in this study and not regional chamber stiffness. However, the earlier studies [22] considered parameters of chamber stiffness which were size dependent and comparisons were not always conducted over common pressure ranges.

After 30 or 50 sec of coronary occlusion, left ventricular systolic function is dramatically depressed with a marked decrease of the ejection fraction due to an increase in end systolic volume. This is clearly related to the large ischemic area as demonstrated by the depression of wall motion shortening which affected specifically the anterior and apical segments. In both groups, a systolic outward displacement of the ischemic segment was observed. Serruys et al [21] showed that the moment of maximal wall displacement for the anterior wall shifted from end systole to early diastole. This late systolic outward displacement of the ischemic segment is probably passive and could be due to the increased inward displacement of the non-ischemic segments. This is similar to the results obtained by Tyberg et al [28] who described the relationship between transient asynergy, myocardial ischemia and alteration in the course of relaxation, and observed that the prolongation of this parameter was seen only upon re-oxygenation. In man, the prolongation of the time constant of the early relaxation phase, is the earliest hemodynamic marker of myocardial ischemia. In both series of patients, marked increases were observed in the time constants of relaxation τ_W, τ_M. By a careful analysis of the left ventricular cineangiogram, Serruys et al [21] showed that these changes accompanied a biphasic wall displacement of the ischemic area after aortic valve closure. The deformation occurring in the ascending limb of the negative dP/dt tracing (Fig. 1) occurred simultaneously with the beginning of the second wave of inward displacement. It should be noted however, that after 50 sec of occlusion (group B), the deformation of peak negative dP/dt generally disappeared.

Indices of chamber and myocardial stiffness employed in this study are dimensionless and therefore are more appropriate for comparison purposes. This has generally not been the case in most previous studies relating to the assessment of chamber stiffness in particular. This fact in addition to the dependence of chamber stiffness on a number of important factors, is the main reason for the difficulty in developing useful and sensitive indices of stiffness that may be applied in the clinical setting.

Although three approaches were employed here for the assessment of myocardial stiffness, these indices also have their limitations. The stiffness constants k and β describe global stiffness and may not be valid in cases of segmental disease as considered in the present study. On the other hand, the radial stiffness constant δ does more closely represent a regional stiffness parameter. However, the possibility exists that pericardial pressure may have been elevated during these procedures and were not accounted for in these or the earlier studies [21, 22]. Thus future studies should include measurements of right atrial pressures [29] enabling one to consider in a semi-quantitative manner, these pericardial effects.

The results of the present studies and those of Serruys and associates [21, 22] have important clinical implications since changes in left ventricular systolic and diastolic function were observed as early as 30 or 50 sec after coronary occlusion. Generally diastolic parameters returned to pre-occlusion values, however, there may be a subset of patients in whom dysfunction persists after completion of the angioplasty procedure. Many more studies therefore need to be conducted and more sophisticated methods for analyzing chamber and myocardial stiffness need to be developed along the lines described by Pasipoularides et al [30].

Appendix 1: Rationale for the development of simple indices of chamber and myocardial stiffness

Employing the theory of elasticity and assuming a spherical geometry for the left ventricle [31], chamber stiffness may be expressed in the form

$$dP/dV = [(4/9) Es - P(V/Vw)]/V(1 + V/Vw).$$

where Es = myocardial stiffness, Vw = left ventricular wall volume, P = the left ventricular diastolic cavity pressure and V = the left ventricular cavity volume.

Normalizing chamber stiffness to Vw, we obtain

$$dP/(dV/Vw) = [(4/9) Es - P(V/Vw)]/(1 + V/Vw)(V/Vw).$$

This parameter is predominantly a function of pressure and the V/Vw ratio and suggests that the dP/(dV/Vw) vs P relation may provide an appropriate index for chamber stiffness.

Normalizing chamber stiffness to the volume V yields

$$dP/(dV/V) = [(4/9) Es - P(V/Vw)]/(1 + V/Vw).$$

This parameter is dominated by myocardial stiffness Es and the dP/(dV/V) vs

P relation may yield an index of myocardial stiffness.

In particular, curve-fitting the pressure-volume data in the forms

$$P = Ae^{\alpha(V/Vw)}; \qquad P = BV^{\beta},$$

we obtain

$$dP/(dV/Vw) = \alpha Ae^{\alpha(V/Vw)} = \alpha P$$

and

$$dP/(dV/V) = \beta BV^{\beta} = \beta P.$$

Thus α and β may be employed as indices of chamber and myocardial stiffness respectively.

Appendix 2: Alternative evaluation of myocardial stiffness constants

Two additional methods for assessing myocardial stiffness are outlined here:

Method 1: Incremental modulus – stress relation

From earlier studies [32], the incremental modulus is given by

$$Einc = (3/2)Dm(d\sigma/dDm)/(2 + Dm^2/Lm^2)ave$$

where

$$\sigma = \sigma_{\theta} - \sigma_{r}$$
$$= P[1 + DL/H(L + D + 2H)]$$

is the difference in circumferential and radial global average stress.

The quantities D and L are respectively the short and long axes of an ellipsoid of revolution, which is the assumed geometry for the left ventricle.

If the stress – diameter ($\sigma - Dm$) data are curve-fit in the form $\sigma = A_d Dm^c$ one obtains

$$Einc = (3/2) \subset Dm(A_d Dm^{c-1})/(2 + Dm^2/Lm^2)ave$$
$$= (3/2) \subset (A_d Dm^c)/(2 + Dm^2/Lm^2)ave$$
$$= K \subset (A_d Dm^c) = K \subset \sigma = k\sigma$$

where $k = (3/2) \subset /(2 + Dm^2/Lm^2)ave$.

The parameter k is the slope of the stiffness vs stress relation and represents an index of circumferential myocardial stiffness.

Method 2: Radial myocardial stiffness

This method has been employed with moderate success in studies on pacing-induced angina in man [33]. Radial myocardial stiffness Er is defined by

$Er = -h(dP/dh)$ where P is the diastolic left ventricular pressure and h is the left ventricular wall thickness. Curve-fitting the pressure-thickness data $(P-h)$ in the form $P = A_h h^{-\delta}$ one obtains $Er = -h(-\delta A_h h^{-\delta-1}) = (A_h h^{-\delta})\delta = \delta P$. Hence δ (the slope of the radial stiffness-pressure relation may be employed as an index of radial myocardial stiffness.

Appendix 3: Evaluation of the time constant τ_M

The pressure-time data from peak negative dP/dt to the time at which pressure decreased to 5 mmHg above end diastolic pressure, were curve-fitted in the form

$$P = a + be^{-\gamma t} \tag{1}$$

where a, b and γ are regression coefficients.

At time $t = 0$ (time of peak negative dP/dt), the pressure P_0 is given by

$$P_0 = a + b. \tag{2}$$

Now τ_M is defined as the time required for P_0 to be reduced by the factor $1/e$ where e is the base of the natural logarithm. Hence τ_M is represented by the relation

$$P_0/e = a + be^{-\gamma\tau_M} \quad \text{(using (1))}$$
$$= (a+b)/e \quad \text{(employing (2))}$$

i.e.

$$e^{-\gamma\tau_M} = [(a+b)/e - a]/b$$
$$= (a+b-ae)/eb.$$

Taking the logarithm of both sides, this yields

$$-\gamma\tau_M = \log[(a+b-ae)/eb]$$

or

$$\tau_M = (1/\gamma) \log[eb/(a+b-ae)]$$

which is the desired result.

References

1. Theroux P, Ross J Jr, Franklin D, Kemper WS, Sasayama S (1976) Regional myocardial function in the conscious dog during acute coronary occlusion and response to morphine, propranolol, nitroglycerine and lidocaine. *Circulation* 53:302–14
2. Heyndrickxs GR, Millard RW, Mc Ritchie RJ, Maroko PR, Vatner SF (1975) Regional myocardial function and electrophysiological alterations after brief coronary artery occlusion in conscious dogs. *J Clin Invest* 56:978–86
3. Pagani M, Vatner SF, Baig H, Braunwald E (1978) Adjustments to brief periods of ischemia and reperfusion in the conscious dog. *Circ Res* 43:83–91
4. Kumada T, Karliner JS, Pouleur H, Gallagher KP, Shirato K, Ross J Jr (1979) Effects of coronary occlusion on early ventricular diastolic events in conscious dogs. *Am J Physiol* 237:H542–9

5. Gaasch WH, Bernard SA (1977) The effects of acute changes in coronary blood flow on left ventricular diastolic wall thickness. An echocardiographic study. *Circulation* 56:593-7

6. Forrester JS, Wyatt HL, Da Luz PL, Tyberg JV, Diamond GA, Swan HJC (1976) Functional significance of regional ischemic contraction abnormalities. *Circulation* 54:64-70

7. Gensini GG, Da Costa BCG (1969) The coronary collateral circulation in living man. *Am J Cardiol* 24:393-400

8. Dwyer EM Jr (1970) Left ventricular pressure. Volume alterations and regional disorders of contraction during myocardial ischemia induced by atrial pacing. *Circulation* 42:1111-1122

9. Mc Laurin LP, Rolett EL, Grossman (1973) Impaired left ventricular relaxation during pacing-induced ischemia. *Am J Cardiol* 32:751-757

10. Barry WH, Brooker JZ, Alderman EL, Harrison DC (1974) Changes in diastolic stiffness and tone of the left ventricle during angina pectoris. *Circulation* 49:255-263

11. Carroll JD, Hess OM, Hirzel HO, Krayenbuehl HP (1983) Exercise induced ischemia: the influence of altered relaxation on early diastolic pressures. *Circulation* 67:521-527

12. Bleifeld W, Mathey D, Hanrath P (1974) Acute myocardial infarction, VI: Left ventricular wall thickness in the acute phase and in the convalescent phase. *Eur J Cardiol* 2:191-198

13. Bertrand ME, Rousseau MF, Lefebvre JM, Lablanche JM, Asseman PH, Carre AG, Lekieffre JP (1978) Left ventricular compliance in acute transmural myocardial infarction. *Eur J Cardiol* 7:179-193

14. Bertrand ME, Rousseau MF, Lablanche JM, Carre AG, Lekieffre JP (1979) Cineangiographic assessment of left ventricular function in the acute phase of transmural myocardial infarction. *Am J Cardiol* 43:472-480

15. Bertrand ME, Lablanche JM, Thieuleux FA (1983) Changes in left ventricular relaxation during transient coronary occlusion in man. *Eur Heart J* 4 (Suppl E): 49

16. Feldman RL, Conti R, Pepine CJ (1983) Regional coronary venous flow responses to transient coronary artery occlusion in human beings. *J Am Coll Cardiol* 2:1-10

17. Rothman MT, Baim DS, Simpson JB, Harrison DC (1982) Coronary hemodynamics during percutaneous transluminal coronary angioplasty. *Am J Cardiol* 49:1615-1622

18. Hauser AM, Vellappilil G, Ramos RG, Gordon S, Timmis GC (1985) Sequence of mechanical electrocardiographic and clinical effects of repeated coronary artery occlusion in human beings. *J Am Coll Cardiol* 5:193-197

19. Das SK, Serruys PW, Van Den Brand M, Domenicucci S, Vletter WB, Roelandt J (1983) Acute echocardiographic changes during percutaneous coronary angioplasty and their relationship to coronary blood flow. *J Cardiovasc Ultrasonogr* 2:269-271

20. Sigwart V, Orbic M, Essinger A, Fisher A, Morin D, Sadeghi H (1982) Myocardial function in man during acute coronary balloon occlusion (abstr). *Circulation* 66 (Suppl II): 86

21. Serruys PW, Wijns W, Van Der Brand M et al (1984) Left ventricular performance, regional blood flow, wall motion and lactate metabolism during transluminal angioplasty. *Circulation* 70:25-36

22. Wijns W, Serruys PW, Slager C et al (1986) Effect of coronary occlusion during percutaneous transluminal angioplasty in humans on left ventricular chamber stiffness and regional diastolic pressure-radius relations. *J Am Coll Cardiol* 7:455-463

23. Kennedy JW, Trendholme SE, Kasser IS (1970) Left ventricular volume and mass from single plane cineangiogram. A comparison of anteroposterior and right anterior oblique methods. *Am Heart J* 80:343-350

24. Ingels N, Daughters G, Stinson E, Alderman E (1980) Evaluation of methods for quantitating left ventricular segmental wall motion in man using myocardial markers as a standard *Circulation* 61:966-972

25. Weiss JL, Fredericksen JW, Weisfeldt ML (1978) Hemodynamic determinants of the time course of fall in canine left ventricular pressure. *J Clin Invest* 58:751-760

26. Mirsky I (1984) Assessment of diastolic function: Suggested methods and future considerations. *Circulation* 69:836-841

27. Gill JL (1978) *Design and analysis of experiments in the animal and medical sciences*, pp 72-5. Vol 3. Ames, Iowa, Iowa State University Press

28. Tyberg JV, Parmley WW, Sonnenblick EH (1969) In vitro studies of myocardial asynchrony and regional hypoxia. *Circ Res* 25:569–579
29. Tyberg JV, Taichman GC, Smith ER, Douglas NWS, Smiseth OA Keon WJ (1986) The relationship between pericardial pressure and right atrial pressure: an intraoperative study. *Circulation* 73:428–432.
30. Pasipoularides A, Mirsky I, Hess OM, Grimm J, Krayenbuehl HP (1986) Myocardial relaxation and passive diastolic properties in man. *Circulation* 74:991–1001
31. Mirsky I, Pfeffer JM, Pfeffer MA, Braunwald E (1983) The contractile state as the major determinant in the evolution of left ventricular dysfunction in the spontaneously hypertensive rat. *Circ Res* 53:767–778
32. Mirsky I, Rankin JS (1979) The effects of geometry, elasticity and external pressures on the diastolic pressure-volume and stiffness-stress relations. How important is the pericardium? *Circ Res* 44:601–612
33. Bourdillon PD, Lorell BH, Mirsky I, Paulus WJ, Wynne J, Grossman W (1983) Increased regional myocardial stiffness of the left ventricle during pacing-induced angina in man. *Circulation* 67:316–323

15. Use of intravenous DSA in the assessment of LV performance during PTCA

MICHAEL S. NORELL and RAPHAEL BALCON

Introduction

PTCA has provided a unique opportunity to study episodes of reversible myocardial ischaemia in man [1]. Although the surface ECG is routinely used in most laboratories to monitor ischaemia during PTCA it has become clear that examination of LV performance is a more sensitive method with which to assess the transient ischaemic changes that occur during balloon coronary occlusion [2].

Previous studies have reported the use of echocardiography [3–6] or direct cine ventriculography [7–9] during PTCA but both of these techniques have limitations during the angioplasty procedure. Echocardiography, although valuable for continuous monitoring and repeated studies, is heavily reliant on patient suitability and images satisfactory for detailed quantitative analysis cannot be obtained in all patients [5, 6]. This disadvantage is avoided with cine ventriculography but this requires a second arterial catheter which increases the invasive nature of the PTCA procedure.

Intravenous DSA has been shown to produce left ventriculograms suitable for quantitative analysis [10–12]. We have used this technique to evaluate LV performance during PTCA [2] and have reviewed our experience of this method for the examination of LV abnormalities that occur during balloon inflation and their relationship to accompanying ECG changes.

Patients

We have studied 52 patients with stable angina who were undergoing elective single vessel PTCA. 45 were male and 7 female, and their mean age was 53 yr (range 39–73). Their regular antianginal medication, which included nitrates, calcium antagonists and beta adrenergic blocking agents, was continued and all had shown ECG evidence of myocardial ischaemia on exercise prior to PTCA.

P.W. Serruys, R. Simon & K.J. Beatt (eds), Percutaneous Transluminal Coronary Angioplasty. ISBN 0-7923-0346-6.
© *1990 Kluwer Academic Publishers, Dordrecht*

Coronary anatomy. 37 patients had single vessel disease (> 70% luminal narrowing), 12 had 2 vessel disease and 3 had 3 vessel disease. In no case was the target vessel occluded (mean stenosis severity = 92%, range 60%–99%). 35 patients had no collateral filling of the arterial segment distal to the target stenosis. In the remaining 17 patients the collateral supply was graded (0–3) according to the extent of retrograde opacification during diagnostic arteriography, using a previously described method [13]. The mean collateral grade was 1.8.

Methods

PTCA procedure. All patients were premedicated with a nitrate and calcium antagonist together with lorazepam or intramuscular papaveretum. PTCA was for LAD stenosis in 37 patients (including 2 with diagonal artery dilatations), right coronary stenosis in 7 and circumflex stenosis in the remaining 8 patients. A mean of 5 balloon inflations per patient were employed (range 2–12) at 8 atmospheres (range 5–12 atm) for 57 secs (range 15–95 sec). The mean total duration of balloon inflation was 162 sec.

ECG monitoring. The standard 12 ECG leads were monitored throughout the procedure. Medicotest (A-50-VS, Cambac) electrodes were used that did not interfere with fluoroscopy. The maximum ST segment alteration (> 1 mm) in any lead was recorded. Mean R wave amplitude was also documented, R wave height in leads V4 to V6 being recorded for 10 consecutive complexes, to allow for respiratory variation.

DSA protocol and analysis. Intravenous digital subtraction ventriculography was performed before and during balloon inflation, and after the PTCA procedure (< 15 min) on 37 patients. The majority of the patients were studied during the third inflation, after 20 sec (28 patients) or after 60 sec (24 patients) of balloon coronary occlusion.

Digital left ventriculograms were acquired following right atrial injection of 40 ml of non-ionic contrast medium (Omnipaque, Nycomed) at 17 ml/sec via a 5 Fr pigtail catheter (Superflow, Cordis) introduced from the right femoral vein. Five to 8 sec were allowed for transit of the contrast bolus through the pulmonary circulation and ventriculograms then obtained in held inspiration in a 30 degree right anterior oblique projecton. Images were acquired at 12.5 frames/sec onto a 256 × 256 pixel matrix using a Siemens Digitron connected online to a Siemens Elema Angioskop D imaging system. Digital informaton was then transferred onto hard disk and then to magnetic tape for later recall and analysis.

End diastolic and end systolic frames were identified and outlined. An area -length method was used for calculation of LV volumes [14] and thereby ejection fraction derived. A previously published method was used to quantify regional wall motion [15] that required the translation of end diastolic and end systolic outlines so that the midpoint of the aortic valve planes were superimposed.

A series of radii were constructed in a clock wise sweep every 8 degrees from the geometric centre of gravity of the end systolic frame to the end diastolic perimeter (Fig 1.). The percentage systolic shortening of each radius was determined and represented on a wall motion plot (Fig. 2). Shortening of radii in each of 5 LV regions were then averaged to give percentage regional shortening. This method of wall motion analysis was felt to be superior to a centre-line method as it did not require the localisation of the LV apex. This can prove difficult in patients with contraction abnormalities in which the apex may become distorted.

Results

Images satisfactory for analysis were obtained in all patients. The only complications of the ventriculographic procedure were transient arrhythmias in

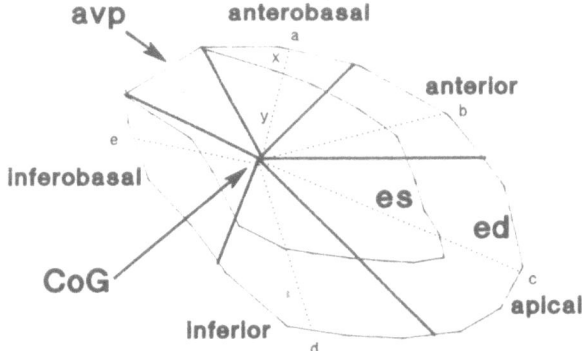

Figure 1. Schematic representation of wall motion analysis method. Sample radii (a–e) are shown for each LV segment. Percentage segmental shortening (e.g. radius a) $= x/x + y \times 100$. CoG $=$ Centre of Gravity of end systolic outline (es); ed $=$ end diastolic outline; avp $=$ aortic valve plane.

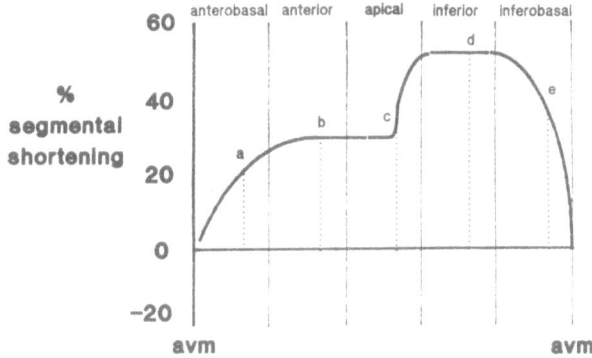

Figure 2. Wall motion plot of percentage shortening of each radius (examples a–e are shown). avm $=$ aortic valve margin.

three patients that occurred during contrast injection. These episodes were shortlived and did not interfere with image analysis.

LV Ejection fraction during PTCA. LV ejection fraction (EF) before PTCA was 73% (mean, range 51%–90%). Regional wall motion (Table 1) for each of the 5 LV segments examined was within a normal range derived in our laboratory from 10 patients with normal LV contraction.

During balloon inflation LVEF decreased by at least 5% in all but one patient (mean fall 73% to 57%, p < 0.001). The fall in LVEF was similar in patients studied during the third inflation compared with those studied during subsequent dilatations. In patients undergoing LAD PTCA the fall in LVEF (19%) was of greater magnitude than that in those having either right (10%, p < 0.05) or circumflex dilatation (8%, p < 0.01).

Regional LV wall motion during PTCA (Table 2). LAD balloon inflation produced reduction in regional shortening of anterobasal, anterior and apical segments (Fig 3). In addition we observed an increase in inferobasal shortening. In contrast right coronary dilation produced abnormalities confined to the inferior and apical segments (Fig 4). Circumflex inflation did not produce a significant change in wall motion in any segment. In the two patients having diagonal PTCA anterior and apical contraction was impaired with an associated increase in inferobasal shortening.

ST segment alteration during PTCA. 32 patients developd ST elevation (mean 3.9 mm) during balloon inflation while 25 developed ST depression (mean 1.9 mm), 24 producing both abnormalities. The fall in LVEF was greater in those with ST elevation than in those without (21% vs 9%; p < 0.001). Furthermore there was a positive correlation between the fall in LVEF and the magnitude of both ST elevation (r = 0.637; p < 0.001) and ST depression (r = 0.396; p < 0.01).

Table 1.   Left ventricular segmental shortening before PTCA.

LV segment	Regional shortening	Normal range
Anterobasal	35 (12)	28–40
Anterior	36 (13)	30–45
Apical	46 (16)	42–62
Inferior	47 (13)	40–58
Inferobasal	8 (13)	0–20

Values = % regional shortening (SD)
LV = left ventricular

Table 2. Percent shortening of left ventricular segments before and during PTCA in patients undergoing left anterior descending, right and circumflex dilatation.

LV seg-ment	LAD (35 patients)			RCA (7 patients)			LCX (8 patients)		
	Pre-PTCA	During PTCA	p	Pre-PTCA	During PTCA	p	Pre PTCA	During PTCA	p
AB	37% (10)	28% (15)	<0.002	33% (14)	30% (12)	NS	27% (15)	22% (14)	NS
A	39 (11)	13 (18)	<0.001	38 (14)	34 (12)	NS	25 (18)	19 (25)	NS
AP	50 (14)	14 (19)	<0.001	44 (19)	38 (20)	<0.02	37 (20)	27 (26)	NS
I	48 (13)	46 (14)	NS	43 (17)	24 (18)	<0.01	52 (11)	41 (14)	NS
IB	8 (13)	25 (17)	<0.001	7 (11)	0 (14)	NS	10 (18)	8 (20)	NS

Values = mean % (SD). AB = Anterobasal; A = Anterior; AP = Apical; I = Inferior; IB = Inferobasal; LV = left ventricular; LAD = left anterior descending; RCA = right coronary artery; LCX = circumflex.

PTCA in single and multivessel disease. Control LVEF was higher in the 37 patients with single vessel disease (75%) than in the 15 with multivessel disease (68%; p < 0.02). During balloon inflation however the fall in LVEF was similar in both groups (16% vs 17% respectively, NS). Similarly the magnitude of ST alteration was no different between these two groups (ST elevation 2.4 mm vs 2.3 mm, NS; ST depression 0.8 mm vs 1.2 mm, NS). In order to assess regional wall motion in these groups we examined only the 35 patients having LAD PTCA (Table 3). There were no differences in segmental contraction between the 27 patients with single vessel disease and the 8 with multivessel disease.

PTCA using 20 or 60 sec balloon inflation. 28 patients were studied after 20 sec of balloon coronary occlusion. Their fall in LVEF (16%) was no different to that seen in the 24 patients studied after 60 sec (15%, NS). Similarly the magnitude of ST deviation was no different between these 2 groups (ST elevation 2.9 mm vs 1.7 mm, NS; ST depression 0.9 mm vs 0.9 mm, NS respectively).

In order to compare differing duration of balloon inflation on regional wall motion we selected only the 27 patients with single vessel disease undergoing LAD PTCA (Table 4). In this group there were no differences in segmental contraction between the 17 patients studied after 20 sec and the 10 patients studied after 60 sec, with the exception of the inferobasal segment. Shortening of this region was enhanced in those examined later in comparison to those studied at an earlier stage of coronary balloon occlusion (37% vs 17% respectively, p < 0.01).

PTCA and LV volumes. The controlled variation in LV volume as a result of

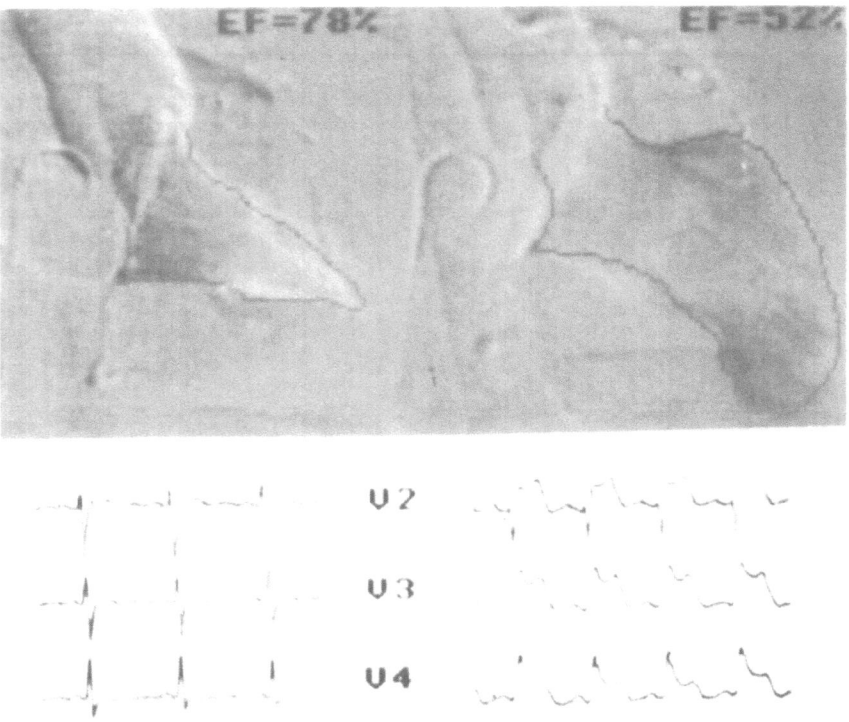

Figure 3. Left ventricular end systolic images, and ECG before (left) and during (right) LAD balloon inflation. Reduction in anteroapical shortening is associated with anterior ST elevation and a reduction in ejection fraction (EF) from 78% to 52%.
Reproduced with kind permission from the British Heart Journal.

ischaemia during balloon inflation allowed us to relate this phenomenon to alteration in ECG R wave amplitude, itself considered to reflect LV volume changes [16]. Thirty patients were examined whose mean control end diastolic and end systolic volumes were 140 ml and 44 ml respectively, and whose mean R wave amplitude was 10.1 mm. During balloon inflation there was an insignificant increase in end diastolic volume of 6% to 148 ml while end systolic volume increased by 73% to 76 ml (p < 0.001). In contrast, R wave amplitude decreased to 8.9 mm (p < 0.001) and there was thus an inverse correlation between this fall and the increase in end systolic volume (r = −0.371; p < 0.05).

PTCA in the presence of collateral supply. 27 patients with single vessel disease undergoing LAD PTCA were studied in order to determine the extent to which the presence collateral vessels on diagnostic arteriography prior to PTCA might influence LV ischaemia during balloon inflation. In this group 12 patients had some degree of collateral supply (mean grade = 1.7) while the remaining 15 had no

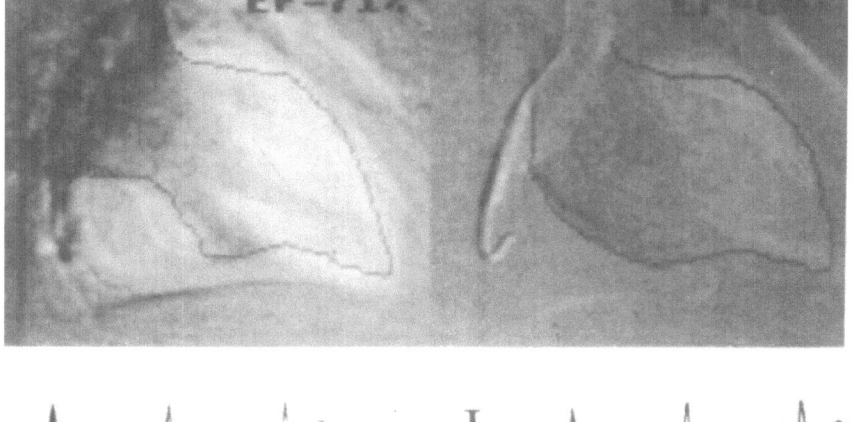

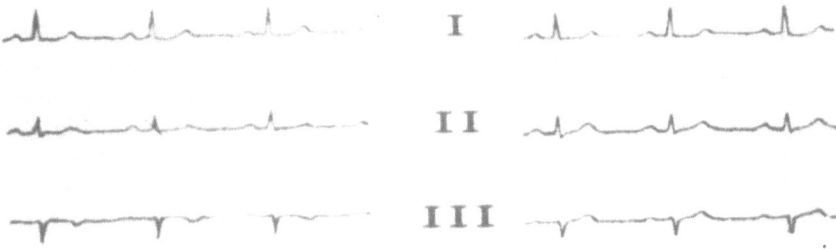

Figure 4. Left ventricular end systolic images and ECG before (left) and during (right) right coronary artery balloon inflation. Reduction in inferobasal shortening is associated with normalisation of a previously inverted T wave in lead III and reduction in ejection fraction (EF) from 71% to 60%.
Reproduced with kind permission from the British Heart Journal.

Table 3. Left ventricular segmental contraction before and during left anterior descending PTCA in patients with single (n = 27) and multivessel disease (n = 8).

LV segment	Pre-PTCA			During PTCA		
	SVD	MVD	p	SVD	MVD	p
Anterobasal	37	36	NS	28	30	NS
	(10)	(11)		(15)	(15)	
Anterior	40	36	NS	15	8	NS
	(10)	(13)		(18)	(16)	
Apical	53	39	NS	17	3	NS
	(10)	(20)		(19)	(13)	
Inferior	48	47	NS	47	43	NS
	(14)	(7)		(14)	(12)	
Inferobasal	7	13	NS	25	24	NS
	(12)	(14)		(20)	(7)	

Values = mean % shortening (SD).
SVD = single vessel disease; MVD = multivessel disease; LV = left ventricular.

Table 4. Effect on LV regional wall motion of 20 (17 pts) or 60 sec (10 pts) balloon inflations.

LV segment	Pre-PTCA			During PTCA		
	20	60	p	20	60	p
Anterobasal	38	36	NS	27	29	NS
	(10)	(9)		(15)	(17)	
Anterior	38	42	NS	17	12	NS
	(11)	(8)		(18)	(19)	
Apical	51	56	NS	19	14	NS
	(11)	(9)		(19)	(21)	
Inferior	45	54	NS	45	51	NS
	(14)	(12)		(12)	(18)	
Inferobasal	4	11	NS	17	37	<0.01
	(9)	(17)		(15)	(20)	

Values = mean % regional shortening (SD).

visible collateral vessels. Control LVEF was similar in the 2 groups (78% vs 74% respectively, NS). During balloon inflation the decrease in LVEF was less in those patients with collaterals (12%) compared to those without (23%, p < 0.01). Using Spearman's rank correlation we also demonstrated an inverse relationship between the fall in LVEF and the grade of collateral supply (r = − 0.446; p < 0.01; Fig 5). ECG changes during balloon inflation were also less marked in patients with collateral vessels. The degree of ST elevation and depression was less in patients with collateral supply (0.9 mm and 0.4 mm respectively) than in those without (4.9 mm, p < 0.001 and 1.4 mm, p < 0.02). As with LVEF there was an inverse correlation between the collateral grade and the degree of both ST elevation (r = − 0.680, p < 0.001; Fig 6) and ST depression (r = − 0.444, p < 0.01).

There was also a difference in regional shortening during PTCA between these 2 groups with apical contraction being better preserved in patients with collaterals than in those without (Table 5).

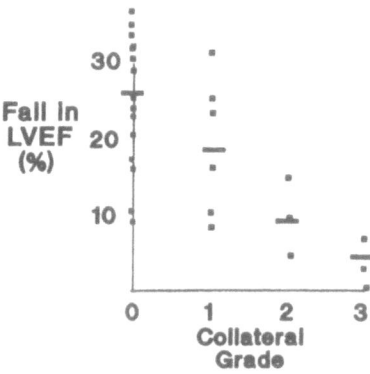

Figure 5. Inverse relationship between the fall in LV ejection fraction (EF) during PTCA and collateral supply (Spearman's rank correlaton). n = 27; r = − 0.446; p < 0.01.

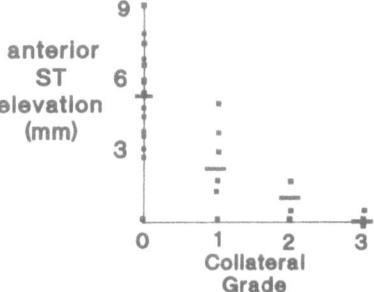

Figure 6. Inverse relationship between degree of anterior ST segment elevation during PTCA and collateral supply (Spearman's rank correlation). n = 27; r = −0.680; p < 0.001.

LV performance after PTCA (Table 6). 37 patients underwent intravenous digital subtraction ventriculography within 15 min of the end of the PTCA procedure. Both LVEF and regional wall motion were similar to that before PTCA.

Discussion

Use of intravenous DSA. We have found intravenous DSA a useful method with which to study LV performance during PTCA. We routinely insert a venous sheath into the femoral vein prior to PTCA and therefore introducing a pigtail catheter into the right atrium from this access did not increase the invasive nature of the procedure. Complications as a result of contrast injection were minor and transient and the use of a non-ionic contrast medium enabled us to acquire three ventriculograms in the majority of our patients.

Table 5. Comparison of % LV regional shortening before and during anterior descending angioplasty in patients without (group 1, n = 15) and with (group 2, n = 12) collateral vessels.

LV segment	Pre-PTCA			During PTCA		
	Group 1	Group 2	p	Group 1	Group 2	p
Anterobasal	37	38	NS	24	33	NS
	(9)	(11)		(13)	(17)	
Anterior	38	42	NS	12	19	NS
	(9)	(11)		(11)	(24)	
Apical	51	55	NS	11	26	<0.05
	(8)	(12)		(14)	(22)	
Inferior	48	48	NS	43	53	NS
	(13)	(15)		(14)	(13)	
Inferobasal	8	5	NS	23	27	NS
	(11)	(14)		(17)	(23)	

Values = mean % shortening (SD).
LV = Left ventricular; PTCA = Coronary Angioplasty.

Table 6. Left ventricular ejection fraction and segmental wall motion before and after PTCA (37 patients).

	Pre-PTCA	Post PTCA	p
LV ejection fraction	74	73	NS
	(9)	(8)	
LV regional shortening			
Anterobasal	37	35	NS
	(11)	(10)	
Anterior	38	36	NS
	(13)	(16)	
Apical	48	45	NS
	(16)	(20)	
Inferior	49	49	NS
	(13)	(17)	
Inferobasal	8	9	NS
	(15)	(15)	

Values = mean % (SD);   LV = left ventricular.

Previous studies have shown that DSA can produce LV images suitable for analysis following central venous administration of contrast and that the results correlate well with those of direct left ventriculography in terms of LV volumes [10, 11] and regional wall motion [12]. Satisfactory images have also been obtained in patients with impaired LV contraction [17], particularly relevant to PTCA, during which LV performance may become markedly impaired. Its less invasive nature has been used to advantage during exercise [18] or atrial pacing [19] and as an outpatient assessment of LV function [20].

Global LV function during PTCA. The decrease in LVEF that we observed in our patients is similar to that seen by others [7–9], however the degree to which this fall is dependent on the vessel undergoing PTCA has not been previously reported. Not surprisingly we were able to demonstrate a greater deterioration in LV performance in patients having LAD PTCA in comparison to those having either right coronary or circumflex lesions dilated.

Regional wall motion during PTCA. Previous studies have documented anteroapical LV dysfunction during LAD PTCA [7] and similarly abnormal inferior wall motion during right coronary PTCA [5]. Our findings support these observations. We were unable to document abnormal wall motion during circumflex PTCA but this may relate to the RAO projection that was used. This does not satisfactorily profile the lateral LV wall and in these cases therefore a LAO projection may have been superior. The effects of diagonal artery dilatation have not been described by others. We demonstrated anterior and apical abnormalities together with augmented enhanced shortening. The augmentation of inferobasal contraction that was also seen during LAD PTCA has been observed previously (8) but is not a universal finding [3, 6]. This phenomenon is thought to relate to mechanical unloading of the nonischaemic segment rather than to a Starling effect secondary to increasing volume or to increased sympathetic drive [21].

Relationship to ST segment alteration. ECG monitoring proved to be a relatively insensitive indicator of myocardial ischaemia during balloon inflation despite the use of a 12 lead system, although this is more sensitive than systems using fewer leads [6]. However, we did show that the magnitude of ST change is related to the degree of LV dysfunction as indicated by the fall in ejection fraction. Recent work suggests that the reliability of ECG monitoring may be enhanced with intracoronary recording [22].

PTCA in single and multivessel disease. We were unable to demonstrate any differences in terms of either global LV performance or ECG change during PTCA in patients with single vessel disease when compared to patients with multivessel involvement. One would anticipate a greater ischaemic burden in the latter group but as ventriculography was performed after only 60 seconds of balloon inflation, it is likely that this may have been too early after coronary occlusion for any difference to become apparent.

Short vs long balloon inflations. ECG and ventriculographic signs of ischemia were no different in patients after 20 sec of balloon occlusion compared to those after 60 sec. It has been well documented that abnormalities in LV contraction following balloon occlusion are apparent after 20 sec [4], but it is unclear to what extent they progress. Previous studies have produced conflicting results with some workers observing the gradual decline in LV performance [5, 6], while other data suggests that once established, the degree of LV dysfunction does not worsen during this time period [9].

It is of interest that we demonstrated enhanced inferobasal shortening after 60 seconds of LAD balloon occlusion which was not apparent after 20 sec. The significance of this finding is not clear but suggests that time may be required before nonischaemic LV segments are recruited.

Alteration in LV volumes during PTCA. The changes in LV volume that we observed are similar to previous findings with little or no increase in end diastolic volume but a marked increase in end systolic volume [7, 9]. We also showed that during PTCA these changes occur independently of R wave. This finding challenges the Brody hypothesis that originally suggested a relationship between these two parameters [16] but is in accord with other studies [23, 24]. Furthermore, previous work suggests that alteration in R wave amplitude during episodes of LV ischaemia is more related to abnormalities of intramyocardial conduction than to changes in LV volume [25].

Functional importance of collateral vessels. Like others [26] we have shown that during balloon occlusion both global and regional LV performance is better preserved in patients with collateral vessels than in those without. Previous work has shown a correlation between the manifestations of ischaemia during PTCA and the extent of collateral supply apparent during balloon inflation [26], but we have shown that this relationship is also valid for the collateral status existing before the procedure.

LV performance after PTCA. We were unable to demonstrate any abnormalities of LV performance after the PTCA procedure. Previous studies have observed hyperfunction, up to 20 sec after balloon deflation, of LV segments rendered ischaemic during balloon occlusion [4, 6]. We did not demonstrate this phenomenon although our post-PTCA study may not have been performed sufficiently soon after the procedure for this to be documented.

Conclusions and clinical implications. Intravenous DSA provides an accurate examination of LV performance during PTCA allowing the consequences of coronary balloon occlusion to be assessed. If long balloon inflations are considered necessary in selected patients undergoing PTCA, this, or other relatively noninvasive methods, may prove valuable in the investigation of techniques designed to ameliorate ischaemia during balloon inflation.

Acknowledgement

Dr M.S. Norell was supported by the British Heart Foundation.

References

1. Serruys PW, Meester GT (eds) (1986) *Coronary Angioplasty: A Controlled Model for Ischaemia.* Dordrecht: Martinus Nijhoff Publishers (DICM 58)
2. Norell MS, Lyons J, Gershlick A et al (1988) Assessment of LV performance during PTCA: A study by intravenous digital subtraction ventriculography. *Br Heart J* 59:419–428
3. Alam M, Khaja F, Brymer J, Marzelli M Goldstein S (1986) Echocardiographic evaluation of left ventricular function during coronary artery angioplasty. *Am J Cardiol* 57:20–25
4. Visser CA, David GK, Kan G et al (1986) Two-Dimensional echocardiography during percutaneous transluminal coronary angioplasty. *Am Heart J* 111:1035–1041
5. Hauser AM, Gangadharan V, Ramos RG, Gordon S, Timmis GC (1985) Sequence of mechanical, electrocardiographic and clinical effects of repeated coronary artery occlusion in human beings: echocardiographic observations during coronary angioplasty. *J Am Coll Cardiol* 5:193–197
6. Wohlgelernter D, Cleman M, Highman HA et al (1986) Regional myocardial dysfunction during coronary angioplasty; evaluation by 2-dimensional echocardiography and 12 lead electrocardiography. *J Am Coll Cardiol* 7:1245–1254
7. Serruys PW, Wijns W, Van der Brand M et al (1984) Left ventricular performance, regional blood flow, wall motion and lactate metabolism during transluminal angioplasty. *Circulation* 70:25–36
8. Doorey AJ, Mehmel HC, Schwarz FX, Kubler W (1984) Amelioration by nitroglycerin of left

ventricular ischaemia induced by percutaneous transluminal coronary angioplasty: assessment by haemodynamic variables and left ventriculography. *J Am Coll Cardiol* 6:267–274

9. Bertrand ME, Lablanche JM, Thieuleux FA (1983) Changes in left ventricular relaxation during transient coronary occlusion in man. *Eur Heart J* 4 (Suppl E):49

10. Norris SL, Slutsky RA, Mancini J et al (1983) Comparison of digital intravenous ventriculography with direct left ventriculography for quantitation of left ventricular volumes and ejection fractions. *Am J Cardiol* 51:1399–1403

11. Tobis J, Nacioglu O, Johnston WD et al (1982) Left ventricular imaging with digital subtraction angiography using intravenous contrast injection and flouroscopic exposure levels. *Am Heart J* 104:20–27

12. Goldberg HL, Borer JS, Moses JW et al (1983) Digital subtraction intravenous left ventricular angiography: comparison with conventional intraventricular angiography. *J Am Coll Cadiol* 1(3):858–862

13. Rentrop KP, Cohen M, Blanke H, Philips RA (1985) Changes in collateral channel filling immediately after controlled coronary artery occlusion by an angioplasty balloon in human subjects. *J Am Coll Cardiol* 5:587–92

14. Sandler H, Dodge HT (1968) The use of single plane angiocardiograms for the calculation of left ventricular volume in man. *Am Heart J* 75:325–34

15. Rickards A, Seabra-Gomes R, Thurston P (1977) The assessment of regional abnormalities of the left ventricle by angiography. *Eur J Cardiol* 5(2):167–82

16. Brody DA (1956) A theoretical analysis of intracavity blood mass influence on the heart-lead relationship. *Circ Res* IV:731–738

17. Nissen SE, Booth D, Waters J et al (1983) Evaluation of left ventricular contractile pattern by intravenous digital subtraction ventriculography: Comparison with cineangiography and assessment of interobserver variability. *Am J Cardiol* 52:1293–1298

18. Goldberg HL, Moses JW, Borer JS et al (1983) Exercise left ventriculography utilizing intravenous digital angiography. *J Am Coll Cardiol* 2:1092–1098

19. Johnson RA, Wasserman AG, Liebhoff RH et al (1983) Intravenous digital left ventriculography at rest and with atrial pacing as a screening procedure for coronary artery disease. *J Am Coll Cardiol* 2:905–10

20. Greenbaum RA, Evans TR (1984) Investigation of left ventricular function by digital subtraction angiography. *Br Heart J* 51:163–167

21. Goto Y, Igarashi Y, Yamada O, Hiramori K, Suga H (1988) Hyperkinesis without the Frank-Staring mechanism in a nonischaemic region of acutely ischaemic excised canine heart. *Circulation* 77:468–477

22. Friedman PL, Shook TL, Kirshenbaum JM, Selwyn AP, Ganz P (1986) Value of the intracoronary electrocardiogram to monitor myocardial ischaemia during percutaneous transluminal coronary angioplasty. *Circulation* 74:330–339

23. Battler A, Froelicher V, Slutsky R, Ashburn W (1979) Relationship of QRS amplitude changes during exercise to LV function and volumes and the diagnosis of coronary artery disease. *Circulation* 60:1004–1013

24. David D, Naito M, Chen C et al (1981) R-wave amplitude variations during experimental myocardial ischaemia: An inadequate index for changes in intracardiac volume. *Circulation*; 63:1364–1371

25. David D, Naito M, Micheloson E et al (1982) Intramyocardial conduction: A major determinant of R wave amptitude during myocardial ischaemia. *Circulation* 65:161–167

26. Cohen M, Rentrop KP (1986) Limitation of myocardial ischaemia by collateral circulation during sudden controlled coronary artery occlusion in human subjects: A prospective study. *Circulation* 74:469–476

16. Two dimensional echocardiography during PTCA

CEES A. VISSER, JACQUES J. KOOLEN, GEORGE K. DAVID and
AREND J. DUNNING

Introduction

More than fifty years ago Tennant and Wiggers were the first to demonstrate that
'the ventricular zone affected by ligation of a large coronary branch not only
appears cyanotic and dilated, but that it seems to alter in its mode of contraction'
[1].

In their classic study they used an optical myograph to evaluate myocardial
wall motion and demonstrated in dogs that ligation of a major coronary artery
resulted within 60 sec in a paradoxical systolic motion of the affected
myocardium.

Since then, the function of ischemic and non-ischemic myocardium has been
studied extensively in animal models by a variety of techniques [2–11], including
M-mode and two-dimensional echocardiography. Similar data in humans on the
effect of transient ischemia on left ventricular function have been limited to
observations during spontaneous or provoked attacks of angina pectoris.
Distante et al performed continuously M-mode echocardiography during both
spontaneous and provoked ischemic attacks [12, 13]. These recordings demonstrated a consistent type of change in cardiac mechanics, both in the ischemic wall
and in the overall ventricular dynamics. As in the animal studies the ischemic wall
in humans may show a paradoxical motion pattern. In addition, left ventricular
diameter increased and chest pain occurred 1 to 3 min after the onset of definite
changes in the ischemic wall. They demonstrated furthermore, that chest pain, the
most common symptom suggestive of ischemia, occurred rather late when
compared to direct ischemic wall motion changes and even to the continuously
monitored ECG.

Using two-dimensional echocardiography Gerson et al. demonstrated, in
a patient with Prinzmetal's angina, akinesia of the previously normally
contracting left ventricular posterior wall during a provoked attack of pain [14].
After administration of nitroglycerine this part of the ventricle showed a hyperkinetic motion pattern. This was in keeping with findings of Distante et al who
also found during some ischemic periods a contractile 'rebound phenomenon' of

P.W. Serruys, R. Simon & K.J. Beatt (eds), Percutaneous Transluminal Coronary Angioplasty. ISBN 0-7923-0346-6.
© *1990 Kluwer Academic Publishers, Dordrecht*

the previously ischemic wall [15]. In these patients with variant angina they demonstrated furthermore, that segmental asynergy was earlier detected than the onset of pain or ST-segment elevation on the ECG.

Percutaneous transluminal coronary angioplasty (PTCA) now provides the unique opportunity to assess more precisely the time course of changes in myocardial wall motion during transient ischemia in humans, and its relation to clinical and electrocardiographic signs of ischemia.

Incidence and time course of asynergy during PTCA

Hauser et al [16] studied 18 patients undergoing PTCA of 22 coronary stenoses. At baseline (i.e. after introduction of the balloon catheter through the coronary stenotic lesion, but prior to balloon inflation), 14 patients had normal wall motion in the territories of 18 stenotic vessels. During PTCA, left ventricular wall motion abnormalities developed in 16 territories; the remaining two patients had no wall motion abnormalities induced during PTCA. One of these patients had a 'highly collateralized' lesion of the left anterior descending artery. In four patients (with four lesions) with at least some degree of wall motion abnormality at baseline, there was an increase in left ventricular dysfunction in two, whereas no changes occurred in the other two, one of these being the only postinfarct patient with a large area of anteroapical akinesis at baseline. If wall motion abnormalities did develop, they usually progressed rapidly from hypokinesis to dyskinesis. The first signs of hypokinesis developed 19 ± 8 sec after balloon inflation. Balloons were kept inflated for 30–60 sec. After deflation, it took 20 ± 8 sec before normalization of wall motion began, and restoration to baseline was always complete 2 min after reperfusion. There were no differences between the first and last inflations (a total of 52 inflations were studied in these 18 patients) as far as time to start of asynergy (19 ± 7 vs 20 ± 8 sec) and time to start of normalization (20 ± 8 vs 15 ± 8 sec) are concerned. Wohlgelernter et al studied 20 patients during PTCA, using computerized quantitative analysis of regional left ventricular wall motion [17]. Profound segmental dysfunction was noted in all patients. The onset of regional dysfunction was 12 ± 5 sec after inflation. After 60 sec of balloon occlusion of the coronary artery, 29% of the patients had severe hypokinesia of the ischemic region and 71% had akinesia or dyskinesia. With deflation there was prompt recovery of regional function, with full recovery at 43 ± 17 sec. They also found no significant differences in time to onset of dysfunction, magnitude of dysfunction or time to complete recovery of function.

We studied the effects of PTCA in 15 patients and evaluated regional wall motion semi-quantitatively [18]. All patients developed new areas of asynergy 8 ± 3 sec after balloon inflation (which was continued for 38 ± 8 sec). Again all degrees of segmental asynergy were encountered from hypokinesis to dyskinesis, but dyskinesis was found only in patients wit stenosis of the left anterior descending artery (8 of 11) and in none of the 5 patients undergoing PTCA of the right coronary artery. This apparent difference was not related to duration of balloon inflation (36 ± 8 vs 34 ± 6 sec). Balloon deflation was followed by complete normalization of wall motion as early as 19 ± 8 sec and was followed in 12 patients by regional hyperkinesis (i.e. the earlier mentioned 'contractile rebound' phenomenon) at 25 ± 7 sec after deflation (Fig. 1). The differences among these studies in onset and disappearance of regional asynergy may be explained by a difference in methodology. We included the first balloon inflation after initial positioning of the uninflated balloon catheter, and this may decrease or interrupt flow in the as yet undilated artery and cloud the true timing of the onset of ischemia. On the other hand, Das et al. demonstrated, using M-mode echocardiography, that reduced wall thickening may be present as early as 8 beats after the fifth inflation [19].

The large majority (12 of 15) of our patients demonstrated hyperkinesis of the previously asynergic segments after balloon inflation. This transient overshoot of contractility, which has been described after dynamic exercise and attacks of variant angina [13, 20, 21] might be explained by reactive hyperemia [22]. In patients with unstable angina, however, wall motion abnormalities may persist after anginal episodes [23]. It is conceivable that duration and intensity of

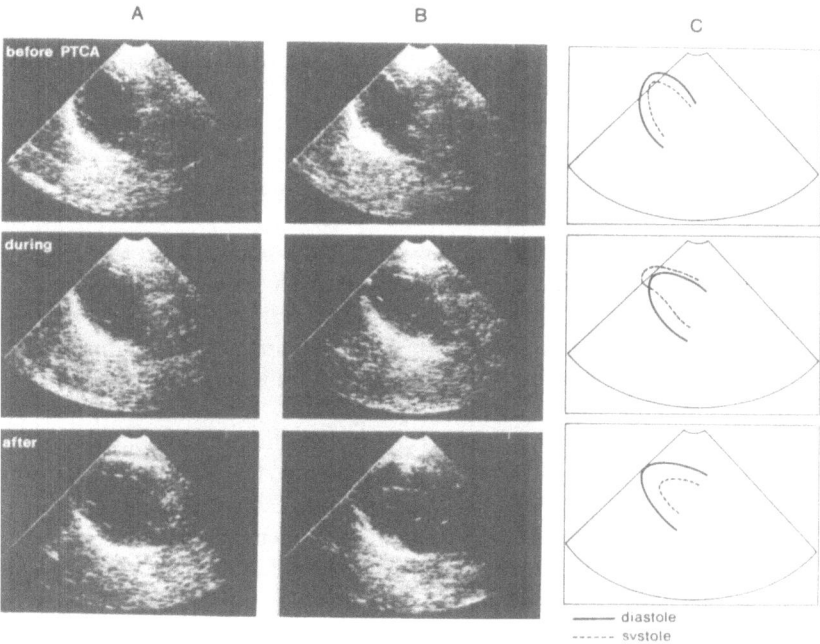

Figure 1. End-diastolic (A) and end-systolic (B) stop frames including endocardial outlines (C) of parasternal long-axis images of the apical area before, during, and after percutaneous transluminal coronary angioplasty (PTCA) of the left anterior descending artery. There is a normal contraction pattern before PTCA. However, during balloon inflation there is a dyskinetic motion pattern of the cardiac apex, which demonstrates hyperkinesis after balloon deflation.

ischemia, as well as myocardial condition at the onset of the ischemic periods highly determine whether the myocardium will only be 'hit' or 'stunned' as suggested by Braunwald and Klover [24].

Although intermittent brief periods of ischemic may have a cumulative effect and may cause myocardial injury in animals, regional myocardial dysfunction is transient in patients undergoing PTCA.

Global left ventricular function and myocardial risk area

Quantitative measurements of left ventricular function were obtained by Hauser et al in only one patient with left anterior descending stenosis whose ejection fraction dropped from 55 to 25% [16].

We used for this purpose a semi-quantitative left ventricular wall motion score, by assigning a numeric value to each of th 13 left ventricular segments according to the degree of asynergy, that is, hypokinesis $+1$, akinesis $+2$, and dyskinesis $+3$. Hyperkinesis was assigned -1 and normokinesis 0.

The effect of 4 occlusions of the left anterior descending artery on this wall motion score in one patient is shown in Fig. 2A. The baseline score is zero and increased during inflation to 8 to 9. After balloon deflation there was, after normalization, an overshoot to values of -5.

Figure 2B shows the wall motion score changes of all 49 ischemic periods recorded in our 15 patients. The mean baseline score of 0.5 ± 1.4 (range 0 to 4) increased up to 6.9 ± 2.2 (3 to 10) and demonstrated after normalization an overshoot of -1.9 ± 1.6 (-5 to $+4$).

Figure 3C apparently demonstrates that occlusion of the left anterior descending artery has a different impact on global left ventricular function than occlusion of the right coronary artery. Baseline wall motion score was not different (1.0 ± 2.0 vs 0.3 ± 1.1). Occlusion of the left anterior descending artery, however, produced a significantly higher wall motion score, 7.9 ± 1.3(6 to 10) vs 4.0 ± 1.3 (3 to 6) (Table 1).

The 'myocardial risk area', i.e. the area of myocardium potentially becoming ischemic during PTCA, and obtained by expressing the number of segments developing any new wall motion abnormality as a percentage of the total number of 13 segments, also demonstrated an apparent difference between occlusion of the left anterior descending and right coronary artery, 34 ± 8 vs 17 ± 4% (Table 1). This is in keeping with preliminary data from Pandian et al [25] who demonstrated, that the 12 patients studied during PTCA developed regional dysfunction involving 29 ± 11% of left ventricular myocardium. Postmortem and in vivo studies on the magnitude of individual coronary vascular beds in humans have indeed demonstrated the difference between the left anterior descending and right coronary artery [26–29]. The importance of collaterals in this respect could not be assessed as only one of the 15 patients studied had collateral vessels and nevertheless developed segmental asynergy.

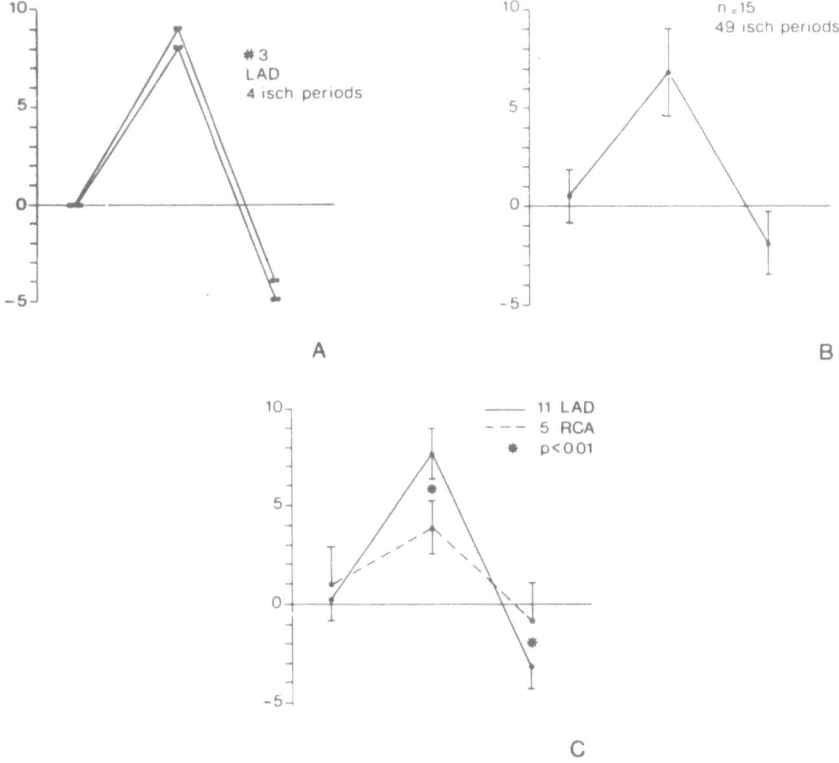

Figure 2.
(A) Wall motion score changes during four balloon inflations of the left anterior descending artery (LAD) in patient no. 3. Baseline score is normal prior to inflation and increases to 8 or 9 during inflation. After deflation an overshoot of the wall motion score is seen to minus 5.

(B) Wall motion score changes of all 49 ischemic periods recorded. Mean baseline score is 0.5 and increases up to 6.9. After deflation an overshoot is seen of minus 1.9.

(C) Wall motion score changes in relation to the involved coronary artery. Inflation of the left anterior descending artery (LAD) produces a significant higher wall motion score than inflation of the right coronary artery (RCA). The postischemic contractile overshoot is also significantly different.

Preliminary data on transesophageal echocardiography in anesthetized patients undergoing PTCA once again demonstrated that both regional and global left ventricular function as well as left ventricular wall stress, is more affected by occlusion of the left anterior descending artery, than by right coronary artery occlusion.

Griffin et al demonstrated more recently, using myocardial contrast perfusion, that regional myocardial enhancement defined the area of dyskinesis following balloon inflation [30]. In every case the area of dyskinesis was confined to the area of contrast enhancement. Furthermore, preliminary studies suggest that,

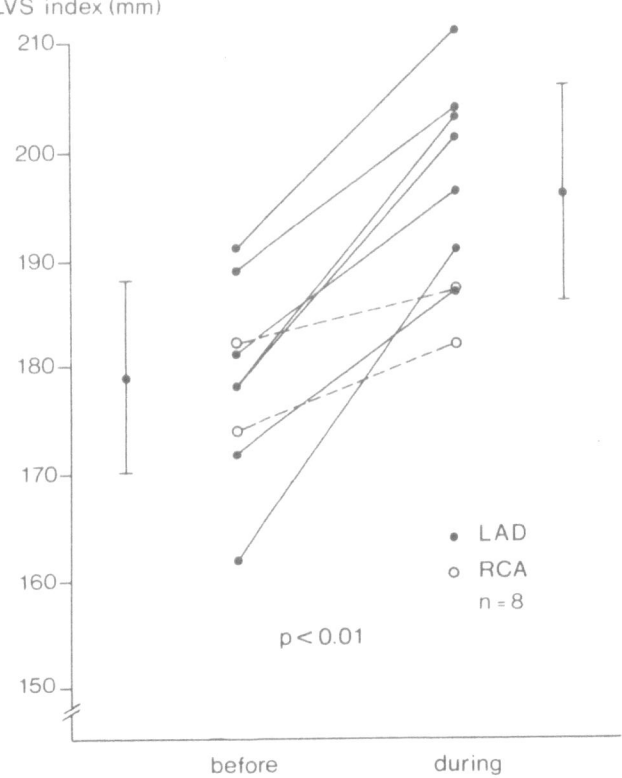

Figure 3. Left ventricular size (LVS) changes of eight patients during angioplasty in relation to the involved coronary artery. There is a significant increase during inflation, which is less pronounced in the two RCA patients undergoing PTCA of the right coronary artery.

using the same technique, regional coronary reserve can be assessed as well as the immediate effects of PTCA on myocardial perfusion [31, 32].

Left ventricular size changes

Using M-mode echocardiography Distance et al [12] demonstrated that the left ventricular diameter increased during provoked or spontaneous attacks of angina. These changes were more pronounced and earlier during systole than during diastole, causing a marked reduction in percentual fractional shortening. The same authors described enlargement and deformation of the left ventricle by two-dimensional echocardiography, showing variable degrees of distortion, such as globular appearance in diastole and an 'hourglass' shape in systole [15]. In addition, an abrupt demarcation between ischemic and non-ischemic zones could

Table 1. Wall motion score and myocardial risk area during PTCA of the right coronary and left anterior descending arteries.

	RCA		LAD
WMS	4.0 ± 1.4	p < 0.01	7.9 ± 1.3
MRA	17 ± 4%	p < 0.01	34 ± 8%

RCA = right coronary artery; LAD = left anterior descending artery; WMS = wall motion score; MRA = myocardial risk area.

be detected, i.e. a clearcut demarcation between an asynergic segment and an adjacent normal or hyperkinetic region. Hauser et al [16] calculated the end-diastolic volume in one patient and noted an increase of 37%. The overall left ventricular size was determined by us by means of three appical views: the two- and four-chamber views and the long-axis view. The endocardial end-diastolic outline of these apical images was traced and measured, and an index of the left ventricular size was obtained by averaging the lengths of these three diastolic outlines.

The effect of ischemia on left ventricular end-diastolic size is shown in Fig. 3. During inflation there is a significant increase of the left ventricular size index from 170 ± 9 up to 196 ± 10 mm (p < 0.01). These changes were less pronounced in patients undergoing PTCA of the right coronary artery.

Animal studies have shown that ischemia may induce increased diastolic fiber length of normal segments of myocardium after coronary occlusion (i.e. Frank-Starling mechanism) [33, 34]. This may be responsible for the diastolic dilation in these patients.

Sequence of ischemic symptoms

Interestingly, both our study [18] and that by Hauser et al [16] demonstrated that regional dyssynergy is the first sign of ischemia to appear, followed by ischemic electrocardiographic changes in 4 of 15 and 8 of 18 patients, respectively. In a more recent study Wohlgelernter et al [17] demonstrated that, using 12-lead electrocardiography, the onset of ischemic electrocardiographic changes invariably lagged behind the onset of wall motion abnormalities, with only 64% of patients showing evidence of ischemia on the 12-lead electrocardiograms at 20 sec of inflation. Furthermore, the last ischemic symptom to appear was angina, which occurred in five of 15 patients in our study. After deflation, ischemic signs disappeared in reverse order (Table 2). The low incidence of angina pectoris as well as the apparently fixed sequence of events was recently also found during dynamic exercise [35]. It seems that angina pectoris is the last ischemic symptom to appear.

Table 2. Time course of onset and disappearance of the echocardiographic, ECG, and clinical signs of ischemia during 11 angioplasty attempts in three patients.

Vessel involved	Onset after balloon inflation			Disappearance after balloon deflation		
	Asynergy	ST shift	Angina	Angina	ST shift	Asynergy
LAD	8	18	24	12	15	25
	10	24	29	10	14	24
	11	20	30	15	15	20
	12	20	33	10	12	24
	10	21	—	—	16	23
LAD	10	24	32	18	18	19
	12	18	27	14	15	21
	8	18	23	12	17	23
	11	19	19	17	19	23
RCA	9	24	25	12	15	21
	14	27	30	10	15	17

All data are expressed in seconds.
LAD = left anterior descending artery; RCA = right coronary artery.

References

1. Tennant R, Wigges J (1935) The effect of coronary occlusion on myocardial contraction. *Am J Physiol* 112:351–361
2. Prinzmetal M, Schwartz LL, Corday E, Spritzler R, Bergman HC, Krueger HE (1949) Studies on the coronary circulation. I. Loss of myocardial contractility after coronary artery occlusion. *Ann Intern Med* 31:429–449
3. Hood WB, Corelli VH, Abelmann WH, Normal JC (1969) Persistence of contractile behaviours in acutely ischemic myocardium. *Cardiovasc Res* 3:249–260
4. Heikkilä J, Tabakin BS, Hugenholtz PC (1972) Quantification of function in normal and infarcted regions of the left ventricle. *Cardiovasc Res* 6:516–531
5. Theroux P, Franklin D, Ross J, Kemper WS (1974) Regional myocardial function during acute coronary artery occlusion and its modifications by pharmacologic agents in the dog. *Circ Res* 35:896–908
6. Kerber RE, Abboud FM (1973) Echocardiographic detection of regional myocardial infarction: an experimental study. *Circulation* 47:997–1005
7. Kerber RE, Marcus ML, Abboud FM (1977) Echocardiography in experimentally induced myocardial ischemia. *Am J Med* 63:21–28
8. Gaasch MH, Bernhardt SA (1977) The effect of acute changes in experimentally induced myocardial ischemia. *Am J Med* 63:29–36
9. Ten Cate FJ, Verdouw PD, Bom AH, Roelandt JR (1979) Effect of coronary artery occlusion and reperfusion on the time course of myocardial wall thickness. In: Lancée CT (ed), *Echocardiology*, pp 111–118 The Hague: Martinus Nijhoff Publishers (DICM1)
10. Pandian NG, Kerber RE (1982) Two-dimensional echocardiography in experimental coronary stenosis. I. Sensitivity and specificity in detecting transient myocardial dyskinesis: comparison with sonomicrometes. *Circulation* 66:597–602
11. Pandian NG, Kieso RA, Kerber RE (1982) Two-dimensional echocardiography in experimental coronary stenosis, II: Relationships between systolic wall thinning and regional myocardial perfuson in severe coronary stenosis. *Circulation* 66:603–611

12. Distante A, L'Abbate A, Maseri A, Landini L, Michelassi C (1979) Echocardiographic changes in vasospastic angina. In: Lancée CT (ed) *Echocardiology*, pp 119–124. The Hague: Martinus Nijhoff Publishers (DICM1)

13. Distante A, Rovai D, Picano E, Moscarelli E, Palombo C, Morales MA, Michelassi C, L'Abbate A (1984) Transient changes in left ventricular mechanics during attacks of Prinzmetal angina: A M-mode echocardiographic study. *Am Heart J* 107:465–471

14. Gerson MC, Nobele RJ, Wann LS, Faris JN, Morris SN (1979) Noninvasive documentation of Prinzmetal angina. *Am J Cardiol* 43:323–334

15. Distante A, Rovai D, Picano E, Moscarelli E, Morales MA, Palombo C, L'Abbate A (1984) Transient changes in left ventricular mechanics during attacks of Prinzmetal angina: a two-dimensional echocardiographic study. *Am Heart J* 108:440–446

16. Hauser AM, Gangadharan V, Ramos RG, Gordon S, Timmis GC (1985) Sequence of mechanical, electrocardiographic and clinical effects of repeated coronary artery occlusion in human beings: echocardiographic observations during coronary angioplasty. *J Am Coll Cardiol* 5:193–197

17. Wohlgelernter D, Cleman M, Ainsley Highman H, Fetterman RC, Duncan JS, Zaret BL, Jaffe CC (1986) Regional myocardial dysfunction during coronary angioplasty: evaluation by two-dimensional echocardiography and 12-lead electrocardiography. *J Am Coll Cardiol* 7:1245–1254

18. Visser CA, David GK, Kan G, Meltzer RS, Koolen JJ, Dunning AJ (1986) Two-dimensional echocardiography during percutaneous transluminal coronary angioplasty. *Am Heart J* 111:1035–1041

19. Das SK, Serruys PW, Brand van den M, Domenicucci S, Vletter WB, Roelandt J (1982) Acute echocardiographic changes during percutaneous coronary angioplasty and their relationship to coronary blood flow. *J Cardiovasc Ultrasonogr* 2:269–271

20. Wann LS, Faris JV, Childress RH, Dillon JC, Weyman AE, Feigenbaum H (1979) Exercise cross-sectional echocardiography in ischemic heart disease. *Circulation* 60:1300–1307

21. Visser CA, Van der Wieken LR, Kan G, Lie KI, Buseman-Sokole E, Meltzer RS, Durrer D (1983) Comparison of two-dimensional echocardiography with radionuclide angiography during dynamic exercise for the detection of coronary artery disease. *Am Heart J* 106:528–534

22. Pagani M, Valuer SF, Haig BR, Braunwald E (1978) Initial myocardial adjustments to a brief period of ischemia and reperfusion in the conscious dog. *Circ Res* 43:83–92

23. Nixon JV, Brown CN, Smitherman TC (1982) Identification of transient and persistent segmental wall motion abnormalities in patients with unstable angina by two-dimensional echocardiography. *Circulation* 65:1497–1503

24. Braunwald E, Klover RA (1982) The stunned myocardium: Prolonged, post-ischemic ventricular dysfunction. *Circulation* 66:1146–1149

25. Pandian MG, Salem DN, Funai JT, Konstam MA, Levine MJ (1984) In vivo assessment of left ventricular risk area during acute, temporary coronary occlusion in humans. Utility of two-dimensional echocardiography during coronary angioplasty (abstr). *Circulation* 77 (Suppl II): II–403

26. Kalbefleish H, Hort W (1977) Quantitative study on the size of coronary artery supply area postmortem. *Am Heart J* 94:183–188

27. Ganz W, Tannera K, Marcus HS, Donosa R, Yoskida S, Swan MJC (1971) Measurement of coronary sinus blood flow by continuous thermodilution in man. *Circulation* 44:181–195

28. Rutishauser W, Noseda G, Bussman W, Prete B (1970) Blood flow measurements through single coronary arteries by roentgen densitometry. *Am J Roentgenol* 109:21–24

29. Klocke F (1976) Coronary blood flow in man. *Prog Cardiovasc Dis* 19:117–166

30. Griffin MB, Timmis ADF, Henderson RA, Sowton E (1987) Contrast perfusion echocardiography: Identification of area at risk of dyskinesis during percutaneous transluminal coronary angioplasty. *Am Heart J* 114:497–502

31. Cheirif J, Zogubi WA, Minor ST, Raizuar AE, Quinoves MA (1978) Assessment of myocardial perfusion and coronary reserve in man by myocardial contrast echocardiography: Effect of coronary angioplasty (abstr). *Circulation* 76 (Suppl IV): IV–504

32. Zotz RJ, Kan B, Brennecke R (1987) Evaluation of PTCA by video-intensitometric analysis of contrast echocardiograms (abstr). *Circulation* 76 (Suppl IV): IV–504

33. Theroux P, Ross J, Franklin D, Kemper WS, Sasayama S (1976) Regional myocardial function in the conscious dog during acute coronary occlusion and responses to morphine, propanolol, nitroglycerin, and lidocaine. *Circulation* 53:302–314
34. Theroux P, Franklin D, Ross J, Kemper WS (1974) Regional myocardial function during acute coronary artery occlusion and its modification by pharmacologic agents in the dog. *Cir Res* 35:896–908
35. Sasishita Y, Koseki S, Matsula M, Tamura T, Yamaguchi L, Ito I (1983) Dissociation between regional myocardial dysfunction and ECG changes during myocardial ischemia induced by exercise in patients with angina pectoris. *Am Heart J* 106:1–8

17. Doppler echocardiographic assessment of left ventricular function during PTCA

ANTHONY C. PEARSON, ARTHUR J. LABOVITZ, MORTON KERN and MICHEL VANDORMAEL

Introduction

Doppler echocardiography has emerged in the last decade as a powerful tool for noninvasively evaluating cardiac blood flow. Previous studies have demonstrated that Doppler evaluation of aortic blood flow could be used to measure stroke volume on a beat-to-beat basis [1–3]. More recently, Doppler has been used to evaluate left ventricular filling and diastolic function [4,5]. Through analysis of mitral inflow velocities, stroke volume [6] and left ventricular filling [7–10] can also be measured on a beat-to-beat basis. This ability to measure left ventricular filling continuously and noninvasively makes the techniques ideal for assessing the effects of percutaneous transluminal coronary angioplasty (PTCA) induced ischemia on left ventricular function. In this study we used Doppler echocardiography to assess the effects of balloon occlusion on left ventricular diastolic function and systolic function in patients undergoing PTCA.

Methods

Patients. Two groups of patients were studied. First, 32 patients undergoing PTCA for clinical indications were studied (Group I). The left anterior descending artery was dilated in 17 patients, the circumflex artery in two and dominant right coronary artery in 13. There were 22 men and 10 women with a mean age of 55 yr (range 36 to 70). Twenty-one had single vessel and 11 had multivessel coronary artery disease. Three patients had electrocardiographic evidence of a prior inferior myocardial infarction, of which two had inferior hypokinesia on the baseline two-dimensional echocardiogram. Additional angiographic, hemodynamic and echocardiographic parameters are summarized in Table 1.

In a Diltiazem administration group of 18 patients (Group II), measurements were made in an untreated state before, during and after balloon inflation (control) and repeated following administration of Diltiazem. The study

P.W. Serruys, R. Simon & K.J. Beatt (eds), Percutaneous Transluminal Coronary Angioplasty. ISBN 0-7923-0346-6.
© *1990 Kluwer Academic Publishers, Dordrecht*

Table 1. Patient characteristics.

Group I		
LVEDP (mmHg)		13.4 ± 8
LVEF (%)		64.4 ± 12
LV end-diastolic diameter (cm/m^2)		2.7 ± 0.3
LA size (cm/m^2)		2.0 ± 0.3
LVSF (%)		33.5 ± 6
Gradient (mmHg)	pre PTCA	61.3 ± 15
	post	16.2 ± 11
Stenosis (%)	pre PTCA	80 ± 11
	post	22 ± 10

LVEDP = left ventricular end diastolic pressure;
LVEF = left ventricular ejection fraction;
LVSF = left ventricular shortening fraction

population consisted of 18 patients selected from those undergoing routine single vessel PTCA with suitable left anterior descending (n = 17) or circumflex coronary artery (n = 1) narrowings (> 60% stenosis by visual estimation of two experienced angiographers).

Coronary angioplasty. PTCA was performed in a routine fashion as previously reported (11) using appropriately sized balloon catheters ranging in diameter from 2.0 to 3.5 mm. After positioning of the balloon catheter, an initial therapeutic inflation was performed with electrocardiographic monotoring only. At least three minutes for reperfusion was allowed before subsequent balloon inflations with Doppler echocardiographic monitoring. Electrocardiographic changes were observed to return to baseline prior to subsequent balloon inflations. Each balloon inflation was maintained for a period of 30 to 90 sec at pressures of five to ten atmospheres. Doppler and two-dimensional echocardiography were performed during the second and third balloon inflations in a random fashion. Time of onset of typical anginal chest pain was recorded.

Diltiazem studies. After the two control ischemic periods were completed, diltiazem, 10 mg bolus, was given intravenously followed immediately with 500 mcg/min continuous infusion. After 15 min, repeat balloon inflations were performed as for the control ischemic periods. Duplicate occlusions prior to and after drug administration demonstrated the reproducibility of ischemic periods on coronary hemodynamics responses.

In this group of patients, mitral inflow recordings and two-dimensional information was available in 12 patients before Diltiazem administration for 60 sec of balloon occlusion. Peak early and peak atrial velocities were recorded as previously described. Two-dimensional echocardiograms were recorded from the apical four-chamber view and ejection fraction calculated using the area-length formula.

Echocardiographic studies. M-mode and two-dimensional echocardiography was performed utilizing a commercially available phased array echo-Doppler system (Hewlett Packard Series 60 or Irex Meridian). After obtaining a baseline M-mode and two-dimensional imaging study in the parasternal long axis, short axis and apical views, the chest was marked prior to the angiographic procedure in order to identify the optimal windows for transducer placement. Two-dimensional short axis images were obtained from the left parasternal region continuously for 30 sec prior to balloon inflation, throughout balloon inflation, and for 30 to 60 sec following balloon deflation. Images were obtained at the low papillary muscle level for procedures involving the left coronary artery and at the tips of the mitral valve leaflets for procedures involving the right coronary artery. Timing of balloon inflation and deflation were recorded directly on video tape. In the Diltiazem study group, these measurements were performed both in the drug free state and following administration of Diltiazem.

Echocardiographic analysis. Baseline studies were evaluated for chamber dimensions and shortening fraction according to the American Society of Echocardiography recommendations. Regional wall motion was analyzed by two experienced observers on a video tape system with real-time, slow-motion and frame-by-frame forward and reverse capabilities. New wall motion abnormalities were defined as new regional left ventricular dysfunction of severe hypokinesia, akinesia, or dyskinesia as compared to the baseline study. Frame markers were utilized to calculate the time elapsed from balloon inflation to onset of segmental dysfunction. In a similar fashion, time to recovery of wall motion abnormalities following balloon deflation was recorded.

Quantitative analysis of global left ventricular systolic function during vessel occlusion was accomplished by calculation of fractional area change by use of an off-line echo-computer system (Franklin Quantic 1200). After identifying end diastolic and end systolic frames, the computer utilizes an automatic edge detection algorithm for locating the endocardial border [12]. The percent area change in the short axis view was then calculated utilizing the formula:

$$\text{Percent area change} = \frac{\text{diastolic area} - \text{systolic area}}{\text{diastolic area}}.$$

These calculations were performed at baseline, 15 and 30 sec during balloon occlusion and 15 sec after balloon deflation.

Doppler studies. Pulsed Doppler echocardiography of mitral inflow was performed from the cardiac apex with the Doppler beam aligned parallel to transmitral flow. The sample volume was placed at the level of the mitral valve annulus and the transducer orientation adjusted for optimal spectral display (highest velocity with least spectral dispersion). Continuous hard copy recordings at paper speeds of 100 mm/sec were obtained for 30 sec prior to balloon inflation, continuously throughout balloon inflation and for 30 sec following balloon deflation with identifying time markers recorded directly on the paper.

Doppler analysis. Doppler measurements were made on a computer interfaced digitizing tablet with custom developed software. Three to 5 consecutive beats were averaged. Analysis of left ventricular filling included measurements of peak early, atrial, and mean diastolic velocities as well as the total velocity integral and its components of early diastolic flow, atrial diastolic flow and 1/3 filling fraction (Fig. 1). In order to assess changes in relative contributions of early and late diastolic velocities, the ratios of early to late peak velocities (E/A), peak early to mean velocity (E/M), and early to late velocity integral (E_i/A_i) were calculated. Decreases in these ratios have been shown to reflect increasing impairment in left ventricular diastolic function [7–10].

As an additional index of global left ventricular systolic function, the stroke integral index was calculated as the product of the total flow velocity integral (sum of early and late velocity integrals) and the heart rate. The flow velocity integral has previously been shown to correlate strongly with stroke volume [1–3]. All measurements were performed at baseline and at 15 sec intervals during and following coronary occlusion.

Electrocardiography. Twelve lead electrocardiograms were obtained using radiolucent precordial electrodes at baseline and at 15 sec intervals during and following coronary occlusion. Electrocardiograms were analyzed for the presence

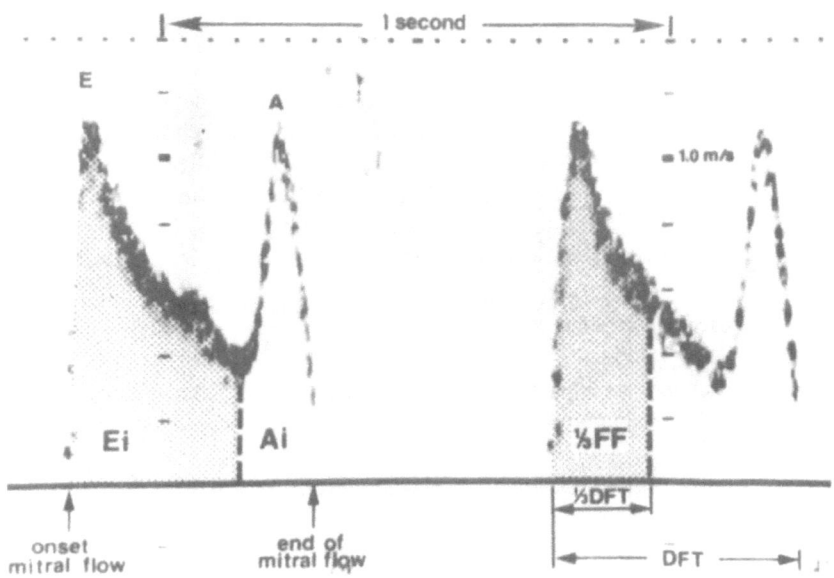

Figure 1. Illustration of Doppler transmitral flow velocity pattern with peak early diastolic (E) and atrial (A) velocity measurements shown. (Left) The area under the flow velocity curves for early diastole (E_1) and atrial systole (A_1) as well as the first third filling fraction (1/3 FF) (Right) were determined as illustrated. DFT = diastolic filling time.

of ST segment elevation compared to baseline. An ischemic response was defined as ST segment elevation equal to or greater than 1 mm at 0.08 sec after the J point occurring in at least 2 leads.

Statistical analysis. Results are presented as mean ± one standard deviation unless otherwise specified. Analysis of variance for repeated measures were applied to assess significant changes in Doppler and echocardiographic indices throughout the procedure. Scheffe's F-test was used to evaluate the significance between measurements during the procedure. Paired and unpaired t tests were utilized where indicated. A probability (p) of <0.05 was considered significant.

Results

Systolic function

Qualitative analysis. New systolic wall motion abnormalities appeared in the region supplied by the occluded coronary artery (anterior or lateral during left anterior descending occlusions, inferior or posterior during right coronary occlusion and posterior or lateral during circumflex occlusions) in 28 of the 32 Group I patients studied. In three patients there was no significant change from baseline wall motion and in one patient two-dimensional images were technically inadequate for analysis. The three patients without changes in systolic wall motion had collateral circulation to the stenotic right coronary artery being dilated. The mean time from coronary occlusion to development of a primary wall motion abnormality was 29 ± 12 sec (range 13 to 53 sec). Following balloon deflation, segmental wall motion returned to baseline in a mean time of 21 ± 8 sec (range 9 to 42 sec).

Quantitative analysis. Following balloon occlusion there was a progressive deterioration of global left ventricular systolic function as evidenced by a fall in the systolic percent area change. This drop became significant at 30 sec (43 ± 9% vs 29 ± 11%, p < 0.01). Patients with left anterior descending occlusion showed a trend toward more extensive left ventricular systolic dysfunction than right coronary artery occlusion (38% ± 21 vs 22% ± 20, p = NS). The fall in stroke integral index, as determined by Doppler, paralleled the drop in systolic percent area change achieving statistical significance at 30 sec following balloon inflation (1104 cm/min to 936 cm/min, p < 0.01) (Fig. 2). By 15 sec post deflation, neither systolic percent area change or stroke integral index was significantly different than baseline.

Diastolic function

Four indices were derived to describe the pattern of ventricular filling during coronary occlusion (Table 2). All four indices showed significant impairment in

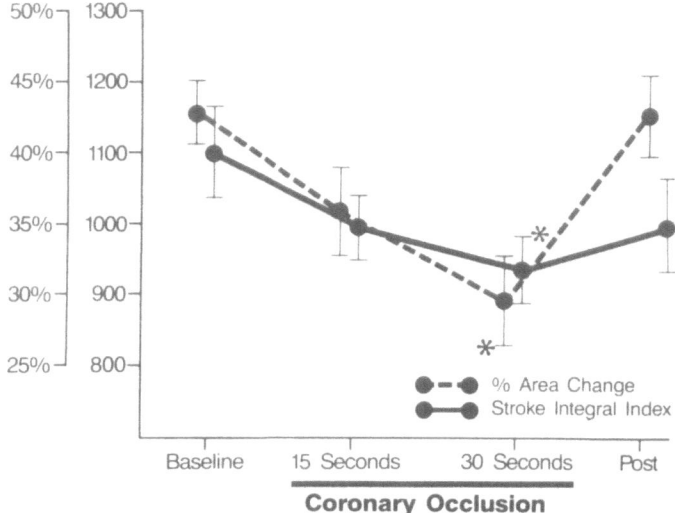

Figure 2. Change in stroke integral index and percent area change following coronary occlusion. Data are expressed as the mean ± SEM (*p < 0.01 versus baseline).

Table 2. Diastolic parameters.

Group I				
		Coronary occlusion		
	Baseline	15 sec	30 sec	Post
E/A	1.11 ± 0.3	0.96 ± 0.3*	0.91 ± 0.2*	1.09 ± 0.3
E/M	1.90 ± 0.4	1.70 ± 0.4*	1.66 ± 0.4*	1.81 ± 0.4
E_i/A_i	1.58 ± 0.7	1.25 ± 0.6*	1.17 ± 0.6*	1.54 ± 0.8
1/3 FF	41 ± 8	38 ± 8*	37 ± 7*	40 ± 8

*p < 0.01 versus baseline.
A = peak atrial diastolic velocity; A_i = late diastolic velocity integral; E = peak early diastolic velocity; E_i = early diastolic velocity integral; M = mean diastolic velocity; 1/3 FF = 1/3 filling fraction; post = 15 sec following balloon deflation. See text.

left ventricular diastolic function to occur within 15 sec of coronary occlusion. In some cases the reversal of the typical early to late diastolic velocity ratios was marked (Fig. 3). There were 28 patients in whom measurements of diastolic filling were available for analysis at baseline and after 15 sec of balloon occlusion. All but two of these patients showed a decrease in the peak early to atrial diastolic filling velocities ratio with coronary occlusion (Fig. 4). The two patients in whom these changes were not seen exhibited decreases in the other Doppler parameters. By 15 sec post deflation, diastolic indices had returned to baseline values.

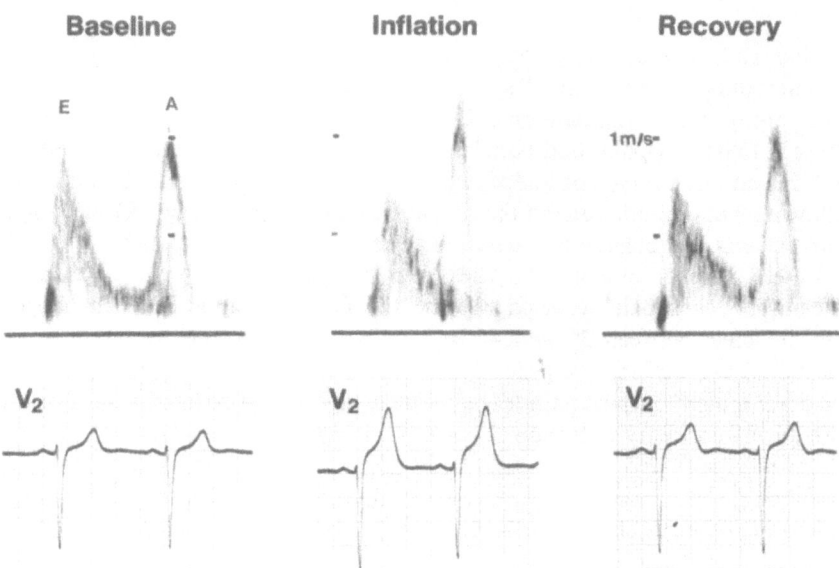

Figure 3. Pulsed Doppler recording of left ventricular inflow velocities with accompanying ECG lead V_2 during left anterior descending coronary artery occlusion (inflation). Note the marked reversal of early (E) and atrial (A) peak velocities and ST segment elevation with coronary occlusion.

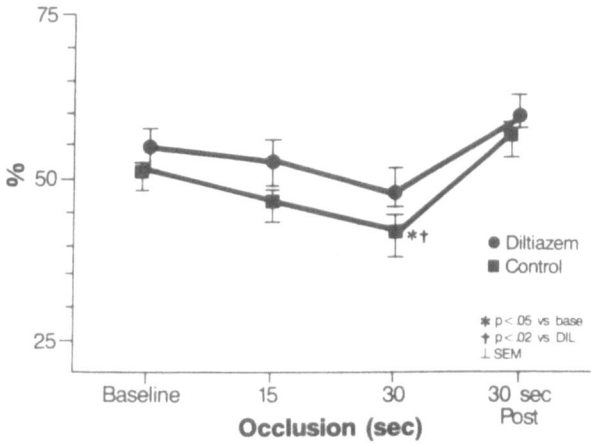

Figure 4. Change in ejection fraction with balloon occlusion during untreated and diltiazem inflations.

Clinical variables

Twelve lead electrocardiograms were available for analysis in 31 of the 32 patients studied. Significant ST segment elevation was noted in all but six of the study group. Following balloon inflation ST segment changes occurred within 15 sec in 15 patients, nine additional patients had ST segment elevation by 30 sec, and one additional patient had significant ST elevation between 30 and 45 sec following balloon inflation. Of the six patients without significant ST elevation, four patients had collateral circulation to the vessel being occluded.

Fifteen patients complained of chest pain following coronary artery occlusion. The onset of chest pain occurred by 15 sec in one individual, by 30 sec in another nine patients, between 30 and 45 sec in three patients and by 60 sec in an additional two patients. In general, the electrocardiographic changes preceded the development of chest pain (Fig. 5). There was no significant change in heart rate during coronary occlusion.

Effects of collateral circulation

Angiographically evident collateral circulation, to the vessel being dilated, was present on diagnostic coronary arteriography in 9 of the 32 patients. The temporal sequence of global systolic and diastolic dysfunction during angio-

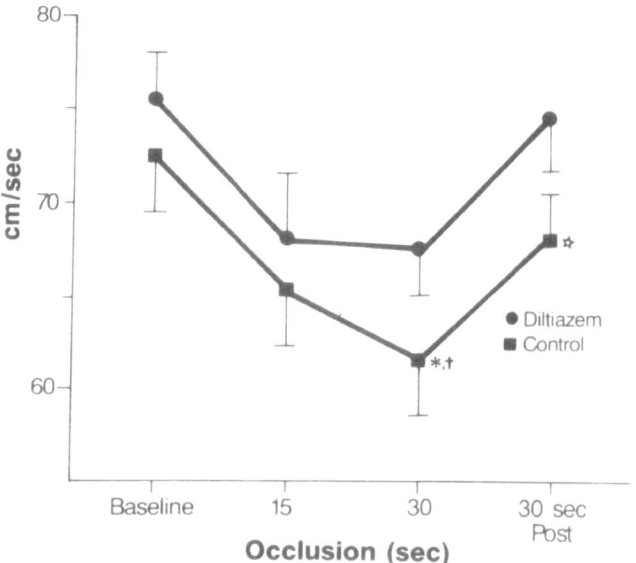

Figure 5. Change in peak early (E) velocity with balloon occlusion during untreated and diltiazem inflations.

plasty was not affected by the presence of collateral circulation. However, in only six of the nine patients with collateral circulation had new segmental wall motion abnormalities during vessel occlusion, whereas all 22 patients without collateral circulation demonstrated new wall motion abnormalities ($p \leqslant 0.05$). Five of the nine patients with collateral circulation did not develop ST segment changes, compared to only one of the patients without collaterals ($p < 0.01$). Angina during vessel occlusion occurred in 44% of the 22 patients with collaterals and 52% of patients without collateral circulation ($p = NS$).

Diastolic filling later after balloon occlusion

In 12 patients prior to Diltiazem administration, filling velocities were available at baseline, 15 and 60 sec following inflation. Table 3 shows the peak E, peak A velocities and ejection fraction response in this group. Peak E velocity dropped by 15 sec and was significantly lower at 60 sec. Peak A velocity, on the other hand, did not drop at 15 sec but by 60 sec was significantly decreased. The ratio of the peak E to peak A, thus, decreased at 15 sec but at 60 sec was higher than at baseline.

Effect of diltiazem on Doppler-echocardiographic measurements

Diltiazem significantly altered the response of diastolic Doppler flow velocities to balloon occlusion (Table 4). At baseline administration of diltiazem did not change heart rate or stroke integral. There was a trend toward a decrease in peak A velocity and an increase in peak E velocity with resulting increases in peak E/peak A and E integral/A integral ratios which did not reach statistical significance. However, there was a significant increase in the one-third filling fraction following diltiazem.

Following balloon occlusion, stroke index decreased significantly in the untreated subjects and by 30 sec the stroke index was significantly lower in the

Table 3. Filling parameters during long inflations.

Group II			
		Coronary balloon occlusion	
	Baseline	15 sec	60 sec
Peak E (cm/sec)	74 ± 19	67 ± 17	64 ± 16*
Peak A (cm/sec)	67 ± 18	66 ± 16	54 ± 14*·**
PE/PA	1.15 ± 0.32	1.06 ± 0.31	1.24 ± 0.44
EF (%)	52 ± 6	46 ± 13	41 ± 14*

*$p < 0.05$ versus baseline; **$p < 0.05$ versus 15 sec.

Table 4. Diastolic parameters during diltiazem and untreated balloon inflations in the ten patients who had all measurements.

		Coronary occlusion			
		Baseline	15 sec	30 sec	30 sec Post
E	Control (10)	72 ± 21	65 ± 20	61 ± 21*	68 ± 17
	Diltiazem (10)	75 ± 16	68 ± 18	67 ± 17	74 ± 13
	p	NS	NS	0.0625	0.0285
A	Control (10)	71 ± 18	67 ± 16	63 ± 15	64 ± 17
	Diltiazem (10)	68 ± 15	68 ± 13	68 ± 16	73 ± 12
	p	NS	NS	NS	0.0262
E/A	Control (10)	1.04 ± 0.27	1.00 ± 0.30	0.99 ± 0.32	1.10 ± 0.26
	Diltiazem (10)	1.2 ± 0.4	1.02 ± 0.22	1.03 ± 0.25	1.03 ± 0.17
	p	NS	NS	NS	NS
SI	Control (10)	1118 ± 325	1047 ± 299	920 ± 290*	974 ± 301*
	Diltiazem (10)	1144 ± 282	1068 ± 287	1022 ± 253*	1109 ± 218
	p	NS	NS	0.0607	0.0171
%AC	Control (9)	43 ± 12	47 ± 16	45 ± 16	39 ± 11
	Diltiazem (9)	37 ± 8	42 ± 10	43 ± 13	41 ± 7.8
	p	0.0195	NS	NS	NS
1/3 FF	Control (10)	41 ± 9	39 ± 10	40 ± 10	42 ± 10
	Diltiazem (10)	45 ± 8	41 ± 10	42 ± 12	42 ± 8
	p	0.0067	NS	NS	NS
HR	Control (10)	73 ± 14	76 ± 14	75 ± 16	73 ± 14
	Diltiazem (10)	72 ± 14	75 ± 14	76 ± 15*	74 ± 13
	p	NS	NS	NS	NS

*$p < 0.05$ versus baseline.
P value is for diltiazem versus control at given measurement interval; SI = stroke integral index; %AC = percent atrial contribution.
Abbreviations as in Table 2.

untreated compared to the diltiazem state (920 ± 29 vs 1012 ± 253 cm/min, $p < 0.05$). This was predominantly due to a drop in flow-velocity integral since the heart rate response to balloon occlusion was unchanged by diltiazem. Left ventricular ejection fraction response to balloon occlusion paralleled the drop in stroke integral index indicating a significant drop in ejection fraction by 30 seconds in the untreated patients. This decline in systolic function was blunted during treatment with diltiazem (Fig. 4).

The response to balloon occlusion of the diastolic function indices, including $E/A/E_i/A_i$, and E/mean was unchanged by diltiazem, with all three showing significant drops by 15 sec. One-third filling fraction which at baseline was significantly higher following diltiazem administration decreased by 15 sec in both diltiazem and baseline states and at 15 sec no difference existed between the two states.

However, analysis of the peak early and peak atrial velocities individually showed differing response to balloon inflation before and after diltiazem administration. At baseline, peak early and peak atrial velocities were unchanged by diltiazem administration, but after 30 sec peak early velocity had markedly and significantly dropped from 72 cm/sec to 61 cm/sec in untreated patients, while remaining unchanged (75 to 67 cm/sec) after diltiazem (Fig. 5). Peak early velocity had dropped in both inflation sequences but remained significantly higher in the diltiazem sequence than the untreated. At 30 sec post inflation the peak early velocity had recurred to baseline values in the diltiazem inflations and the untreated inflations had a significantly lower value than diltiazem inflations. Peak atrial velocity, in contrast was essentially unchanged at 15 and 30 sec after inflation in both treated and diltiazem sequencies. Thirty seconds post inflation the peak velocity was significantly higher in the diltiazem inflations than control.

Discussion

Temporal sequence of ventricular dysfunction

This study confirms that the ischemic response to transient coronary artery occlusion involves both systolic and diastolic left ventricular dysfunction, and that diastolic impairment occurs early and preceeds the development of new segmental wall motion abnormalities. Following balloon inflation, diastolic filling indices revealed a significant reversal of early to late filling patterns within 15 sec of vessel occlusion. Two independent markers of global left ventricular systolic function (1) percent area change, reflecting left ventricular ejection fraction and (2) stroke integral index, a measure of cardiac output, however, did not exhibit significant decreases until 30 sec after coronary artery occlusion. Electrocardiographic ST segment elevation occurred before systolic dysfunction (similar to diastolic dysfunction) while angina accompanied or followed the development of wall motion abnormalities. Systolic and diastolic indices showed rapid recovery following balloon deflation and were not significantly different from baseline by 15 sec after balloon deflation.

Comparison with previous studies

Systolic function. As early as 1935, Tennant and Wiggers [13] recognized that early systolic dysfunction occurs following coronary artery ligation. Pandian, using two-dimensional echocardiography, observed systolic wall thinning within 30 sec of coronary occlusion in the open chest dog [14–15]. While these findings cannot be directly extrapolated to the description of segmental wall motion abnormalities during coronary angioplasty, the temporal relationship is similar to the present study. Likewise, the mean time of approximately 30 sec from balloon inflation until onset of left ventricular regional dysfunction is similar to that reported in previous echocardiographic studies [16–18] in which both qualitative and semi-quantitative assessment of regional left ventricular function was performed utilizing two-dimensional echocardiography. Visser [17] observed changes in systolic function to occur much earlier (mean = 8 sec), however, in that study the first inflation was used in the analysis. We have observed systolic left ventricular dysfunction to occur with occlusion of the artery by the guidewire or the uninflated balloon catheter alone, prior to the first inflation, and have acquired our data after the first dilatation accordingly. It has been suggested that intermittent episodes of ischemia may result in 'stunned myocardium' or prolonged periods of myocardial systolic dysfunction [19]. The rapid return to baseline of new systolic wall motion abnormalities demonstrated here (usually within 30 sec) indicate that the brief periods of coronary occlusion occurring during PTCA do not result in such a phenomena. In addition, although the patient subset is small, the presence of angiographically apparent collateral circulation appeared to offer some protection during vessel occlusion.

Diastolic function. Several studies have suggested that left ventricular diastolic dysfunction may be a more sensitive marker of coronary ischemia than systolic dysfunction [20–24]. Aroesty [24] reporting on a group of patients with coronary artery disease and pacing induced ischemia, found diastolic impairment, as assessed by pressure volume curves, most often preceed systolic left ventricular dysfunction. Bonow et al [21, 22], utilizing radionuclide angiography, reported improvement in left ventricular diastolic filling following coronary angioplasty in patients with normal left ventricular systolic function. Differences in diastolic function following revascularization were evident at rest, while differences in systolic function were only evident with exercise. Wijns and coworkers [25] demonstrated significant impairment of left ventricular compliance, measured by the elastic constant of chamber stiffness, at 20 sec following coronary occlusion in patients undergoing PTCA. Doorey [26] found the rate of pressure decline during early diastole (tau) to be markedly prolonged (indicating abnormal relaxation) during balloon angioplasty with hemodynamic recovery evident by 20 sec following balloon deflation.

The changes in left ventricular filling we have recorded during induction of ischemia are particularly interesting in light of recent work from our laboratory and others indicating that impaired relaxation and impaired compliance have contrasting effects on left ventricular filling [27–29]. Our research involving simultaneous high-fidelity left ventricular pressure measurements, M-mode echocardiography and Doppler recording of left ventricular inflow has demonstrated that patients with impaired relaxation have lower peak early velocities and peak early to peak atrial ratios whereas patients with impaired compliance have lower peak atrial velocities with higher peak early to atrial ratios. The rapid drop in peak early velocity seen following balloon inflation is consistent with an early effect of ischemia on left ventricular relaxation. Impaired left ventricular relaxation is probably the earliest manifestation of ischemia [30–32]. Serruys et al [32] have shown abnormal relaxation occurring on average at 17 sec following balloon occlusion. The blunting and delayed drop in peak early velocity seen following diltiazem administration is consistent with an amelioration of the impaired relaxation due to calcium-channel blockade. Since wall motion abnormalities were noted on average following 29 sec of balloon occlusion, the diastolic filling parameters recorded at 30 sec post inflation undoubtedly reflect both the effects of impaired systolic function and the previously noted impaired relaxation. The net result is a drop in stroke volume which is manifested as a reduced stroke integral index. The trend toward reduced peak atrial velocity noted at 30 sec, especially in untreated inflation sequences is probably secondary to reduced stroke volume. Diltiazem prolongs the time to onset of ischemic wall motion abnormalities during PTCA, thus preserving systolic function at 30 sec [33] and resulting in higher stroke integral index at 30 sec inflation.

At 60 sec post inflation, the ratio of peak early to atrial velocities increases back towards and in some cases may exceed baseline values. This is due to the drastic drop in peak atrial velocities at 60 seconds. These findings are similar those of Bowman et al [34]. This group found no sigificant change in PE/PA values at 60 sec of balloon inflation compared to baseline in 26 patients undergoing PTCA. The explanation for this normalization of filling may lie in the increase in left ventricular end diastolic pressure which occurs during ischemia. The elevated left ventricular end diastolic pressure may present a greater afterload to atrial emptying resulting in atrial failure at 60 seconds of balloon occlusion. In addition, impaired compliance would also contribute to this normalization.

Acknowledgements

We are grateful for the expert technical assistance of the technicians and nurses of the cardiac catheterization laboratory and Susan Buenger Johnson in the preparation of this manuscript.

References

1. Ihlen H, Myhre E, Amlie JP, Forfang K, Larsen S (1985) Changes in left ventricular stroke volume measured by Doppler echocardiography. *Br Heart J* 54:378–83
2. Labovitz AJ, Buckingham TA, Habermehl K, Nelson J, Kennedy HL, Williams GA (1985) The effects of sampling site on the 2-dimensional echo Doppler determination of cardiac output. *Am Heart J* 109:327–332
3. Goldberg SJ, Sahn DJ, Allen HD, Valdes-Cruz LM, Hoenecke H, Carnahan Y (1982) Evaluation of pulmonary and systemic blood-flow by 2-dimensional Doppler echocardiography using fast fourier transform spectral analysis. *Am J Cardiol* 50:1394–1400
4. Pearson A, Labovitz AJ, Windhorst D, Williams GA, Kennedy HL (1987) Assessment of diastolic filling in normal and hypertrophied hearts: Comparison of Doppler echocardiography and M-mode echocardiography. *Am Heart J* 113:1417–1425
5. Pearson AC, Goodgold H, Labovitz AJ (1988) Comparison of pulsed Doppler echocardiography

and radionuclide angiography in the assessment of left ventricular filling. *Am J Cardiol* 61:446–454

6. Lewis JF, Kuo LC, Nelson JG, Limacher MC, Quinones MA (1984) Pulsed Doppler echocardiographic determination of stroke volume and cardiac output: Clinical validation of two new methods using the apical window. *Circ* 70:425–431

7. Spirito P, Maron BJ, Bonow RO (1986) Noninvasive assessment of left ventricular diastolic function: Comparative analysis of Doppler echocardiographic and radionuclide angiographic techniques. *J Am Coll Cardiol* 7:518–526

8. Rokey R, Kuo LC, Zoghbi WA, Limacher MC, Quinones MA (1985) Determination of parameters of left ventricular diastolic filling with pulsed Doppler echocardiography: Comparison with cineangiography. *Circ* 71:543–550

9. Takenaka K, Dabestani A, Gardin JM, Russell D, Clark S, Allfie A, Henry WL (1986) Pulsed Doppler echocardiographic study of left ventricular filling in dilated cardiomyopathy. *Am J Cardiol* 58:143–147

10. Snider AR, Gidding SS, Rocchini AP, Rosenthal A, Dick M, Crowley DC, Peters J (1985) Doppler evaluation of left ventricular diastolic filling in children with systemic hypertension. *Am J Cardiol* 56:921–926

11. Vandormael VG, Chaitman BR, Ischinger T, Aker UT, Harper M, Hernandez J, Deligonul U, Kennedy HL (1985) Immediate and short-term benefit of multilesion coronary angioplasty: Influence of degree of revascularization. *J Am Coll Cardiol* 6:983–991

12. Collins SM, Skorton DJ, Geiser EA, Nichols JA, Conetta DA, Pandian NG, Kerber RE (1984) Computer-assisted edge detection in two-dimensional echocardiography: Comparison with anatomic data. *Am J Cardiol* 53:1380–1387

13. Tennant R, Wiggers LJ (1935) The effect of coronary occlusion on myocardial contractions. *Am J Physiol* 112:351–361

14. Pandian NG, Kerber RE (1982) Two-dimensional echocardiography in experimental coronary stenosis, I: Sensitivity and specificity in detecting transient myocardial dyskinesis: comparison with sonomicrometers. *Circ* 66:597–602

15. Pandian NG, Kieso RA, Kerber RE (1982) Two-dimensional echocardiography in experimental coronary stenosis, II: Relationship between systolic wall thinning and regional myocardial perfusion in severe coronary stenosis. *Circ* 66:603–611

16. Hauser AM, Gangadharan V, Ramos RG, Gordon S, Timmis GC, Dudlets P (1985) Sequence of mechanical, electrocardiographic and clinical effects of repeated coronary artery occlusion in human beings: Echocardiographic observations during coronary angioplasty. *J Am Coll Cardiol* 5:193–197

17. Visser CA, David GK, Kan G, Romijn KH, Meltzer RS, Koolen JJ, Dunning AJ (1986) Two-dimensional echocardiography during percutaneous transluminal coronary angioplasty. *Am Heart J* 111:1035–1046

18. Alam M, Khaja F, Brymer J, Marzelli M, Goldstein S (1986) Echocardiographic evaluation of left ventricular function during coronary artery angioplasty. *Am J Cardiol* 57:20–25

19. Braunwald E, Kloner RA (1982) The stunned myocardium: prolonged, post ischemic ventricular dysfunction. *Circ* 66:1146–1149

20. Carroll JD, Hess OM, Hirzel HO, Turina M, Krayenbuehl HP (1985) Left ventricular systolic and diastolic function in coronary artery disease: Effects of revascularization on exercise-induced ischemia. *Circ* 72:119–129

21. Bonow RO, Kent KM, Rosing DR, Lipson LC, Bacharach SL, Green MV, Epstein SE (1982) Improved left ventricular diastolic filling in patients with coronary artery disease after percutaneous transluminal coronary angioplasty. *Circ* 66:1159–1167

22. Bonow RO, Vitale DF, Bacharach SL, Frederick TM, Kent KM, Green MV (1985) Asynchronous left ventricular regional function and impaired global diastolic filling in patients with coronary artery disease: reversal after coronary angioplasty. *Circ* 71:297–307

23. Lewis JF, Verani MS, Poliner LR, Lewis JM, Raizner AE (1985) Effects of transluminal coronary angioplasty on left ventricular systolic and diastolic function at rest and during exercise. *Am Heart J* 109:792–798

24. Aroesty JM, McKay RG, Heller GV, Royal HD, Als AV, Grossman W (1985) Simultaneous assessment of left ventricular systolic and diastolic dysfunction during pacing-induced ischemia. *Circ* 71:889–900
25. Wijns W, Serruys PW, Slager CJ, Grimm J, Krayenbuehl HP, Hugenholtz PG (1986) Effect of coronary occlusion during percutaneous transluminal angioplasty in humans on left ventricular chamber stiffness and regional diastolic pressure-radius relations. *J Am Coll Cardiol* 7:455–463
26. Doorey AJ, Mehmel HC, Schwarz FX, Kubler W (1985) Amelioration by nitroglycerin of left ventricular ischemia induced by percutaneous transluminal coronary angioplasty: Assessment by hemodynamic variables and left ventriculography. *J Am Coll Cardiol* 6:267–274
27. Stoddard MF, Pearson AC, Kern MJ, Ratcliff J, Labovitz AJ (1988) Influence of left ventricular chamber stiffness and relaxation on diastolic filling. *Eur Heart J* 9:169
28. Stoddard MF, Pearson AC, Labovitz AJ, Kern MJ, Mrosek DG (1987) Sensitivity and specificity of Doppler for assessing abnormalities of left ventricular relaxation and stiffness. *Transactions of the Association for Academic Minority Physicians* 1:14A
29. Stoddard MF, Pearson AC, Labovitz AJ, Kern MJ (1988) Effects of preload reduction on pulsed Doppler indices of left ventricular filling. *Clinical Research* 36:321A
30. Sigwart V, Grbic M, Essinger A, Fisher A, Morin D, Sadeghi H (1982) Myocardial function in man during acute coronary balloon occlusion. *Circ* 66:86
31. Bertrand ME, Lablanche JM, Thieuleux FA (1983) Changes in left ventricular relaxation during transient coronary occlusion in man. *Eur Heart J* 4:49
32. Serruys PW, Wijns W, van den Brand M (1984) Left ventricular performance, regional blood flow, wall motion and lactate metabolism during transluminal angioplasty. *Circ* 70:25–36
33. Kern MJ, Deligonul U, Gabliani G, Labovitz A, Vandormael M, Woodruff R, Chernoff S. (1988) Systemic and coronary hemodynamic effects of intravenous diltiazem in patients during transient myocardial ischemia
34. Bowman LK, Cleman MW, Cabin HS, Zaret BL, Jaffe CC (1988) Dynamics of early and late left ventricular filling determined by Doppler two-dimensional echocardiography during percutaneous transluminal coronary angioplasty. *Am J Cardiol* 61:541–545

18. Ejection filling and diastasis during transluminal occlusion in man

Consideration on global and regional left ventricular function

PATRICK W. SERRUYS, FEDERICO PISCIONE, WILLIAM WIJNS,
CEES SLAGER, PIM DE FEYTER, MARCEL VAN DEN BRAND,
PAUL G. HUGENHOLTZ and GEERT T. MEESTER

Introduction

An extensive literature exists describing the acute changes in hemodynamics and left ventricular function following coronary occlusion in animals [1-4]. Much less, however, is known in man. Extrapolating results from animals to man is potentially difficult, since, in man preexisting atherosclerotic coronary disease and a unique distribution of collateral circulation [5-7] may influence findings.

Until recently the measurement in man of left ventricular geometry and hemodynamics early after an abrupt occlusion of a major coronary artery has not been feasible. Percutaneous transluminal coronary angioplasty (PTCA) however, now provides a unique opportunity to study the time course of these variables during the transient interruption of coronary flow in the balloon occlusion sequence in patients with single vessel disease and without angiographically demonstrable collateral circulation [8-10].

Study population and protocol

After a preliminary study to confirm the absence of effects of nonionic contrast media (metrizamide-Amipaque®) on left ventricular function, permission was obtained from the Thoraxcenter Ethics Committee to perform left ventricular angiography during balloon inflation at PTCA. All patients involved in the study gave informed consent and no complications related to the research procedure occurred. Fourteen patients with coronary artery disease undergoing PTCA, with the following selection criteria, were studied:

1. isolated, obstructive lesion of one coronary artery (10-left anterior descending; 3-right coronary; 1-left circumflex), without angiographically demonstrable collateral circulation.
2. normal left ventricular wall motion at rest, as determined at prior diagnostic catheterization.
3. no intraventricular conduction abnormalities on the resting ECG.

P.W. Serruys, R, Simon & K.J. Beatt (eds), Percutaneous Transluminal Coronary Angioplasty. ISBN 0-7923-0346-6.
© *1990 Kluwer Academic Publishers, Dordrecht*

Four patients had mild essential hypertension and an elevated left ventricular end-diastolic pressure (≥ 25 mmHg). Standard antianginal therapy was allowed until the day of the study.

During the PTCA procedure the number of transluminal occlusions performed per patient was 4.9 ± 2.2 (mean ± SD). The average duration of each occlusion was 51 ± 12 s (mean ± SD) and the total occlusion time during the whole procedure was 252 ± 140 s (mean ± SD).

Left ventricular pressure was recorded during ventriculography (30° right anterior oblique view at 50 frames/s) carried out before balloon dilatation, at a mean occlusion time of 20 s during the second dilatation, at a mean occlusion time of 48 s during the fourth dilatation and at a mean of 12 min after the last dilatation. Angiography during the fourth dilatation was performed in only 10 patients. A total of 3 to 10 occlusions were performed and the duration of balloon inflation ranged from 15 to 75 s. Each consecutive balloon inflation was made only when end-diastolic pressure and left ventricular pressure-derived isovolumic parameters of contractility and relaxation, which were available on-line during the procedure [11, 12], had returned to basal values. Care was taken to maintain uniform patient position relative to X-ray equipment during sequential angiograms which were performed with the breath held in shallow inspiration.

Methods

Analysis of pressure derived indices during systole and diastole

Left ventricular pressure was measured with a Millar micromanometer catheter and digitized ag 250 samples/s. Combined analog and digital filtering resulted in an effective time constant of less than 10 msec. This employed an updated version of the beat-to-beat program described previously [11, 12].

Peak LV pressure, LV end-diastolic pressure, peak negative dP/dt, peak positive dP/dt and the relation between dP/dt/P and P linearly extrapolated to $P = 0$ (V_{max}) were computed on line after a data acquistion of 20 s.

A new technique has been implemented for the off-line beat-to-beat calculation of the relaxation parameters [13], using a semilogarithmic model:

$P(t) = P_0 e^{-t/T}$ The P_0 and T parameters are estimated from a linear least squares fit of $LnP = -t/T + LnP_0$, starting from the time of peak $-dP/dt$.

(a) fit of first 40 msec	($n = 8$), Tau_1, bi-exponential [13]
(b) fit after the first 40 msec	($n = 8$), Tau_2, bi-exponential [13]
(c) fit of all points	($n = 8$), T, mono-exponential

Isovolumic relaxation period was defined as the time interval between the aortic valve closure and the mitral valve opening. This later was defined during left ventriculography, as occurring in the last frame preceding the entry of non-opacified blood into the left ventricle form the left atrium. The left ventricular pressure corresponding to this frame was considered to reflect left atrial pressure [14].

Analysis of regional and global left ventricular function

Ejecting dynamics. A complete cardiac cycle was analyzed frame by frame from each angiogram. The ventricular contours were automatically detected by an analysis system [15] and the instantaneous volume calculated according to Simpson's rule. End-diastolic and end-systolic volumes, cardiac index, stroke index and ejection fraction and the derivative of me relative to time (dV/dt) were derived. End-diastolic (ED) pressure was defined at that point on the pressure trace at which the derivative of the pressure first exceeded 200 mmHg/s [11] and in all cases coincided with the maximal measured LV volume.

End-systole (ES) was defined, with reference to the pressure tracing, at the occurrence of the dicrotic notch of the central aortic pressure. To analyze the regional left ventricular function, the computer generated a system of coordinates along which the left ventricular wall displacement is determined frame by frame in 20 segments (Fig. 1). The definition of the 20 segmental coordinates was derived from the mean trajectories of endocardial sites in 23 normal individuals [16] and generalized as a mathematical expression amenable to automatic data processing [17, 18].

Segmental volume was computed from the local radius (R) and the height of

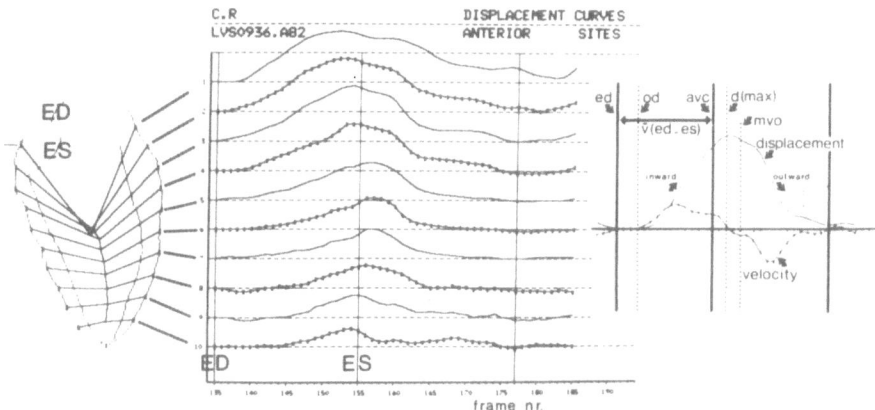

Figure 1. End-diastolic and end-systolic left ventricular contours, as detected by the automated analysis system. On these silhouettes is superimposed a system of coordinates along which segmental left ventricular wall displacement is detected. Left ventricular wall velocity – first derivative of wall displacement – is derived from these data. Abbreviations: ed: end-diastole; es: end-systole; od: onset of displacement; v(ed-es): mean ejection phase wall velocity; d(max): maximal inward wall displacement; mvo: mitral valve opening.

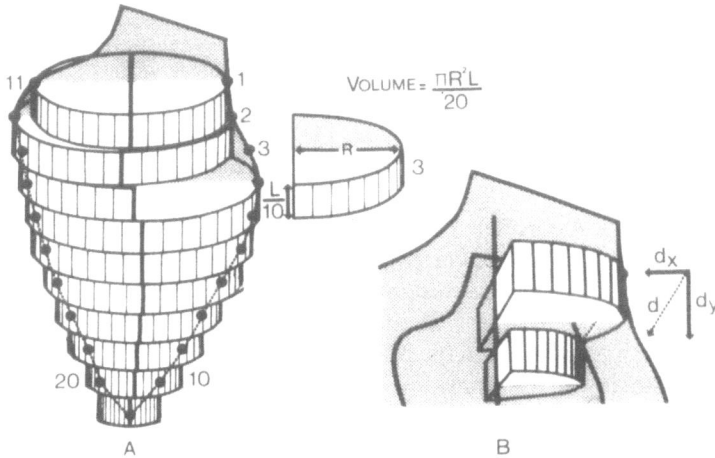

Figure 2. Method for computing regional contribution to ejection fraction (CREF): volume of each segment (slice volume) is computed according to the formula shown in the figure. The systolic volume change is derived from the regional displacement and is mainly a consequence of the decrease of radius (R) of a half slice, which is expressed by the x-component (dx) of the displacement vector (d). L: left ventricular long axis length extending from base to apex.

each segment (1/10 of left ventricular long axis length L) according the formula: $1/20 \, \Pi R^2 L$, when normalized for end-diastolic volume, the systolic segmental volume change can be considered as a parameter of regional pump function (Fig. 2). During systole this parameter expresses quantitatively the contribution of a particular segment to global ejection fraction, termed regional contribution to global ejection fraction or CREF [17]. The sum of the values for all 20 segments equals the global ejection fraction.

Segmental wall velocity was computed as the first derivative of the instantaneous displacement function. Mean ejection phase wall velocity (V) for each segment was calculated from end-diastole to end-systole (V_{ed-es}), (Fig. 1).

Filling dynamics. Peak segmental inward and outward velocity was calculated as the first derivative relative to time of the segmental wall displacement after a 3 point smoothing function had been applied to the data (Fig. 1). Peak ejection rate was taken as the lowest dV/dt after end-diastole; peak global filling rate as the peak dV/dt after mitral valve opening and the time to peak filling rate was the time interval between the aortic valve closure and the peak dV/dt. The time interval was measured between the occurrence of the globak peak filling rate and the peak velocity of segmental outward displacement (Fig. 3). We defined $\Sigma\Delta t_1$ as the sum of the absolute values of the time differences between global peak filling rate and peak velocity of segmental outward displacement; $\Sigma\Delta t_1/Dt$ was $\Sigma\Delta t_1$ normalized for diastolic time. We defined $\Sigma\Delta t_2$ as the sum of the absolute values of the time differences between aortic valve closure and peak segmental inward displacement (Fig. 3) and $\Sigma\Delta t_2/ET$ was $\Sigma\Delta t_2$ normalized for ejection time. The

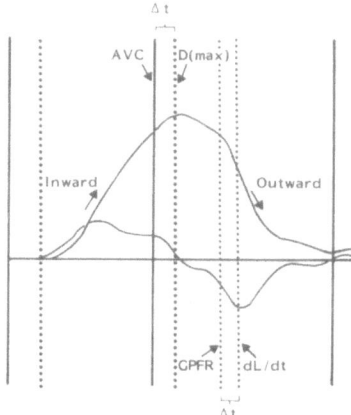

Figure 3. Segmental wall displacement and its first derivative are superimposed to show the temporal relationship between inward and outward phases with the aortic valve closure (AVC). The time intervals (Δt) between AVC and the maximal inward wall displacement (Dmax) and between the occurrence of global peak filling rate (GPFR) and the peak velocity of outward displacement (dL/dt) were measured in every segment.

terms $\Sigma\Delta t_1$, $\Sigma\Delta t_1/Dt$; $\Sigma\Delta t_2$, $\Sigma\Delta t_2/ET$ are thus indexes reflecting variations in the synchrony of ventricular filling and contraction respectively.

Diastasis. This part of the study includes the 10 patients (1 female and 9 males) who underwent a percutaneous transluminal coronary angioplasty of a left anterior descending coronary artery stenosis. One of the 10 patients was excluded because the small number of available data points due to a higher heart rate precluded analysis of the diastolic function. Thus simultaneous left ventricular pressure and volume were obtained after a median occlusion of 20 s (range 15–27) during the second dilatation in 9 patients and after a median occlusion of 48 s (range 46–59) during the fourth dilatation in five.

In this subset of patients study, the length of the 20 segmental radii defined by the model was measured frame by frame and among them, was selected for analysis six radii located either in the core of the ischemic segment (anterior, antero lateral and apical radius), or in the non ischemic segment (anterobasal and posterobasal radius), as well as the interior radius immediately adjacent to the ischemic segment (Fig. 4). The linear correlation coefficients between repeated measurements of radius length in 20 patients ranged from 0.96 to 0.99 (SEE = 0.4 to 1.4%) for the same operator and from 0.91 to 0.99 (SEE = 0.4 to 2.3%) for two different operators.

For the evaluation of the global chamber stiffness, the left ventricular pressure (P) and volume (V) data obtained every 20 msec starting at the lowest diastolic pressure and ending at the end-diastolic pressure were fitted by a simple elastic model: $P = \alpha e^{\beta V} + C$, where α = intercept (mmHg), β = constant of elastic chamber stiffness and C = baseline pressure (mmHg). The three constants of this equation

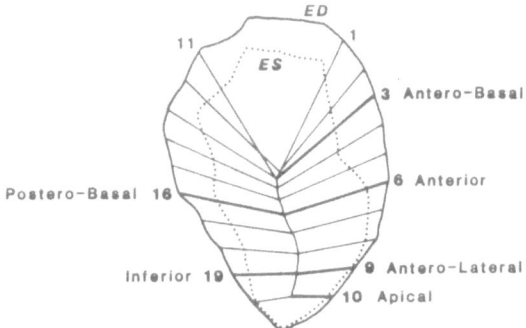

Figure 4. The end-diastolic (ED) and end-systolic (ES) contours of a left ventriculogram during transluminal occlusion are displayed with the system of 20 radii along which regional wall displacement was determined. For the analysis of regional diastolic function, we selected radius 6, 9 and 10 within the ischemic zone; radius 3 and 16 within the nonischemic zone as well as radius 19 in the adjacent inferior zone.

(α, β, C) were determined using an iteration procedure until the best non-linear curve fit was obtained [19].

For the evaluation of the regional chamber stiffness, the left ventricular pressure and the segment radius length (L) data were fitted in a similar way for each of the six $(1, 2, \ldots n)$ analyzed segmental radii: $P = \alpha_n e^{\beta} n^L + C_n$, where β_n represents the regional elastic stiffness constant for a given radius. The same approach was applied previously by others to pressure-length relations obtained either by ultrasonic subendocardial crystals [20] or by contrast ventriculography [21, 22].

Statistical analysis. Results are given for all patients and the subgroup analysed after 50 s occlusion either as mean $\pm$ standard deviation or as median values using analysis of variance for repeated measurements. Comparisons between pre-angioplasty, post-angioplasty and 20 s occlusion conditions were performed in 10 patients. The data obtained before angioplasty, after 50 s occlusion and after angioplasty were compared in the appropriate subgroup of 5 patients. In both cases, when overall significance was found, multiple comparisons were used to delineate which paired comparisons were significantly different at the 0.05 level.

The relationship between peak filling rate and the regional indexes reflecting asynchrony of contraction and filling were analyzed by regression analysis.

Results

Global left ventricular function during systole and diastole

Volumes, pressures and derived parameters measured before, during and after transluminal occlusion are listed in Table 1a and 1b. There was no important change in heart rate during the PTCA procedure. The pattern of change in peak LVP, LVEDP, peak + dP/dt, and V_{max}, however, suggests a progressive depression in myocardial mechanics without any indication of an early peak (Fig. 5).

In contrast, within four or five beats after occlusion, a deformation appeared in the ascending limb of the negative dP/dt curve (Fig. 6) and in the next ten seconds this deformation in the negative dP/dt curve gradually increased so that the irregularity in the negative dP/dt curve reached the same height as peak $-$dP/dt which has progressively decreased to its nadir. In the next 20–50 s, peak $-$dP/dt began to return towards control levels with a resolution of the irregularity in the ascending limb of $-$dP/dt. At 50 s, peak $-$dP/dt recovered to 77% of the preocclusion value and the deformity was no longer present.

This deformation of the negative dP/dt signal at the early phase of the occlusion means that the time course of left ventricular pressure decay deviates substantially from the mono-exponential model usually proposed and it means also that asynchronous contraction or relaxation may be involved at the very beginning of the transluminal occlusion. Therefore bi-exponential fitting of the pressure curve was computed during the isovolumic relasation, primarily on the basis that the pressure curve when plotted on semilogarithmic paper was noted to follow two straight lines rather than the one predicted by the mono-exponential mode.

The first half of Table 1b summarizes the results of the relaxation parameters. The behaviour of the two time constants (Tau_1, Tau_2) during PTCA is illustrated in Fig. 5.

An example of the frame to frame analysis of left ventricular volume before and during ischemia induced by balloon inflation is shown in Fig. 7 with its derivative (dV/dt). The global indexes of the ejection phase decreased during the two periods of coronary occlusion; the ejection fraction fell from 61% to 54% over 20 s ($p < 0.005$) and from 62% to 48% ($p < 0.005$) over 50 s, this reduction being mainly due to the increase in end-systolic volume over 20 s (from 31 ± 9 ml/m^2 to 37 ± 9; $p < 0.005$) and 50 s (from 29 ± 7 ml/m^2 to 41 ± 9; $p < 0.005$). Consequently the stroke volume was significantly decreased from 50 ± 11 ml/m^2 to 44 ± 12 ($p < 0.05$) during the first period of occlusion and from 49 ± 11 ml/m^2 to 39 ± 14 ($p < 0.05$) during the second. A slight but not significant reduction in peak ejection rate was observed over 20 s but after 50 s it was decreased from 255 ± 106 ml/m^2 to 185 ± 61 ($p < 0.05$) (Fig. 8). Normalization for end-diastolic volume and stroke volume did not render the change in peak ejection rate at 20 s significant. In parallel to the prolongation of Tau_1 and Tau_2. The isovolumic relaxation period increased from 71 ± 18 msec to 85 ± 16 ($p < 0.05$) over 20 s are from 77 ± 18 msec to 80 ± 17 ($p = NS$) over 50 s. The left ventricular pressure in the time of mitral valve opening increased from 19 ± 5 mmHg to 23 ± 8 ($p = NS$) over 20 s and from 18 ± 3 mmHg to 25 ± 6 ($p < 0.05$) over 50 s. Peak filling rate was reduced from 311 ± 85 ml/sec to 234 ± 82 ($p < 0.05$) after 20 s of ischemia (Fig. 4) and from 296 ± 84 ml/s to 225 ± 93 ($p < 0.05$) after 50 s. When normalized for stroke volume, peak filling rate was unchanged after 20 and 50 s of occlusion, whereas after normalization for end diastolic volume it was significantly decreased after 20 (from 4 ± 1 EDV/sec to 3 ± 0.8; $p < 0.05$) and 50 s (from $3.7 \pm$

Table 1a. Global *systolic* before PTCA, 20 and 50 s after the onset of occlusion

Variables	Before PTCA	
	Total group n = 14	Subgroup n = 9
Heart rate, bpm	62 ± 16	59 ± 18
End-diastolic volume ml/m²	81 ± 15	79 ± 14
End-systolic volume ml/m²	31 ± 9	29 ± 7
Stroke volume ml/m²	50 ± 11	49 ± 11
Ejection fraction %	61 ± 8	62 ± 6
Mean systolic ejection rate (ml/s)	129 ± 24	127 ± 24
Peak ejection rate (ml/s)	251 ± 97	255 ± 106
Time to peak ejection rate (msec)	172 ± 44	175 ± 50
Peak ejection rate (SV/s)	5 ± 1	5.4 ± 1
Peak ejection rate (EDV/s)	3 ± 0.8	3.3 ± 0.9
End systolic pressure (mmHg)	95 ± 18	92 ± 22
Peak LVP, mmHg	154 ± 30	151 ± 35
Peak +dP/dt, mmHg⁻¹	1403 ± 304	1356 ± 257
Vmax, s⁻¹	39 ± 9	40 ± 8

LVP = left ventricular pressure; dP/dt = rate of change of pressure; V_{max} = maximal velocity

Table 1b. Global *diastolic* function before PTCA, 20 and 50 s after the onset of occlusion

Variables	Before PTCA	
	Total group n = 14	Subgroup n = 9
Tau₁ (msec)	55 ± 8	55 ± 6
Tau₂ (msec)	44 ± 7	43 ± 7
IRP msec	71 ± 18	77 ± 18
MVO pressure (mmHg)	19 ± 5	18 ± 3
MVO volume (ml/m²)	37 ± 9	35 ± 7
Peak filling rate (ml/s)	311 ± 83	296 ± 84
Time to peak filling rate (msec)	128 ± 20	133 ± 22
Peak filling rate (SV/s)	6.5 ± 1	6 ± 0.9
Peak filling rate (EDV/s)	4 ± 1	3.7 ± 0.8
Pmin (mmHg)	10 ± 5	8 ± 3
Volume at Pmin (ml/m²)	51 ± 13	48 ± 11
MRVI (ml/s)	179 ± 82	198 ± 78
EDP mmHg	22 ± 8	18 ± 6
EDV ml/m²	81 ± 15	79 ± 14

Tau₁ and Tau₂ = time constant of relaxation (biexponential fitting), Tau₁ fit of the first 40 msec, Tau₂ fit after 40 msec; IRP = isovolumic relaxation period; MVO = mitral valve opening; Pmin = minimal left ventricular diastolic pressure; MRVI = mean rate of volume and after PTCA.

20 s occlusion Total group n = 14	50 s occlusion Subgroup n = 9	After PTCA Subgroup n = 9	Total group n = 14
61 ± 13	62 ± 14	63 ± 11	64 ± 11
81 ± 15	81 ± 16	78 ± 11	77 ± 11
37 ± 9*	41 ± 9*	26 ± 15	27 ± 7°
44 ± 12°	39 ± 14°	52 ± 10	50 ± 9
54 ± 8*	48 ± 12*	66 ± 6	64 ± 7
125 ± 32	116 ± 67	165 ± 48	147 ± 27
222 ± 69	185 ± 61°	248 ± 77	240 ± 68
172 ± 56	153 ± 34	170 ± 88	166 ± 76
5 ± 0.7	5 ± 0.9	5 ± 0.6	4.7 ± 0.6
2.7 ± 0.5	2.3 ± 0.5*	3.2 ± 0.5	3 ± 0.5
90 ± 19	98 ± 24	91 ± 15	90 ± 14
142 ± 29	145 ± 37	148 ± 25	147 ± 21
1312 ± 320	1278 ± 317	1442 ± 384	1412 ± 333
39 ± 9	34 ± 10°	43 ± 12	42 ± 11

of the contractile element (dPdt/P linearly extrapolated to P = 0).

and after PTCA.

20 s occlusion Total group n = 14	50 s occlusion Subgroup n = 9	After PTCA Subgroup n = 9	Total group n = 14
79 ± 17*	68 ± 16*	56 ± 7	54 ± 7
51 ± 8°	59 ± 8*	45 ± 8	45 ± 9
85 ± 16°	80 ± 17	77 ± 16	71 ± 15
23 ± 8	25 ± 6°	19 ± 5	21 ± 6
41 ± 9°	45 ± 10*	30 ± 6	31 ± 8
234 ± 82°	255 ± 93°	297 ± 117	277 ± 109
145 ± 38	151 ± 26	130 ± 18	126 ± 23
5.9 ± 1	6 ± 2	5.8 ± 0.8	5.7 ± 1
3 ± 8°	2.8 ± 0.7*	3.8 ± 0.9	3.6 ± 1
11 ± 4	16 ± 6*	8 ± 5	8 ± 4
53 ± 10	55 ± 10	45 ± 11	45 ± 9
98 ± 78*	104 ± 69*	161 ± 131	138 ± 113
22 ± 7	29 ± 5*	21 ± 5	20 ± 6
81 ± 15	81 ± 16	78 ± 11	77 ± 11

inflow during the time interval between MVO and Pmin; EDP = end-diastolic pressure; EDV = end-diastolic volume. °p < 0.05; *p < 0.005 (compared with before PTCA, paired Student t test).

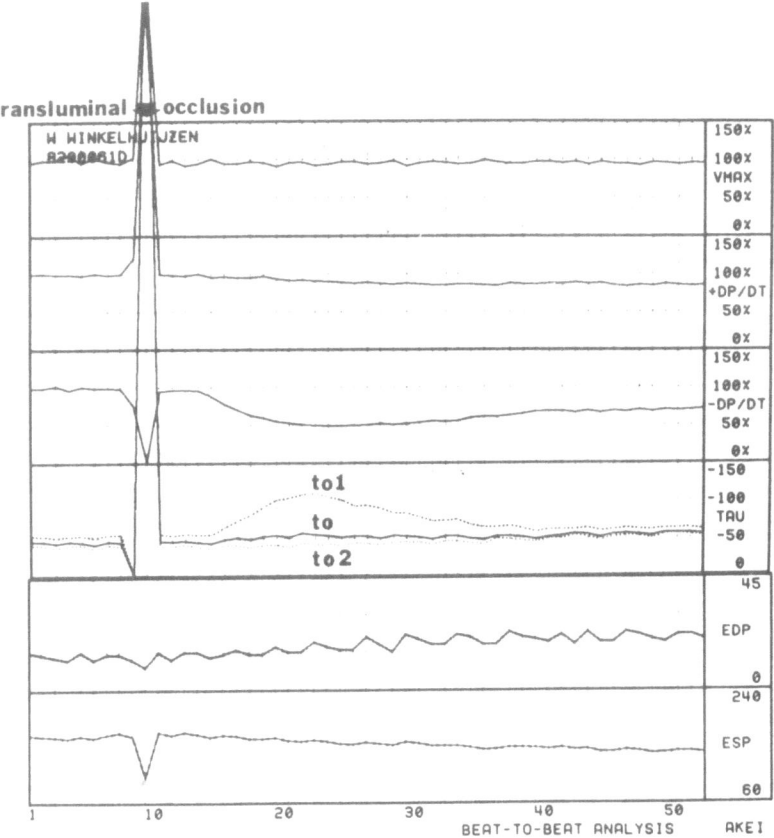

Figure 5. Hemodynamic measurements in a patient during percutaneous transluminal coronary angioplasty. From top to bottom, maximal velocity of the contractile elements (Vmax), peak – and + dP/dt expressed as a percentage of control values, the time constants of relaxation To_1 dashed line, To solid line, To_2 dotted line (scale 50 msec), end-diastolic pressure (EDP, scale 15 mmHg), peak systolic pressure (ESP, scale 60 mmHg, with 60 mmHg offset). The break in the data at beat 10 corresponds in inflation of the PTCA balloon.

0.8 EDV/sec to 2.8 ± 0.7; $p < 0.005$). The mean rate of volume inflow, measured during the early filling period between the mitral valve opening and the occurrence of minimal diastolic pressure, declined significantly both at 20 (from 179 ± 82 ml/sec to 98 ± 78; $p < 0.005$) and 50 s (from 198 ± 94 ml/sec to 104 ± 69; $p < 0.005$) from the onset of occlusion.

The left ventricular volume at the lowest diastolic pressure as well as at end-diastole did not change significantly during and after angioplasty while the lowest diastolic ($p < 0.05$) and the end-diastolic ($p < 0.01$) pressures were increased in the subgroup of patients studied after 50 s of anterior descending coronary artery occlusion. The increase in pressure relative to volume during transluminal

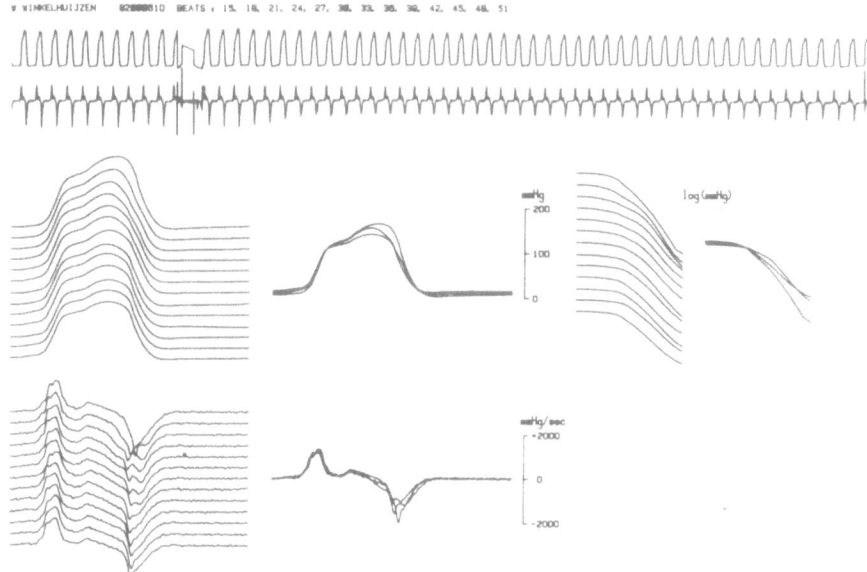

Figure 6. Effects of coronary artery occlusion on left ventricular pressure (mmHg) and + and −dP/dt (mmHg/sec). The break in the recording at beat 15 corresponds in inflation of the balloon. On the left hand side are displayed the left ventricular pressure and + and −dP/dt of individual beats (15, 18, 21, and so forth) while the natural logarithm of the pressure is shown on the right-hand side. Notice decrease in −dP/dt associated with an irregularity in the upstroke of the negative dP/dt curve. After 30 s (beat 42) peak −dP/dt starts to return toward a more normal shape of the signal.

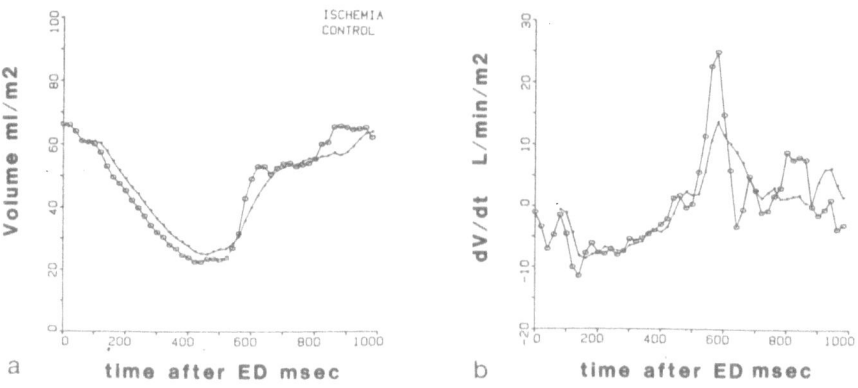

Figure 7. (a) Left ventricular volume curves for the same patient, derived from angiographic volumes every 20 msec throughout a complete cardiac cycle, before and during transluminal occlusion. (b) Instantaneous left ventricular volume derivative (dV/dt) curves for the same patient, measured every 20 msec throughout a complete cardiac cycle, before and during transluminal occlusion. During ischemia a decrease in peak dV/dt was observed.
ED = end-diastole.

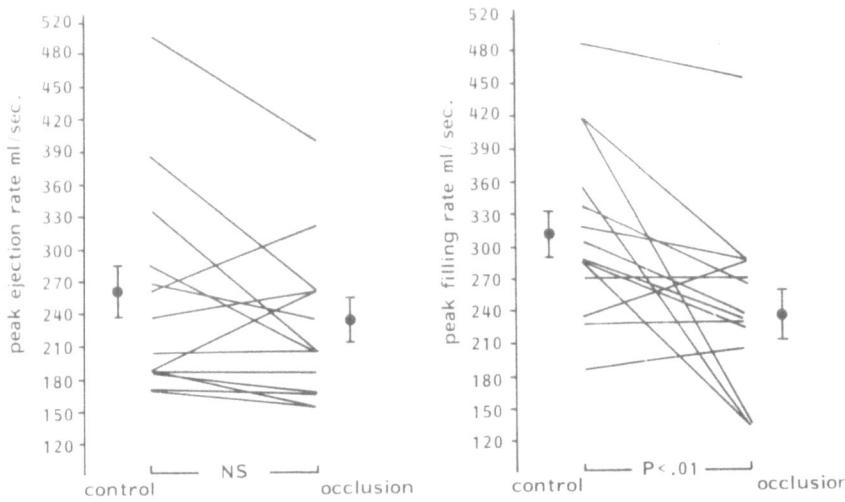

Figure 8.   Individual and mean changes (± SEM) in peak ejection rate and peak filling rate during transluminal occlusion (20 msec). Only the peak filling rate showed a significant decrease during the early phase of coronary occlusion.

occlusion resulted in an upward shift of the entire pressure-volume relation, as shown for two representative patients (patient 2 and 7) in Fig. 9. In only two instances (patient 6 and 9), we observed a shift downward and to the right of the pressure-volume relation.

The calculated parameters of global chamber stiffness showed a similarly increased constant of elastic stiffness (β) after 20 as well as after 50 s of occlusion (Table 2). The baseline pressure (C) increased significantly (p < 0.01) only after 50 s of coronary occlusion. No change in the intercept (α) was observed (Table 2). All patients but one showed an increase in chamber stiffness during coronary occlusion which, after the procedure, returned to values not significantly different from the pre-angioplasty value. However, the post-angioplasty elastic constant remained higher than the control value in five instances. This is further illustrated in Fig. 9 as the pressure-volume relation obtained after the procedure is nearly superimposed on the control curve in patient 2 (Fig. 9A) whereas the post-angioplasty curve remains shifted upwards in patient 7 (Fig. 9B).

Regional indexes of left ventricular ejection and filling and region:
pressure-radius length relations

The profound effect of a 20 s occlusion of the left anterior descending artery (LAD) on left ventricular wall motion and its time sequence is shown in Fig. 10. The delay in onset of displacement with respect to end-diastole as well as the timing relationship between the aortic valve closure and the occurrence of the

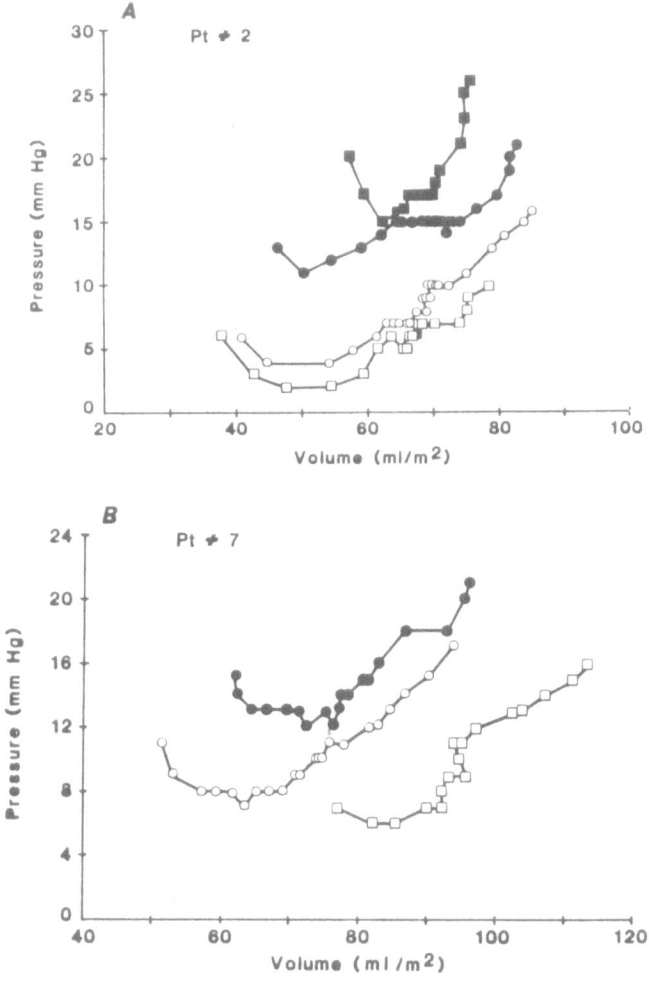

Figure 9. Diastolic pressure-volume relation in two representative patients. Note the upward shift of the relation during coronary occlusion. In patient 2, the post-angioplasty relation returned towards control while it remains shifted upwards in patients 7 (respectively Figs 9A and 9B). Open squares = pre angioplasty; close circles = 20 s occlusion; closed squares = 50 s occlusion; open circles = post angioplasty.

maximal wall displacement is illustrated in Fig. 10. The onset of displacement of the anterior and inferior wall was no significantly affected after 20 s of LAD occlusion. On the contrary, the moment of maximal wall displacement for the anterior wall shifted from end-systole to early diastole. The anterolateral segment (no 6 and 7) and the apical segment (no 9 and 10) of the anterior wall, as well as the apical segment (no 20 and 19) of the inferior wall appeared to be most affected.

Table 2. Global left ventricular chamber stiffness (simple elastic model).

	α Intercept mmHg	β Constant of elastic stiffness	Γ Baseline pressure mmHg
all patients (n=9)	NS	*	NS
PRE	4.6±4.9	0.0273±0.017	−1.4±9.5
20 s occlusion	1.2±3.3	0.0621±0.026*	5.2±8.3
POST	1.2±1.5	0.0529±0.037	2.8±4.7
subgroup (n=5)	NS	**	**
PRE	5.3±5.9	0.0214±0.007	−5.8±7.4
50 s occlusion	0.2±0.3	0.0605±0.015*	9.4±2.7**
POST	1.9±1.8	0.0396±0.027	0.8±5.6

Values are mean ± 1 s.d.; overall and paired (versus PRE angioplasty) significance values are given.
* = p<0.05; ** = p<0.01.

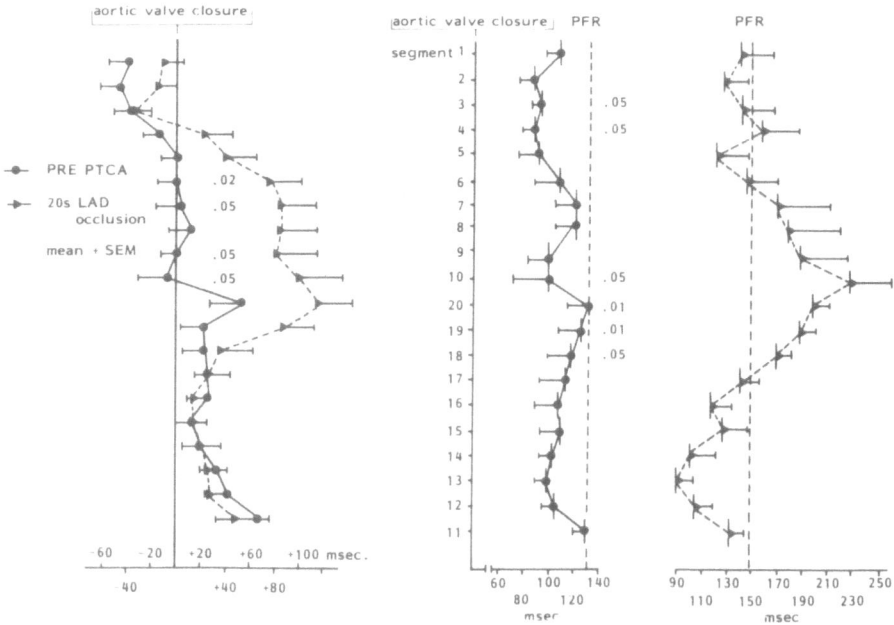

Figure 10. Left panel: Time relationship between aortic valve closure and the occurrence of maximal inward wall displacement before and after 20 msec of occlusion of the left anterior descending artery. Right panel: Time relationship between aortic valve closure and the occurrence of peak velocity of segmental outward displacement before and after 20 s of occlusion of the left anterior descending artery.
PFR = global peak filling rate.

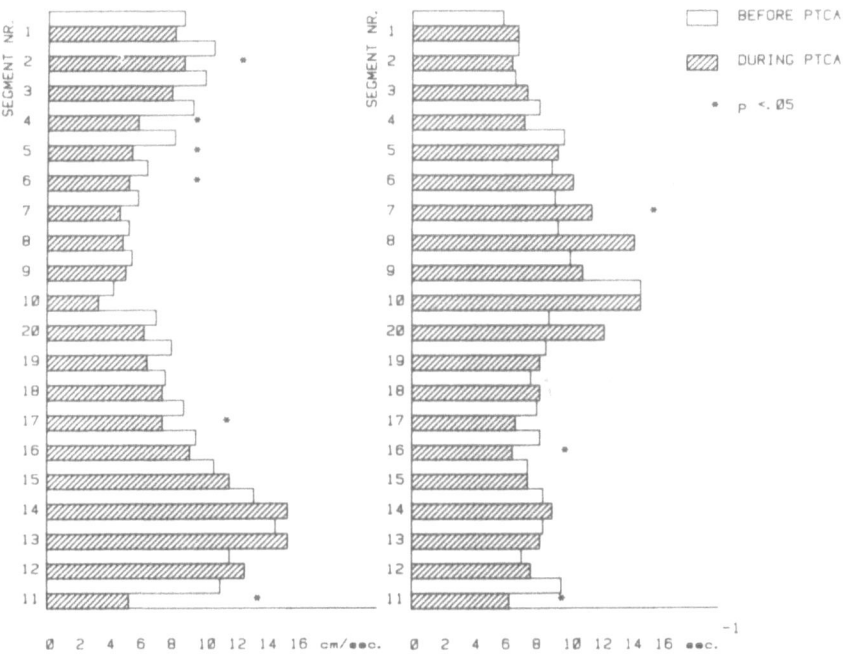

Figure 11. Left panel: Mean changes in peak velocity of segmental outward displacement (dL/dt in 10 anterior and 10 posterior segments before and during occlusion of the left anterior descending artery. Right panel: Mean changes in the ratio dL/dt/maximal outward displacement in 10 anterior and 10 posterior segments before and during occlusion of the left anterior descending artery.

Parallel to this shift in peak inward wall displacement a delay was observed in the occurrence of peak velocity of outward displacement (dL/dt) with respect to aortic valve closure, particularly in the apical region (segments 10 and 20 in Fig. 10) and the absolute value of the dL/dt was reduced in the ischemic segments (Fig. 11). In the non-ischemic, segments a compensatory increase in dL/dt was observed. In order to test whether this decrease in the absolute value of dL/dt was in fact intrinsically related to a reduction in the amplitude of the peak outward displacement, we normalized segmental dL/dt for the corresponding value of maximal outward displacement. After normalization we observed an increase in the ischemic segments while no major changes were apparent in the nonischemic segments (Fig. 11). Therefore a relationship between the asynchrony of segmental dL/dt and the reduction of global peak filling rate was sought by measuring the sum of the absolute values of the time differences from global peak filling rate to the occurrence of peak dL/dt in each of the 20 segments ($\Sigma \Delta t_1$). This sum increased significantly during both the first (from 572 ± 194 msec to 940 ± 264; $p < 0.005$) and the second occlusion (from 546 ± 198 msec to 842 ± 224; $p < 0.005$, as well as $\Sigma \Delta t_1 / Dt$, thus indicating an asynchrony in filling (Table 3). To

Table 3.   Measurement of regional asynchrony in inward and outward wall displacement before PTCA, 20 and 50 s after the onset of occlusion and after PTCA.

Variables	Before PTCA	Occlusion	After PTCA
All patients (n = 14)		20 s	
$\Sigma\Delta t_1$ msec	572 ± 194	$940 \pm 264^*$	645 ± 355
$\Sigma\Delta t_2$ msec	965 ± 348	$1442 \pm 314^*$	978 ± 281
$\Sigma\Delta t_1$/diastolic time	1.1 ± 0.7	$1.8 \pm 0.8^*$	1.2 ± 0.6
$\Sigma\Delta t_2$/ejection time	2.6 ± 0.9	$4.2 \pm 0.9^*$	2.8 ± 0.8
Subgroup (n = 9)		50 s	
$\Sigma\Delta t_1$ msec	546 ± 198	$842 \pm 224^*$	495 ± 179
$\Sigma\Delta t_2$ msec	948 ± 415	$1472 \pm 370^{**}$	985 ± 171
$\Sigma\Delta t_1$/diastolic time	1.3 ± 0.8	$1.9 \pm 1^*$	1.3 ± 0.7
$\Sigma\Delta t_2$/ejection time	2.8 ± 0.7	$4.5 \pm 0.9^{**}$	3 ± 0.9

$^{**}p < .05$; $^*p < .005$ (compared with before PTCA, paired Student t test).

$\Sigma\Delta t_1$ = sum of the time intervals between global peak filling rate and peak velocity of segmental outward displacement (dL/dt).

$\Sigma\Delta t_2$ = sum of the time intervals between aortic valve closure and segmental peak inward displacement.

elucidate whether the decrease in global peak filling rate was related to the asynchrony in regional peak filling rate rather than to other causes we correlated global peak filling rate with $\Sigma\Delta t_1$ and found a significant negative correlation ($r = -0.68$; $p < 0.001$), demonstrating that a greater degree of asynchrony was associated with a reduction in peak filling rate (Fig. 12). To determine whether the asynchrony in regional filling was an isolated phenomenon or the effect of a temporal nonuniformity in inward wall displacement, we quantified this systolic nonuniformity by measuring the time relationship between end-systole

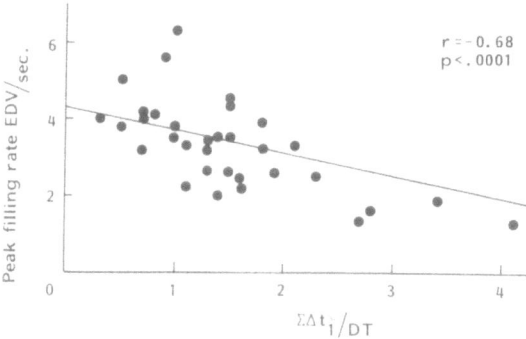

Figure 12.   The negative correlation between the global normalized peak filling rate and the $\Sigma\Delta t_1$/Diastolic time as an index of segmental asynchrony in filling, in patients with left anterior descending artery disease.

and the occurrence of the segmental peak inward displacement. The sum of the absolute time differences between aortic valve closure and the peak regional inward wall displacement ($\Sigma\Delta t_2$) was used as an index of systolic asynchrony, and during coronary occlusion both $\Sigma\Delta t_2$ and $\Sigma\Delta t_2/ET$ increased in the same fashion as $\Sigma\Delta t_1$ and $\Sigma\Delta_1/Dt$ (Table 3). In addition, we found a significant correlation ($r = 0.66$; $p < 0.001$) between $\Sigma\Delta t_2$ and $\Sigma\Delta t_1$ (Fig. 13) suggesting an interdependence between the asynchrony of contraction and the anormalities of filling dynamics. This temporal interdependence between inward and outward wall displacement is illustrated in Fig. 5. Further supportive evidence for the interrelationship between contraction and filling was given by the significant negative correlation between the global peak filling rate and $\Sigma\Delta t_2$ ($r = -0.73$; $p < 0.001$) (Fig. 14). Thus the greater the asynchrony in the pattern of contraction

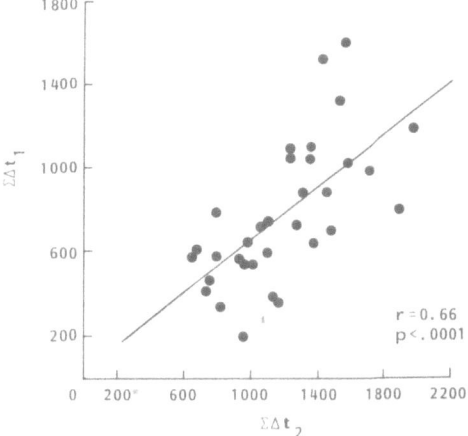

Figure 13. The correlationship between the $\Sigma\Delta t_1$ as a index of segmental asynchrony in filling and the $\Sigma\Delta t_2$ as an index of segmental asynchrony in contraction.

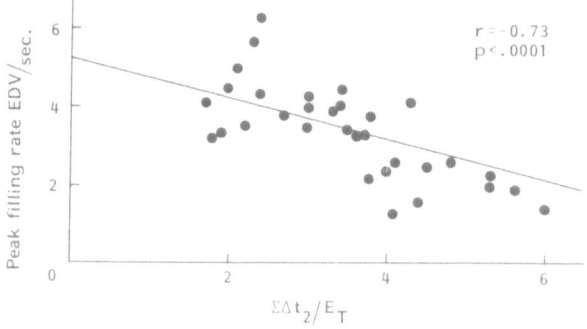

Figure 14. The negative correlation between the global normalized peak filling rate and the $\Sigma\Delta t_2$/Ejection time as an index of segmental asynchrony in contraction, in patients with left anterior descending artery disease.

the greater the decrease in peak filling rate. All these data indicate that the asynchrony in the occurrence of the regional filling with subsequent decreases in peak filling rate, reflects nonuniformity of left ventricular contraction and occurs within 20 s of the onset of ischemia. To further elucidate the dynamic interplay between asynchrony in contraction and abnormalities in early diastolic phase we correlated $\Sigma\Delta t_2$ with parameters of the relaxation phase and these latter parameters with the peak filling rate. A significant correlation was observed between $\Sigma\Delta t_2$ and Tau_1 ($r = 0.75$, $p < 0.0001$) and between Tau_1 and the duration of isovolumic relaxation period ($r = 0.58$; $p < 0.0001$). On the other hand no correlation or only weak correlations were observed between parameters of the relaxation phase and peak filling rate (Table 4).

Table 4. Correlation between parameters of left ventricular relaxation and filling.

Comparison	Correlation coefficient	p value
Tau_1-PFR	−0.33	0.06
Tau_2-PFR	−0.152	0.37
IRP-PFR	−0.53	0.009
MVO*-PFR	−0.23	0.2

* = pressure;
PFR = peak filling rate;
For other legends see Table 1b.

Regional pressure-radius length relation

There was no significant difference during the procedure in the length at end-diastole of the various segmental radii. Plots of the left ventricular pressure against a representative radius within the ischemic segment (radius 6, 9 or 10) are shown in Fig. 15. During occlusion, the slope of the pressure-radius length relation increased; this was often accompanied by an upward shift. The post-angioplasty curves showed either a return towards the control relation or remained parallel to the curves during occlusion. The latter was mainly observed in patients 4, 6, 7 and 9, all of whom had persistent global increased chamber stiffness after the procedure, as mentioned earlier.

These relations were fitted with the same elastic model used for calculation of the global chamber stiffness. The changes in the constant of regional chamber stiffness (β_n) showed a marked and persistant increased stiffness in the ischemic segment as well as in the adjacent inferior segment (radius 19). The regional stiffness in the non-ischemic segments was not significantly affected by the coronary occlusions (Table 5). There were also no significant changes in the non linear elastic constant (β_n). Similar shifts in the baseline pressure (C) as for the global diastolic function were observed since the same left ventricular pressure data were used for both calculations of global and regional chamber stiffness.

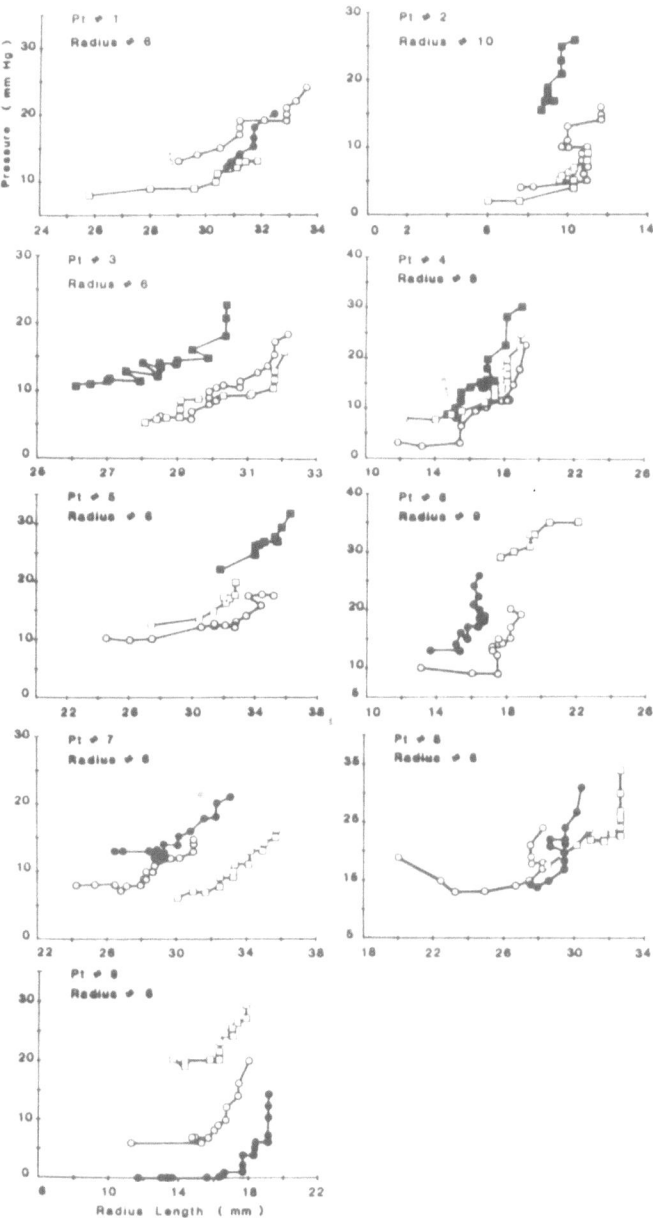

Figure 15. Plots of left ventricular pressure against the radius length in the ischemic zone. During occlusion, the slope of this relation increased as compared to pre-angioplasty. The increased slope was mostly accompanied by an upward shift. The post-angioplasty curves showed either a return towards the control relation or remained parallel to the curves observed during occlusion (patient 4, 6, 7, 9). Symbols as in Figure 9.

Table 5. Regional left ventricular chamber stiffness (β_n).

Zone	Non-ischemic		Ischemic		Adjacent inferior	Non-ischemic postero-basal
	antero-basal	anterior	antro-lateral	apical		
Radius	3	6	9	10	19	16
All patients (n = 9)	NS	NS	*	NS	NS	NS
PRE	1.59	3.92	3.11	2.93	2.76	4.03
20 s occlusion	3.03	4.03	5.63	4.97	6.59	5.01
POST	2.73	2.59	6.45*	7.16	5.98	3.64
Subgroup (n = 5)	NS	NS	+	+	+	NS
PRE	1.59	3.45	2.81	1.09	1.52	2.59
50 s occlusion	4.13	4.81	5.39	6.16	7.56*	5.54
POST	1.98	3.71	5.59	7.16	6.93	4.35

β_n = constant of regional elastic stiffness; given are median values; overall and paired (versus PRE angioplasty) p values are given; * = p 0.05, + = p 0.01, + = the statistical significance was borderline at the 0.05 level.

Discussion

Myocardial ischemia, transient asynergy and altered relaxation

The earliest (1 to 15 s after occlusion) and most sensitive hemodynamic indicator of regional perfusion deficit proved to be an impairment in early relaxation, with extreme prolongation of Tau_1, the time constant of the early relaxation phase. If the premise of the two time constant models previously described [13], is correct, then the early change in Tau_1 with constant Tau_2 represent an exacerbation in the asynchrony of relaxation.

This is illustrated by the change in negative dP/dt and wall displacement induced by a 20 s coronary occlusion (Fig. 16). Within four or five beats after occlusion, a distinct deformation appears in the ascending limb of the negative dP/dt curve and in the next ten seconds this deformation reaches the same height as peak $-dP/dt$ which in the meantime has progressively decreased to its nadir. Accompanying this change in negative dP/dt, the ischemic segments exhibit a biphasic inward-outward wall displacement that occurs after valve closure and peak negative dP/dt. During the remainder of relaxation and rapid filling the ischemic segments display a second wave of inward wall displacement. The beginning of this second wave of inward wall displacement in early diastole corresponds closely in time to the irregularity in dP/dt. In the same way, the peak inward displacement of the control segment is consistently observed near the notching in the dP/dt. Shortly after this point, the pressure ceases to have a relaxation time constant Tau_1 and abruptly switches to Tau_2. On the other

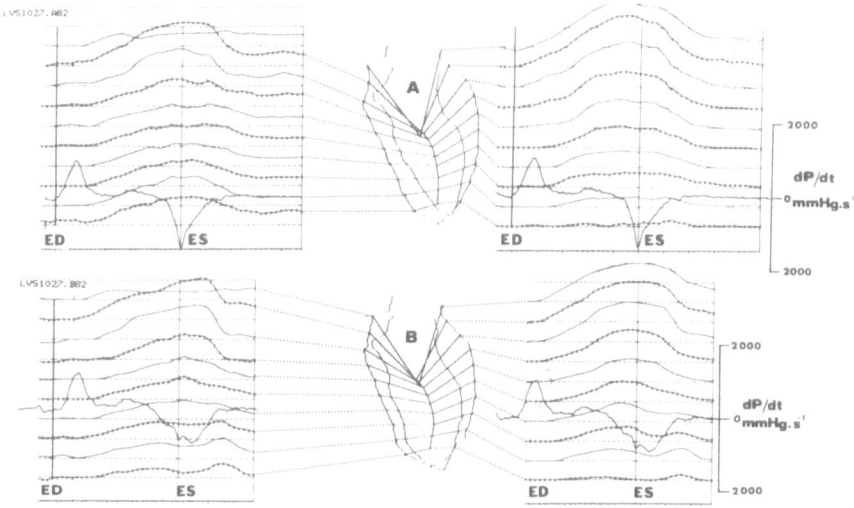

Figure 16. Left ventricular wall displacement studied in twenty separate segments, ten in the anterior (right) and ten in the infero posterior wall (left). A typical example of the relation between segmental wall displacement and dP/dt curve is observed before PTCA (A) and after 20 s (B) of left anterior descending artery occlusion: after 20 s of occlusion, the notch in the dP/dt curve corresponds to a second wave of inward wall displacement in the antero- and infero-apical segments.

hand, after 50 s of occlusion the majority of the ischemic segments were a kinetic exhibiting an increased regional stiffness, whereas Tau_1, the time constant of the early relaxation phase tended to return toward less abnormal values. At 50 s, the deformity in $-dP/dt$ was no longer present.

The connection between transient asynergy, myocardial ischemia and alteration in the time course of relaxation was pointed out as early as 1969 by Tyberg et al. [23] who designed an experimental model consisting of two papillary muscles in series; they demonstrated that when one muscle of the pair was hypoxic, but still contracting, it was disturbing the time course of the total tension fall generated by the two muscles, much more than when one of the muscles in series was not contracting at all and infinitely stiff [23]. More recent studies in conscious animals after experimental coronary occlusion have indicated that ventricular dyssynchrony due to late systolic contraction and relaxation in different regions can produce marked effects on the linearity and maximal rate of pressure fall in the left ventricle [2, 23–25]. The time course and magnitude of changes in global parameters of left ventricular function following coronary occlusion in our patients are similar to those previously reported in conscious animals after experimental coronary occlusion [1, 2, 25]. Progressive and gradual decreases in parameters of systolic function accompanied very early changes in the rate of left ventricular pressure decay. The biexponential approximation of the isovolumic pressure fall is consistent with an asynchrony of regional myocardial contraction or relaxation [13]. Changes in parameters of isovolumic pressure fall were most pronounced during the first half of occlusion and slightly less at the end of occlusion. In our study one of the earliest change in epicardial wall motion was a decrease in the extent of shortening while velocity of early shortening was maintained. These results are similar to the earliest changes of motion of left ventricular mid-wall ultrasonic crystals during ischemia in conscious dogs as reported by Pagani et al. [1].

Our angiographic observation suggest that a similar phenomenon occur in the intact human heart during acute ischemia. At 20 s, the late systolic outward displacement of the ischemic segment is probably passive and due to a simultaneously increased and active inward displacement of the non-ischemic segments. Conversely the early diastolic inward displacement of the ischemic segments must correspond to an accelerated outward displacement of the normal segment. Ultimately the ischemic zone after 20 s of ischemia appears to act as an additional elastic element, in series with the actively contracting and relaxing non-ischemic segment. This mechanism is consistent with the model of LV pressure relaxation recently proposed by our group [13] which assumes that the observed time constant Tau_1 results from the combined action of that fraction of the myocardium in the process of relaxing and the remaining fraction in which relaxation has not yet been iniated.

After 40 s of ischemia, despite paradoxical lengthening (epicardial wall motion) throughout systole, early diastolic shortening was still observed consistent with a markedly diminished yet persistent tension becoming manifest only after a decline in the load imposed upon the region by the remainder of the effectively contracting ventricle.

Uncoordinated segemental contraction as a cause of impaired filling dynamics

Variability in the temporal sequence of regional left ventricular contraction in normal subjects has been previously observed and attributed to variations in the sequence of electrical activation or to other factors playing an important role in determining ventricular geometry such as ventricular volume and fiber orientation [26, 27]. In patients with coronary artery disease, the completion of ejection was found to be delayed whereas the onset of ejection was not and the severity of coronary and artery disease was positively correlated with the persistence of these contraction abnormalities into early diastole [28]. During spontaneous angina, a significant prolongation of left ventricular ejection time with an accompanying shortening of diastole has also been observed [29]. All these observations dictate that studies of relaxation and filling in early diastole should be correlated with the pattern of contraction.

Determinants of filling dynamics. It has been suggested that the peak filling rate is dependent on the rate of left ventricular relaxation and on the left atrial pressure [30]. Under normal conditions the relaxing left ventricle produces a rapid change in the atrio-ventricular pressure gradient, which is the driving force for the inflow [31]. Thus a prolonged relaxation phase, as observed during acute ischemia, causes a delay in the development of the atrio-ventricular pressure gradient, and consequently, a greater left atrial pressure is required to open the mitral valve. In fact we observed a consistent delay in the relaxation rate occuring 20 s after the onset of ischemia and concomitantly both the isovolumic relaxation period and the left atrial pressure required for mitral valve opening increased. The significant relationship existing between $\Sigma \Delta t_2$ and Tau_1 and between this latter parameter and the duration of the isovolumic relaxation period suggests that, during acute ischemia, the atrio-ventricular dynamic interplay occurring during the early diastole is affected by the asynchronous left ventricular contraction. Yellin et al. [30], demonstrated in the dog that under conditions of similar left atrial pressure at valve opening, the prolongation of the time constant of relaxation decreases the rate and amplitude of filling whereas under conditions of similar left ventricular pressure during relaxation, an increase of left atrial pressure increases the amplitude of early filling. Thus the lack of correlation between peak filling rate and any single parameters of the relaxation phase, such as time constants of relaxation, isovolumic relaxation period of mitral valve opening pressure was expected since these latter parameters, during acute ischemia, are changing in opposite direction.

A decrease in peak filling rate has been extensively reported in patients with coronary artery disease with or without previous myocardial infarction. Until recently no data were available in the literature regarding the relationship between global and regional left ventricular filling. Yamagishi et al. [32] investigated this relationship using radionuclide angiography in normal subjects and in patients with left anterior descending coronary artery disease without previous myocardial infarction and found differences in peak filling rate differentiating normals from those with coronary artery disease. To explain this difference they analyzed regional filling dynamics and identified that asynchrony in regional filling was a major determinant of decrease in peak filling rate. The sum of the absolute time differences between the global and regional peak filling rate was inversely correlated to the global peak filling rate and proposed as an index of asynchrony in diastolic filling. More recently Bonow et al. [33] studied with radionuclide angiography the relationship between regional left ventricular diastolic asynchrony and global diastolic filling, before and after PTCA in patients with single vessel coronary artery disease. Before PTCA impaired global diastolic filling was found and was related to regional variations in the timing of left ventricular relaxation and filling determined by variations in phase among sectors and by regional quadrant analysis. In addition, they demonstrated a negative correlation between the magnitude of global peak filling rate and the extent of regonal asynchrony. Reevaluation one day to one month after PTCA showed an improvement of the above mentioned changes in diastolic global and regional function.

Role of the asynchronous contraction. In the present study, we demonstrated that ischemia occurring early during coronary occlusion severely alters filling dynamics and that the major determinant of this change is asynchrony in regional filling. This diastolic asynchrony was secondary to a nonuniformity of inward wall displacement but the crucial question remains whether this diastolic asynchrony was a direct, intrinsic manifestation of altered relaxation properties of the myocardium (inactivation) or a consequence of dysfunction of the contractile properties of the myocardium (activation) [34, 35].

Effect of coronary occlusion on left ventricular chamber stiffness and regional diastolic pressure-radius relations

The third major finding of the present study was that ischemia induced by complete occlusion of the left anterior descending coronary artery increased the regional chamber stiffness of the ischemic anterior wall, even during an occlusion as short as 20 s. Parallel to this increase in regional stiffness, the global stiffness of the left ventricle increased significantly. In experimental studies [36–38], an increase in global chamber stiffness was only seen when the area rendered ischemic was large, such as during acute occlusion of the left anterior descending coronary artery.

The baseline pressure (constant C) increased slightly from -1.4 to 5.2 mmHg 20 s and from -5.8 to 9.4 mmHg 50 s after acute coronary occlusion (Table 2). This increase in baseline pressure reflects the upward shift of the diastolic pressure-volume relation during coronary occlusion, which was thus 6.6 mmHg after 20 s and 15.2 mmHg after 50 s.

Twelve minutes after the end of the procedure including repeated (3 to 10) and brief (15 to 75 s) occlusions. The parameters of global and regional systolic function were back to normal, as shown from the indices of isovolumic contraction, relaxation and segmental wall motion [39]. In contrast, the parameters of regional diastolic function were still abnormal (Table 5) while the constant of global chamber stiffness and the baseline pressure remained slightly elevated. This suggests the persistance of post-ischemic diastolic abnormalities while complete recovery of systolic function and relaxation has already occurred.

Significance of the upward shift in pressure-volume and pressure-radius relations

The significance of the upward shift in the pressure-volume and/or pressure-radius length relations is still the subject of controversy. In the various previous studies [21, 22, 36–41], this shift was attributed to any or a combination of the following factors: changes in intrinsic diastolic myocardial stiffness, delayed left ventricular relaxation, loss of elastic recoil due to ventricular asynergy, changes in right ventricular loading conditions, effects of the pericardium and coronary perfusion. A limitation of the present study is that we cannot address directly these specific issues. For instance, fitting of the pressure-volume relation by a simple elastic model, as we did, does not allow one to infer that the intrinsic diastolic properties of the myocardium were affected by acute coronary occlusion since this would require analysis of left ventricular stress and strain [42]. Heretofore, regional wall thickness measurements are needed which cannot be obtained accurately at 20 msec intervals from the left ventricular angiocardiograms. Also, the strain data should be normalized for a reference unloaded muscle length, i.e. at a transmural pressure of 0 mmHg and this cannot be obtained easily during cardiac catheterization in man.

As far as extrinsic factors are concerned, we feel that the coronary perfusion, or the so-called 'erectile effect', is not likely to account for the increased stiffness in the core of the ischemic segment.

During coronary occlusion of the left anterior descending artery, inflation of the dilatation balloon results on average in a 44% decrease in regional blood flow [43], hereby reducing the myocardial wall blood volume. Likewise, the post-angioplasty measurements were obtained at a time where any increased myocardial turgor due to reactive hypermia had worn off [43]. Interestingly, the increase in regional stiffness observed in the adjacent inferior segment could be related to an increased turgor as the collateral flow to that area might increase during left anterior descending occlusion [44].

Comparison with animal models of acute low-flow ischemia

Coronary angioplasty mimics the experimental coronary occlusion in the animal laboratory and induces transient acute low-flow ischemia. In this animal model, Hess et al. [22] showed that 'myocardial wall stiffness is increased during complete coronary occlusion when there is systolic thinning of the ischemic wall'. In these conscious chronically instrumented dogs, the ischemic alteration in the intrinsic diastolic properties of the muscle resulted in an upward shift of the pressure-volume control curve. They observed an average 27% increase in diastolic wall stiffness which compares well with the 35% increase in global chamber stiffness after 50 s of anterior descending coronary artery occlusion in the present data. It is worth mentioning that in the animal study, the upward shift of the pressure-volume curve was prevented by inferior vena caval obstruction. This emphasizes the modulating role of the right ventricular loading conditions and the ventricular interaction, which can offset the increase in pressure.

Thus, the observed changes in global and regional diastolic chamber stiffness are in accordance with previous experimental work [20, 22, 37] demonstrating an increase in the myocardial stiffness during coronary occlusion.

Mechanism of increased myocardial stiffness. The mechanism by which ischemia increases the myocardial stiffness remains speculative and may depend on the pathophysiology [36] and the duration [45] of a given ischemic condition. In the acute coronary occlusion model [22, 37], systolic overstretch of the akinetic muscle fibers by adjacent non ischemic myocardium was thought to be responsible for the diastolic thinning of the ischemic wall and the increase in resting muscle length. This 'creep' effect causes the ischemic myocardium to operate at a higher point on the pressure-sarcomere length relation, and thus, at an increased stiffness level. Although we observed no significant changes in end-diastolic volume throughout the procedure, it cannot be excluded that 'creep' actually occurred. Echocardiographic evidence of wall thinning during angioplasty and during attacks of variant angina supports this hypothesis [8, 46]. The other major mechanism refers to the concept of residual diastolic actin-myosin-interaction [47]. An increase in cytosolic ionic calcium and a decrease in adenosine triphosphate available for cross bridge dissociation could result in the presence of an abnormal myocardial 'tone', This mechanism is unlikely after prolonged occlusion since the ischemic segment becomes akinetic or dyskinetic and systolic cross bridge formation is probably minimal or absent. However, after 20 s occlusion, we observed asynchrony and late shortening of the ischemic wall [43, 45], which were shown to affect the stiffness of a rat heart trabeculae [48]. Also, the persistant abnormalities in diastolic function seen after the procedure could be related to an abnormal myocardial 'tone' despite normalization of the rate of relaxation. As recently emphasized [21, 36], such failure of complete myofilament inactivation implies a reduced extent of relaxation which is not necessarily synonymous to a reduced rate of relaxation, as measured from the time constant of isovolumic left ventricular pressure decay.

Finally, it should be realized that the increase in calculated stiffness constant could also be related to an increase resistance to early filling. It was shown recently in humans that early diastolic filling can be kept normal during ischemia despite delayed relaxation and loss of elastic recoil (increase in end-systolic volume) by increasing the left atrial driving pressure [49]. Under these conditions, the diastolic properties of the myocardium would be better characterized by a visco elastic model rather than by a simple elastic stress-strain relation [50, 51].

We used a simple elastic model because the present angiocardiographic data did not allow proper quantitation of the strain rates, which are essential for determining diastolic viscous effects. Therefore, our calculated stiffness constant includes both elastic and viscous forces. Interestingly, we found similar increases in the constant of elastic chamber stiffness after 20 and 50 s of occlusion while left ventricular asynchrony and late shortening of the ischemic wall were observed only at 20 s. This decreased chamber stiffness observed only at 20 s may only be apparent and related more to an increase in viscous resistance to early filling, although asynchrony and late shortening have been shown to affect the stiffness of rat heart [51].

Conclusion: PTCA is an ischemic model?

Early wall motion during acute ischemia: how to interpret?

Recently we evaluated the beat to beat myocardial shortening changes accompanying acute coronary occlusion in one patient undergoing PTCA of a coronary artery bypass graft in whom pairs of epicardial wall markers had been placed at the time of his original cardiac surgery [45]. Their motion reflecting epicardial transverse shortening was characterized, in ischemic myocardium, by the early appearance of a late systolic lengthening followed by an early diastolic shortening (Fig. 17). We referred to this biphasic motion as the 'W' phenomenon due to its morphologic characteristics, transient duration, and frequency of appearance in studies of endocardial wall thickness motion during regional ischemia. This polyphasic wall motion pattern appears to be similar to that described by Wiegner et al. [48] who studies the interaction of normal and hypoxic myocardial muscles in series. They identified a biphasic pattern of motion of the hypoxic muscle analogous to that observed in the ischemic region of the intact left ventricle (Fig. 18). The early lengthening phase of the hypoxic muscle was attributed to a premature onset of force decline and the second late shortening phase was ascribed to either a persisting contractile force of the muscle or a manifestation of stored force from elastic recoil of previously stretched passive muscle elements. Furthermore they indicated the possible negative role of late shortening on filling dynamics. Similar types of wall motion abnormalities have been described in animals [1, 2, 4, 52] and during chronic ischemia in man [53, 54]. In our angiographic study, the frame by frame analysis of the anterior wall displacement during brief occlusion of left anterior descending artery also showed a variety of biphasic wall motion pattern. As shown in Fig. 19, after 17 s of occlusion, some of the segments adjacent to the ischemic area exhibited the 'W' phenomenon, while the segment located in the core of the ischemic area exhibited a late inward wall displacement in early diastole. This phenomenon was mirrored by an accelerated outward displacement of the normal segment. Ultimately the interaction between ischemic and nonischemic segments results in segmental asynchrony in the occurrence of peak velocity of outward displacements. Since this parameter reflects the segmental peak filling rate, an asynchrony in segmental outward displacement corresponds to the asynchrony in the filling phase with consequent changes in the global peak filling rate.

In summary, out study demonstrates that short periods of ischemia, induced by balloon inflation, cause an early disruption of the normal sequence of inward-outward segmental displacement in the ischemic segments. This phenomenon is characterized by an early lengthening occurring during late systole with late shortening occurring during early diastole. These data in part confirm an 'asynchronous contraction' occurring during brief periods of ischemia [55] and, in particular, demonstrate the close relationship existing between uncoordinated contraction and the impairment of filling dynamics.

Are there clinical implications in chronic ischemia?

A possible relationship between the resting wall motion abnormalities with chronic ischemia and those transiently observed during acute ischemia is suggested by the work of Sasayama et al. [54] who recently demonstrated an inward motion of left ventricular ischemic segments accompanied by an outward

A

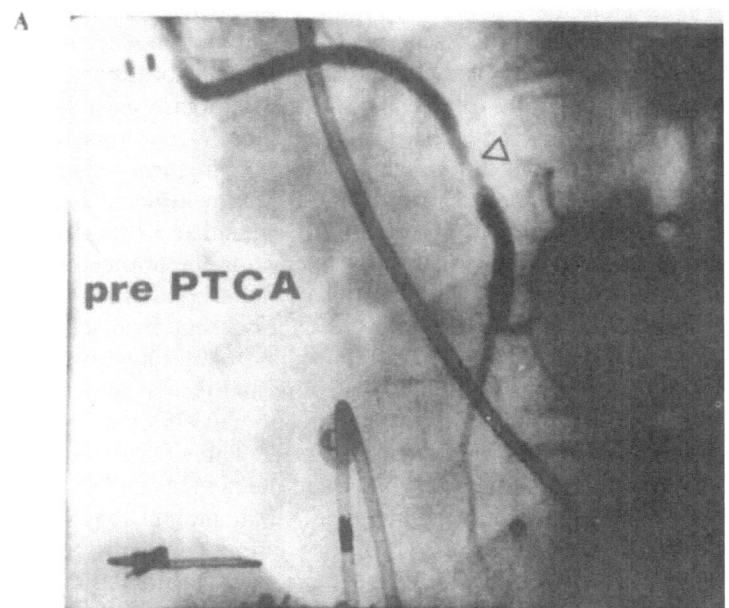

B

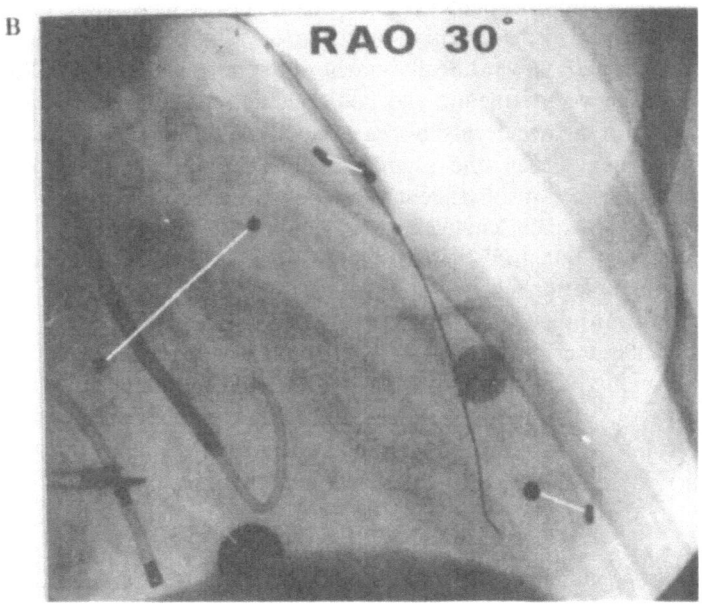

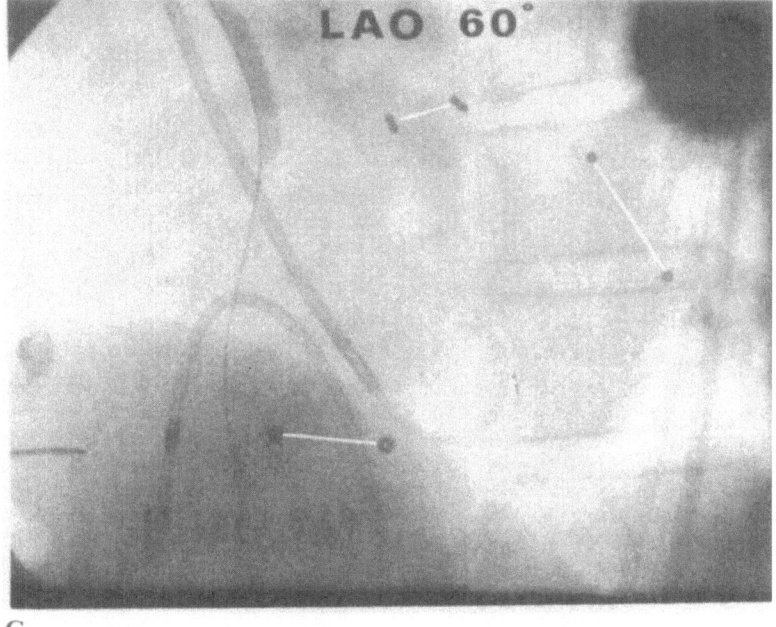

C

EPICARDIAL MARKER PAIR SHORTENING

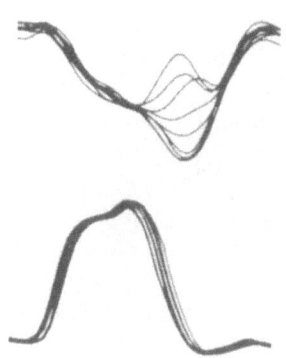

D LEFT VENTRICULAR PRESSURE

Figure 17. Angiogram of left anterior descending bypass graft stenosis and markers before PTCA (A). Frames B and C show the inflated angioplasty catheter in place, respectively in RAO and LAO 60°. In D changes in epicardial marker pair shortening in region of bypass graft and left ventricular pressure during graft occlusion. The 'W' phenomenon (see text) is evident.

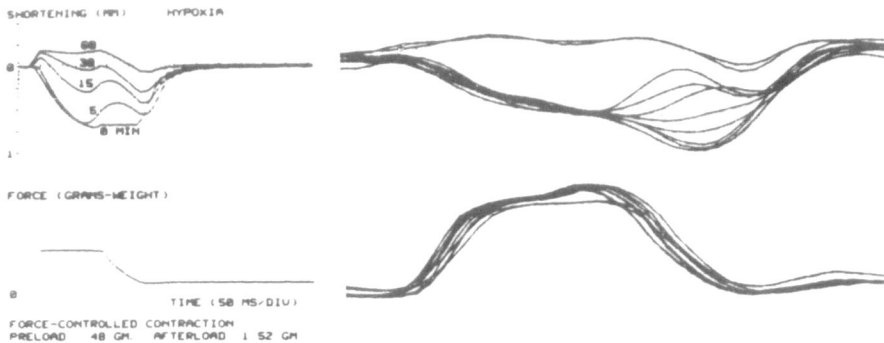

Figure 18. Left panel: Interaction between a muscle subjected to hypoxia for 60 min (length record in upper panel) and a 'normal' muscle (force record in lower panel). The earliest change is a premature onset of lengthening (5 min) and as hypoxia progress, there is less total shortening; by 60 min the hypoxia muscle demonstrates 'systolic' lengthening which coincides with the period of force development in the normal muscle. During the period of force decline (normal muscle, below), the hypoxic muscle manifests late systolic shortening. Right panel: Beat by beat changes in epicardial marker pair shortening in region of bypass graft and left ventricular pressure with graft occlusion. Within 6–8 beats after occlusion, marker pair showed abnormal late systolic lengthening and early diastolic shortening. Paradoxical systolic expansion is evident after 40 s of occlusion.

motion of normal segments during isovolumic relaxation in patients with chronic angina. This motion was attributed to both persisting contractile activity and elastic recoil of passive elements within the ischemic muscle. In these patients, however, a late systolic expansion of ischemic segments preceding early diastolic contraction was not observed.

Whether a relationship exists between abnormal left ventricular relaxation and left ventricular rapic diastolic filling is uncertain. In patients with coronary artery disease, a prolongation of the monoexponential time constant of relaxation has been shown to correlate with an increase in minimal left ventricular pressure and inversely correlate with early diastolic ventricular inflow rate and inflow volume [14]. Increases in the time constant of isovolumic relaxation have also been associated with an increase in the left ventricular diastolic constant of elastic chamber stiffness during exercises induced angina [49].

Are there clinical implications for the PTCA procedure?

We can conclude that repeated complete coronary occlusions of the left anterior descending coronary artery in conscious man are associated with profound alterations in diastolic chamber stiffness which persist well after restoration of myocardial blood flow and a normal systolic function. Further work is needed to document the time course of the recovery to a normal regional diastolic function

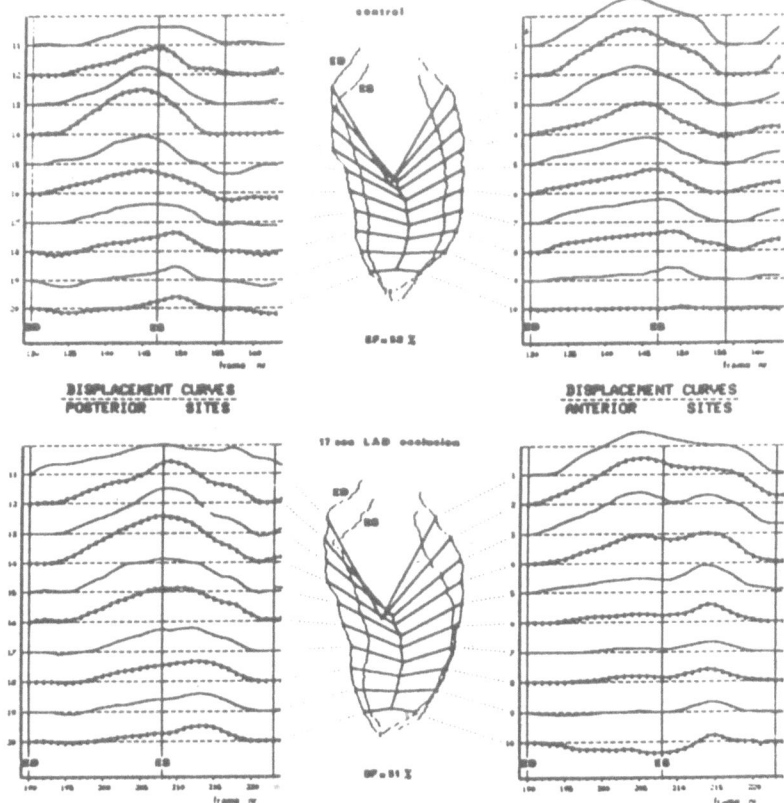

Figure 19. Left ventricular wall displacement in 10 anterior (right) and 10 inferoposterior (left) segments. After 17 s of occlusion of the left anterior descending (LAD) artery, a biphasic pattern of contraction is observed in the anterior segments, while the apical segments (anterior and inferoposterior) show a late inward wall displacement occuring in the early diastole. In the non ischemic segments an accelerated outward displacement is observed.

and to address the responsible derangement of subcellular metabolism as the mechanisms of the observed abnormalities are not yet fully understood.

From the clinical point of view, many factors have contributed to increasing the extent and severity of iatrogenic ischemia during angioplasty: longer balloon inflation time, dilatation of multiple lesions during a single setting and inclusion of patients with unstable angina or impaired left ventricular function. This has prompted studies attempting to modify ischemic changes induced by balloon inflation by means of various intervention [9, 56, 57].

Along with our previous studies [43, 45], the present data suggest that the analysis of diastolic function may prove a sensitive tool in assessing the possibly deleterious effects of repeated coronary occlusions during angioplasty and could be a useful end point in evaluating the efficacy of 'cardioprotective' interventions.

Acknowledgements

The authors wish to thank Gusta Koster and Anja van Huuksloot for typing this manuscript. The illustrations were prepared with great care by Mary Lee Griswold.

References

1. Pagani M, Vatner S, Brig H, Braunwald E (1978) Initial myocardial adjustments to brief periods of ischemia and reperfusion in the conscious dog. *Circ Res* 43: 83–91
2. Kumada T, Karliner JS, Pouleur H, Gallagher KP, Shirato K, Ross J (1979) Effects of coronary occlusion on early ventricular diastolic events in conscious dogs. *Am J Phys* 237: H542–H549
3. Gaasch WH, Bernard SA (1977) The effects of acute changes in coronary blood flow on left ventricular end-diastolic wall thickness. An echocardiographic study. *Circulation* 56: 593–597
4. Forrester JS, Wyatt HL, de Luz PL, Tyberg JV, Diamond GA, Swan HJC (1976) Functional significance of regional ischemic contraction abnormalities. *Circulation* 54: 65–70
5. Rentrop KP, Cohen M, Blanke H, Phillips RA (1985) Changes in collateral filling immediately after controlled coronary artery occlusion by an angioplasty balloon in human subjects. *JACC* 5: 587–592
6. Probst P, Zangl W, Pachinger O (1985) Relation of coronary arterial occluson pressure during percutaneous transluminal coronary angioplasty to presence of collaterals. *Am J Cardiol* 55: 1264–1269
7. Meier B, Luethy P (1984) Coronary wedge pressure as predictor of recuitable collateral arteries. *Circulation* 70 (Suppl II): 266
8. Das SK, Serruys PW, van den Brand M, Domenicucci S, Vletter WB, Roelandt J (1983) Acute echocardiographic changes during percutaneous coronary angioplasty and their relationship to coronary blood flow. *J Cardiovasc Ultrasonography* 2: 269–71
9. Serruys PW, van den Brand M, Brower RW, Hugenholtz PG (1983) Regional cardioplegia and cardioprotection during transluminal angioplasty, which role for nifedipine? *European Heart Journal* 4: 115–21
10. Sigwart U, Grbic M, Payot M, Goy JJ, Essinger A, Fischer A: Ischemic events during coronary artery balloon obstruction. In: Rutishauser W, Roskamm H (eds) *Silent Myocardial Ischemia.* Berlin-Heidelberg-New York-Tokyo: Springer Verlag, pp 29–36
11. Meester GT, Bernard, N, Zeelenberg C, Brower RW, Hugenholtz PG (1975) A computer system for real time analysis of cardiac catheterization data. *Catheterization and Cardiovasculr Diagnosis* 1: 112–23
12. Meester GT, Zeelenberg C, Bernard N, Gorter S (1974) Beat to beat analysis of cardiac cathetherization data. In: *Computers in Cardiology.* Los Angeles: IEEE Computer Society 63–65
13. Brower RE, Meij S, Serruys PW (1983) A model of asynchronous left ventricular relaxation predicting the bi-exponential pressure decay. *Cardiovasc* 17: 482–488
14. Fioretti P, Brower RW, Meester GT, Serruys PW (1980) Interaction of left ventricular relaxation and filling during early diastole in human subjects. *Am J Cardiol* 46: 197–203
15. Slager CJ, Reiber JHC, Schuubiers JCH, Meester GT (1978) Contouromat – a hardwired left ventricular angio processing system. Design and application. *Comp Biomed Res* 11: 431–502
16. Slager CJ, Hooghoudt TEH, Reiber JCH, Booman F, Meester GT (1980) Left ventricular contour segmentation from anatomical landmark trajectories and its application to wall motion analysis. In *Computers in Cardiology.* Los Angeles: IEEE Computer Society, 347–350
17. Hooghoudt TEH, Slager CJ, Reiber JHC, Serruys PW, Schuurbiers JCH, Meester GT, Hugenholtz PG (1980) 'Regional contribution to global ejection fraction' used to assess the applicability of a new wall motion model to the detection of regional wall motion in patients with asynergy. In: *Computers in Cardiology.* Los Angeles: IEEE Computer Society, 253–56

18. Slager CJ, Hooghoudt TEH, Serruys PW, Reiber JHC, Schuubiers JCH (1982) Automated quantification of left ventricular angiograms. In: Short MD et al. (eds) *Physical Techniques in Cardiological Imaging.* Bristol: Hilger A Ltd, 163–72

19. Hess OM, Grimm J, Krayenbuehl HP (1979) Diastolic simple elastic and viscoelastic properties of the left ventricle in man. *Circulation* 59: 1178–87

20. Theroux P, Franklin D, Ross J Jr, Kemper WS (1974) Regional myocardial function during acute coronary artery occlusion and its modification by pharmacologic agents in the dog. *Circulation Res* 35: 896–908

21. Sasayama S, Nonogi H, Migazaki S, Sakurai T, Kawai C, Eiko S, Kuwahara M (1985) Changes in diastolic properties of the regional myocardium during pacing-induced ischemia in human subjects. *J Am Coll Cardiol* 5: 599–606

22. Hess OM, Koch R, Bamert C, Krayenbuehl HP (1980) Regional wall stiffness during acute myocardial ischemia in the canine left ventricle. *Eur Heart J* 1: 435–43

23. Tyberg JV, Parmley MW, Sonnenblick EH (1969) In vitro studies of myocardial asynchrony and regional hypoxia. *Circulation* 25: 569–79

24. Theroux P, Ross J Jr, Franklin D, Covell JW, Bloor CM, Sasayama S (1977) Regional myocardial infarction in the unanaesthetized dog. *Circ Res* 40: 158–65

25. Theroux P, Ross J Jr, Franklin D, Kemper WS, Sasayama S (1976) Regional myocardial function in the conscious dog during acute coronary occlusion and responses to morphine, propranolol, nitroglycerine and lidocaïne. *Circulation* 53: 202–14

26. Clayton PD, Bulawa WF, Klausner SC, Urie PM, Marshall HW, Warner HR (1979) The characteristic sequence for the onset of contraction in the normal human left ventricle. *Circulation* 59: 671–679

27. Klausner SC, Blair TJ, Bulawa WF, Jeppson GM, Jensen RL, Clayton PD (1982) Quantitative analysis of segmental wall motion throughout systole and diastole in the normal human left ventricle. *Circulation* 65: 580–590

28. Holman LB, Wynne J, Idione J, Neill J (1980) Disruption in the temporal sequence of regional ventricular contraction. I: Characteristic and incidence in coronary artery disease. *Circulation* 61: 1075–1083

29. Ferro G, Piscione F, Carella G, Betocchi S, Spinelli L, Chiariello M (1984) Systolic and diastolic time intervals during spontaneous angina. *Clin Cardiol* 7: 588–592

30. Yellin EL, Yoran C, Sonnenblick EH, Frater RWM (1980) The relation between left ventricular relaxation and early diastolic filling in the intact dog heart. *Eur Heart J* 1 (Suppl B): 179–180

31. Yellin EL, Peskin C, Yoran C, Koeningsberg M, Matsumoto M, Laniado S, Mc Queen D, Shore D, Frater RWM (1981) Mechanism of mitral value motion during diastole. *Am J Physiol* 214: H389–H400

32. Yamagishi T, Ozaki M, Kumada T, Ikezono T, Shimizu T, Furutami Y, Yamaoka H, Ogawa H, Matsuzaki M, Matsuda Y, Arima A, Kusukawa R (1984) Asynchronous left ventricular diastolic filling in patients with isolated disease of the left anterior descending coronary artery: assessment with radionuclide ventriculography. *Circulation* 69: 933–942

33. Bonow RO, Vitale DF, Bacharach SL, Frederick TM, Kent KM, Green MV (1985) Asynchronous left ventricular regional function and impaired global diastolic filling in patients with coronary artery disease: reversal after coronary angioplasty. *Circulation* 71: 297

34. Brutsaert DL, Housemans PR, Goethals MA (1980) Dual control of relaxation: its role in the ventricular function in the mammalian heart. *Circ Res* 47: 637–652

35. Brutsaert DL, Rademakers FE, Sys SV (1984) Triple control of relaxation: implications in cardiac diseases. *Circulation* 69: 190–196

36. Paulus WJ, Grossman W, Serizawa T, Bourdillon PD, Pasipoularides A, Mirsky I (1985) Different effects of two types of ischemia on myocardial systolic and diastolic functions. *Am J Physiol* 248: H719–28

37. Hess OM, Osakada G, Lavelle JF, Gallagher KP, Kemper WS, Ross J Jr (1983) Diastolic myocardial wall stiffness and ventricular relaxation during partial and complete coronary occlusion in the conscious dog. *Circulation Res* 52: 387–400

38. Grossman W, Serizawa T, Carabello BA (1980) Studies on the mechanism of altered left ventricular diastolic pressure-volume relations during ischemia. *Eur Heart J* (Suppl A): 141–7
39. Bourdillon PD, Lorell BH, Mirsky I, Paulus WJ, Wynne J, Grossman W (1983) Increased regional myocardial stiffness of the left ventricle during pacing-induced angina in man. *Circulation* 67: 316–23
40. Shirato K, Shabetai R, Bhargava V, Franklin D, Ross J Jr (1978) Alteration of the left ventricular diastolic pressure segment length relation produced by the pericardium: effects of cardiac distension and afterload reduction in conscious dogs. *Circulation* 57: 1191–98
41. Serizawa T, Carabello BA, Grossman W (1980) Effect of pacing-induced ischemia on left ventricular diastolic pressure-volume relations in dogs with coronary stenoses. *Circulation Res* 46: 430–9
42. Glantz SA, Parmley WW (1978) Factors which affect the diastolic pressure-volume curve. *Circulation Res* 42: 171–180
43. Serruys PW, van den Brand M, Mey S, Slager CJ, Schuurbiers JCH, Hugenholtz PG, Brower RW (1984) Left ventricular performance, regional blood flow, wall motion and lactate metabolism during transluminal angioplasty. *Circulation* 70: 25–36
44. Wahr DW, Ports TA, Botvinick EH, Dae M, Schechtman N, Huberty J, Hattner RS, O'Connell JW, Turley K (1985) The effects of coronary angioplasty and reperfusion on distribution of myocardial flow. *Circulation* 72: 334–43
45. Jaski BE, Serruys PW (1985) Epicardial wall motion and left ventricular function during coronary graft angioplasty in humans. *J Am Coll Cardiol* 6: 695–700
46. Distante A, Rovai D, Picano E, Moscarelli E, Palombo C, Morales MH, Michelassi C, L'Abbate A (1984) Transient changes in left ventricular mechanics during attacks of Prinzmetal's angina. *Am Heart J* 107: 465–72
47. Nayler WG, Williams A (1978) Relaxation in heart muscle: some morphological and biochemical considerations. *Eur J Cardiol* 7 (Suppl): 35–50
48. Wiegner AW, Allen GJ, Bing OHL (1978) Weak and strong myocardium in series: implications for segmental dysfunction. *Am J Physiol* 235 (6): H776–83
49. Carroll JD, Hess OM, Hirzel HO, Krayenbuehl HP (1983) Dynamics of left ventricular filling at rest and during exercise. *Circulation* 68: 59–67.
50. Rankin JS, Arentzen CE, McHale PA, Ling D, Anderson RW (1977) Viscoelastic properties of the diastolic left ventricle in the conscious dog. *Circulation Res* 41: 37–45
51. Pouleur H, Karliner JS, Le Winter MM, Covell JW (1979) Diastolic viscous properties of the intact canine left ventricle. *Circulation Res* 45: 410–9
52. Heijndrick GR, Millard RW, McRitchie RJ, Maroko PR, Vatner SF (1975) Regional myocardial function and electrophysiological alterations after brief coronary artery occlusion in conscious dogs. *J Clin Invest* 56: 978–85
53. Gibson DJ, Prewitt TA, Brown DT (1976) Analysis of left ventricular wall movement during isovolumic relaxation and its relation to coronary artery disease. *Brit Heart J* 38: 1010–1019
54. Sasayama S, Nonogi H, Fujita M, Sakurai T, Wakabayashi A, Kawai C, Eiho S, Kuwahara M (1984) Analysis of asynchronous wall motion by regional pressure length loops in patients with coronary artery disease. *JACC* 4: 256–267
55. Gaasch WH, Blaustein AS, Bing OHL (1985) Asynchronous (segmental early) relaxation of the left ventricle. *JACC* 5: 891–897
56. Doorey AJ, Mehmel HC, Schwartz FX, Kübler W (1985) Amelioration by nitroglycerin of left ventricular ischemia induced by percutaneous transluminal coronary angioplasty: assessment by hemodynamic variables and left ventriculography. *J Am Coll Cardiol* 6: 267–74
57. Mc Donald FM, Fuchs M, Kreuzer J, Höpp HW, Heinen A, Arnold G, Heymans L, Hirche HJ, Hombach V (1985) Hemodynamic and antiarhythmic protective effects of intracoronary perfusion during percutaneous transluminal coronary angioplasty. *Eur Heart* 6: 284–93

19. Myocardial ischemia during PTCA: Consequences and treatment strategies

ANDREW ZALEWSKI, MICHAEL SAVAGE and SHELDON GOLDBERG

Transluminal coronary angioplasty is not only an effective method of myocardial revascularization but also a valuable tool for the investigation of ischemia induced by the transient interruption of epicardial coronary blood flow [1, 2]. The electrocardiographic, hemodynamic, and metabolic consequences of relatively brief periods of coronary occlusion during PTCA have been characterized and will be reviewed in the first section of this chapter. Following this, we will discuss investigations designed to assess the efficacy of various anti-ischemic pharmacologic agents in the setting of controlled myocardial ischemia induced by balloon occlusion. Finally, the effects of a variety of mechanical interventions designed to reduce ischemia will be reviewed.

Research into these therapeutic modalities may provide us with insights into the mechanisms of action of various measures aimed at reducing myocardial ischemia. In addition, the safety and efficacy of the technique of coronary angioplasty might be enhanced if the myocardium could be reliably protected from the stress of ischemia induced by the balloon occlusion. If this were possible, then PTCA could be applied in higher risk clinical settings. Furthermore, the success rate of PTCA could perhaps be improved if the myocardium could be protected during very prolonged balloon inflations: a certain number of flow limiting intimal disruptions might be salvaged by extended inflation times. Another potential benefit of 'protected' very prolonged balloon inflation could be a reduced rate of restenosis, but this remains uncertain. Finally, the use of effective myocardial protection during PTCA might help reduce the extent of myocardial necrosis following failed PTCA procedures.

Consequences of balloon induced coronary occlusion

The degree of ischemic response during balloon occlusion varies with the individual patient and depends on several factors, including the amount of myocardium at risk and the degree of collateralization to the vessel being dilated [3, 4].

P.W. Serruys, R. Simon & K.J. Beatt (eds), Percutaneous Transluminal Coronary Angioplasty. ISBN 0-7923-0346-6.
© *1990 Kluwer Academic Publishers, Dordrecht – Printed in the Netherlands.*

Baseline   **Occlusion**

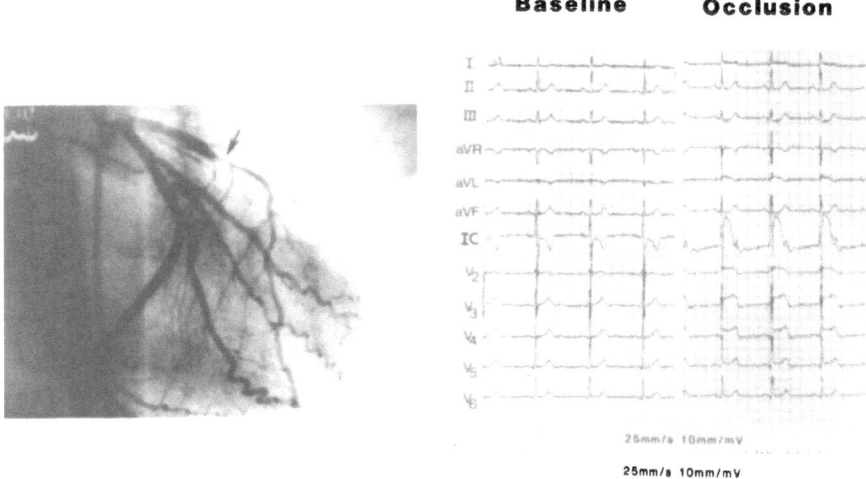

(A) Electrocardiographic changes accompanying balloon occlusion of a left anterior descending stenosis. The surface electrocardiogram shows ST elevation in the precordial leads paralleling the changes on the intracoronary (IC) electrogram. ST elevation on the surface electrocardiogram occurred in 84% of patients who exhibited regional transmural ischemia.

Baseline   **Occlusion**

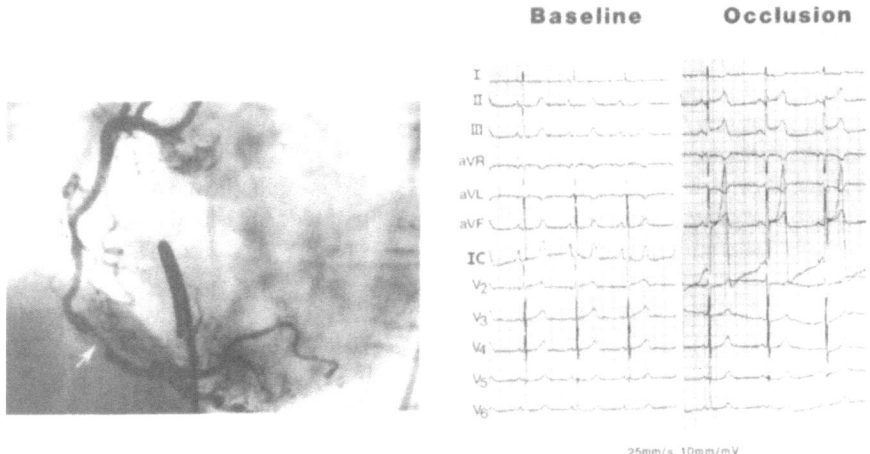

(B) The electrocardiographic changes occurring with occlusion of the right coronary artery. Surface ST elevation occurred in 92% of patients with regional transmural ischemia.

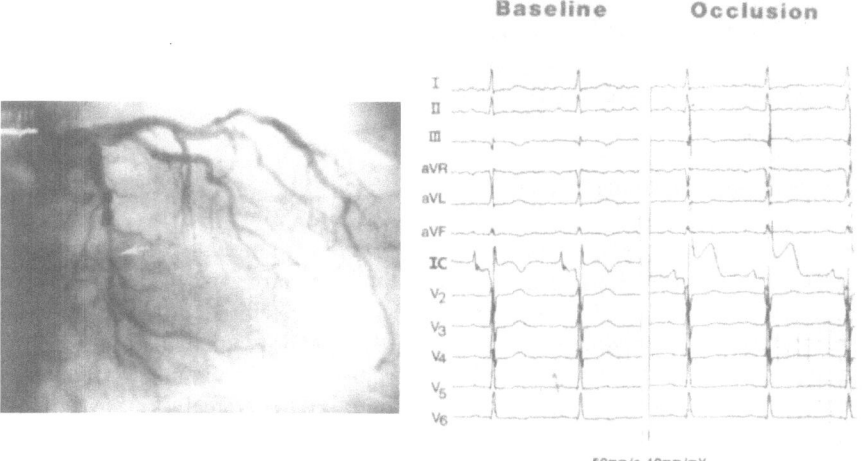

(C) Occlusion of the left circumflex coronary artery has different electrocardiographic consequences. Surface ST elevation occurred in only 32%; either no ST changes or precordial ST depression were common.

Figure 1.   The electrocardiographic changes accompanying PTCA of the 3 regional beds. From Berry et al, *Am J Cardiol* 63:21–26, 1989. Reprinted with permission.

Electrocardiographic changes

We recently examined the electrocardiographic responses to balloon occlusion of each of the 3 coronary beds during PTCA in patients undergoing routine coronary angioplasty [5]. The most common finding was the rapid development of ST segment elevation usually within 30 sec of interruption of coronary blood flow. Using simultaneous intracoronary and surface recordings, we defined transmural ischemia as ST elevation of at least 0.1 mV on the regional (intracoronary) electrocardiogram and demonstrated that ST elevation occurred in 21 of 25 patients (84%) during balloon occlusion of the left anterior descending (Fig. 1A). Similarly, during right coronary artery occlusion, ST elevation occurred in 11 of 12 patients (92%) with local electrocardiographic changes (Fig. 1B). In contrast, when the left circumflex coronary artery was occluded, surface ST elevation occurred in only 6 of 19 patients (32%) who demonstated regional transmural ischemia (Fig. 1C). From this study, we concluded that ST elevation frequently occurred during transient occlusion of the left anterior descending and right coronary artery beds; however, surface ST elevation was a relatively uncommon finding during left circumflex occlusion. During left circumflex occlusion, the most frequent findings are either no important repolarization change or precordial ST segment depression.

The electrocardiographic changes resolve very rapidly with balloon deflation, with return toward baseline usually within 30–60 sec. In fact, persistence of electrocardiographic abnormalities after balloon deflation should alert the physician that flow limitation is present.

Left ventricular functional changes

In a series of elegant experiments [6], Serruys et al demonstrated that coronary occlusion during PTCA in patients resulted in the rapid transient development of left ventricular relaxation abnormalities which were closely followed by systolic dysfunction. In similar studies using echocardiographic measurements, Wohlgelernter et al [7] also showed the development of regional systolic wall motion abnormalities within 12 sec, which progressed to severe dyskinesis within one minute of coronary artery occlusion.

A graphic demonstration of the electrocardiographic wall motion and left ventricular hemodynamic changes is illustrated in Fig. 2.

The effect of PTCA on coronary hemodynamics has been characterized as well. During left anterior descending occlusion, there is a fall in great cardiac vein flow; subsequent balloon deflation results in a marked hyperemic response which

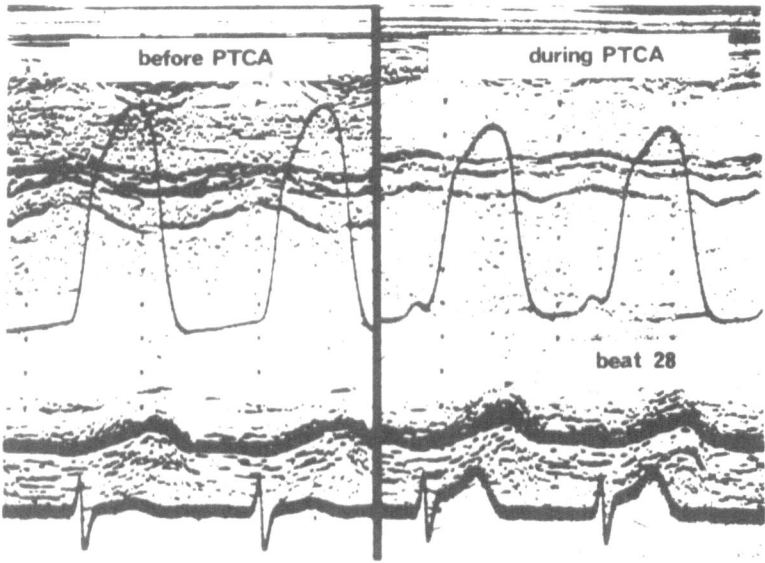

Figure 2. Simultaneous electrocardiographic, echocardiographic, and left ventricular pressures recorded before and during balloon inflation of the left anterior descending coronary artery. Note the rapid development of ST elevation accompanied by depressed systolic septal contraction and drop in left ventricular systolic and rise in left ventricular diastolic pressures.
From Serruys et al, *Eur Heart J* 4(Suppl C): 115, 1983. Reprinted with permission.

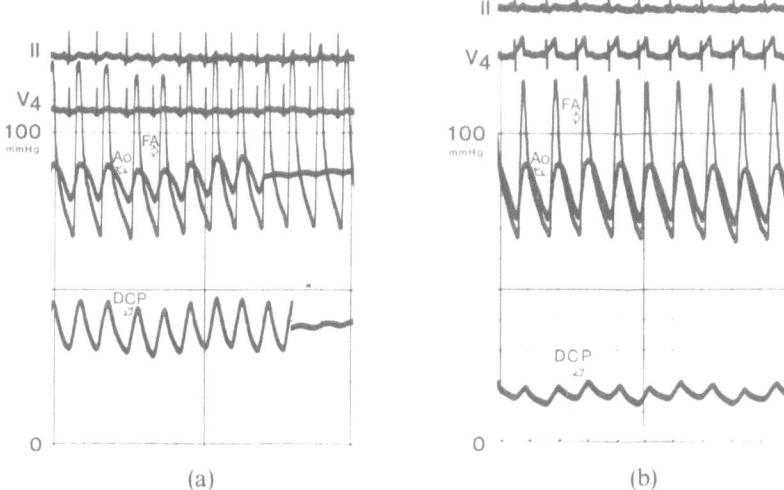

Figure 3. Electrocardiogram and systemic arterial and distal coronary pressures during balloon occlusion of the left anterior descending in a patient with (A) and without (B) collateral vessels. Note the ST elevation in (B) with a distal occluded pressure (DCP) of approximately 16 mmHg. Contrast this with the situation in (A) when there is absence of injury current and the DCP is approximately 38 mmHg.

diminishes in magnitude with subsequent inflation-deflation cycles [6, 8, 9, 10]. Concomitant with balloon inflation, there is a drop in distal coronary pressure as measured through the dilatation catheter. Distal occluded pressures below 25 mmHg are usually associated with transmural injury current and absent or poorly developed collaterals. Distal occluded pressures of > 35 mmHg are associated with less of an ischemic response on the surface electrocardiogram and a well developed collateral circulation supplying the occluded vessel (Fig. 3).

Accompanying the changes in the electrocardiogram, left ventricular function and coronary hemodynamics, is a change over from aerobic to anaerobic metabolism which is reflected by lactate production as measured in coronary sinus blood [6]. Of great practical clinical importance, is the fact that all of the above mentioned markers of balloon induced ischemia return to baseline shortly after balloon deflation. Multiple inflation–deflation cycles do not seem to have a cumulative deleterious effect in patients undergoing PTCA.

Pharmacologic agents designed to protect the ischemic myocardium

Several classes of drugs have been tested in the clinical setting of PTCA in attempts to limit the degree of ischemia induced during abrupt transient occlusion of an epicardial coronary artery.

Nitroglycerin

The efficacy of nitroglycerin has been assessed during both intravenous and intracoronary administration with mixed overall results. Thus, Doorey et al [11] reported a significant delay in the time to onset of angina and electrocardiographic changes in patients undergoing PTCA who had been treated with 200 µg of intravenous nitroglycerin. The time to onset of angina and time to development of ST segment shifts was increased from 29 ± 3 sec to 58 ± 6 sec and from 30 ± 3 sec to 62 ± 8 sec, respectively. The authors did not demonstrate improvement in left ventricular wall motion, but detected less displacement of the left ventricular pressure volume relation with inflations which were done after nitroglycerin administration. This effect is demonstrated in Fig. 4. Conflicting results were reported in another study in which the investigators failed to show a beneficial effect of intravenous nitroglycerin in reducing ischemia when given just before left anterior descending coronary artery occlusion [12].

The efficacy of intracoronary nitroglycerin in reducing ischemia during PTCA was tested by Kern et al [13]. These authors compared data from 2 matched balloon occlusion periods in 17 patients undergoing left anterior descending PTCA. After administration of 200 µg of intracoronary nitroglycerin, there was a reduction in mean arterial pressure and an increase in basal coronary blood flow, and no change in coronary occlusion pressure during ischemia. Intra-

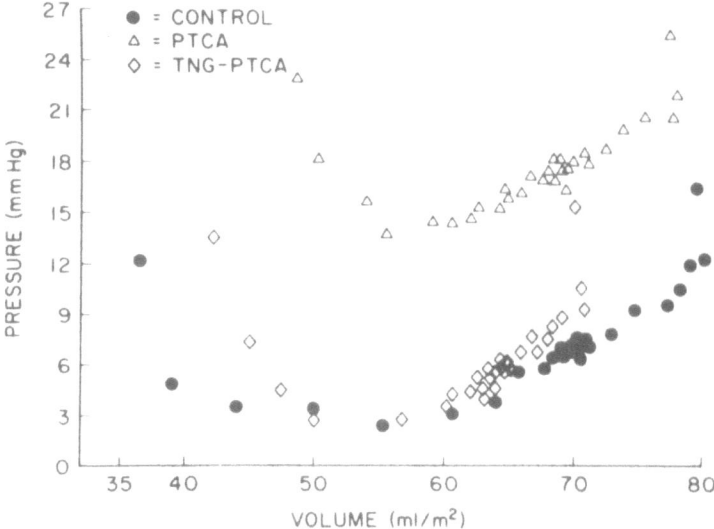

Figure 4. Protective effect of intracoronary nitroglycerin on the left ventricular pressure-volume relation during left anterior descending PTCA. During balloon inflation, there is typical upward displacement of the left ventricular pressure-volume relation compared to the baseline state. After intracoronary nitroglycerin pretreatment, the displacement in the pressure-volume loop is attenuated. From Doorey et al, *J Am Coll Cardiol* 6:267, 1985.

coronary nitroglycerin did not attenuate the degree of ischemic ST segment shift after 1 min of coronary artery occlusion.

Beta adrenergic blocking agents

Previous studies of beta adrenergic blockers have demonstrated that they reduced the degree myocardial injury as judged by the extent of ST segment elevation during acute myocardial infarction [14]. Feldman et al [15] tested *intravenous* propranolol in a dose of 0.1 mg/kg in patients undergoing left anterior descending coronary angioplasty. In that study, there was a mixed response with 6 of 16 patients showing no reduction in ischemia, while 10 patients demonstrated the delayed development of chest pain and electrocardiographic changes. Surprisingly, there was no difference in the heart rate response in responders vs nonresponders. In addition, the response to intravenous propranolol did not seem to depend on the presence of angiographically visible collateral blood flow to the left anterior descending coronary artery.

The effect of *regional* propranolol administration on ameliorating myocardial ischemia was tested in a randomized study of 21 patients undergoing elective PTCA [16]. All patients underwent two control inflations with measurements made of time to development of ST elevation $\geqslant 0.1$ mV and the degree of ST elevation at 60 sec of coronary artery occlusion. Heart rate and arterial pressure were also recorded. After the second balloon inflation, patients were randomly assigned to receive either intracoronary saline or intracoronary propranolol (average dose 1.1 mg). Following this, a third inflation was carried out and the aforementioned indices were again measured. The results can be summarized as follows: There was a uniformly beneficial response to intracoronary propranolol with the time to ST elevation increasing from 19 ± 4 sec to 53 ± 9 sec ($p < 0.001$). In contrast, there was no prolongation in time to ST elevation in the placebo treated control patients. Similarly, intracoronary propranolol decreased the degree of ST segment elevation from 0.23 ± 0.06 mV to 0.12 ± 0.04 mV ($p < 0.005$) during 60 sec of occlusion. Interestingly, there was no significant effect of intracoronary propranolol on heart rate or systolic arterial pressure. These findings indicate that the beneficial anti-ischemic effect of propranolol was mediated by a local protective effect of the drug. An example of the salutory effect of regional propranolol administration is shown in Fig. 5, while the overall findings are summarized in Figs 6 and 7. The clinical utility of intracoronary propranolol to achieve a more prolonged inflation is demonstrated in Fig. 8.

Calcium channel antagonists

Serruys et al tested the efficacy of intracoronary nifedipine administration during routine angioplasty [8]. Administration of 0.2 mg of intracoronary nifedipine resulted in a significant negative inotropic effect as judged by as peak negative

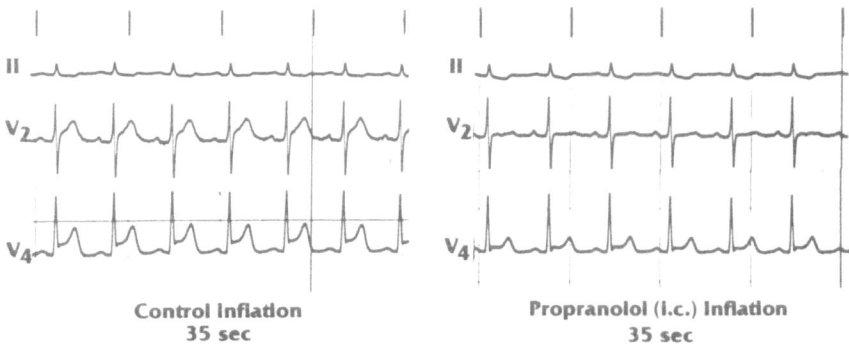

Figure 5. The protective effect of intracoronary propranolol during balloon angioplasty. The electrocardiographic response at 35 sec of a control balloon inflation is shown in the *left* panel. After intracoronary propranolol, (1 mg), there is marked reduction of the injury current for the same occlusion time (right panel).
From Zalewski et al, *Circulation* 73:734, 1986. Reprinted with permission.

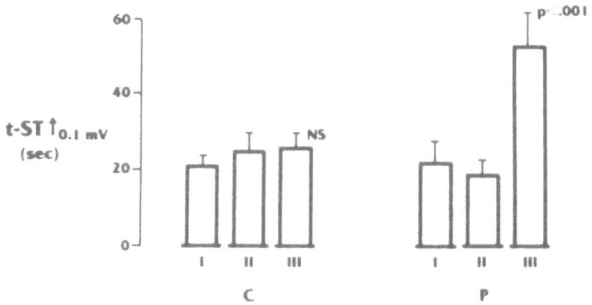

Figure 6. Time to development of ST elevation for 3 inflations in the patients assigned to intracoronary placebo (left) vs. intracoronary propranolol (right). Note the marked prolongation of time to ST elevation in patients assigned to intracoronary propranolol.
From Zalewski et al, *Circulation* 73:734, 1986. Reprinted with permission.

dp/dt. In addition, the magnitude of reduction of systolic left ventricular performance was similar to the effect of a 45 sec control balloon inflation. However, the degree of myocardial ischemia as judged by coronary sinus lactate production was less for inflations performed after nifedipine pretreatment. These findings suggested that a nifedipine induced decrease in myocardial oxygen consumption resulted in a protective effect of the drug on the affected myocardium.

Kern et al [13] found no significant prolongation in the time to development of ischemic electrocardiographic changes when nifedipine 10 mg sublingual was used during left anterior descending PTCA in 9 patients.

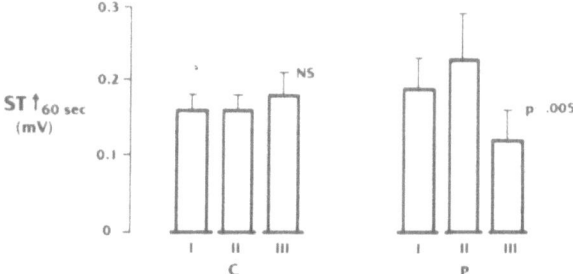

Figure 7. Amelioration of ischemic injury after intracoronary propranolol administration. Note reduced magnitude of ST elevation for the balloon occlusion after intracoronary propranolol administration compared with control.
C = control; P = propranolol.
From Zalewski et al, *Circulation* 73:734, 1986. Reprinted with permission.

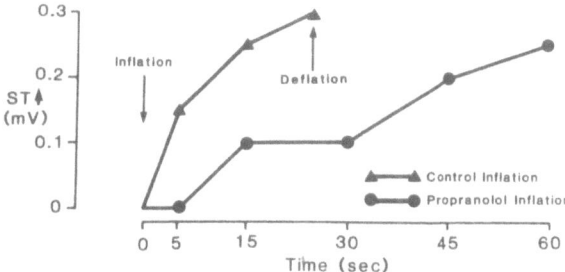

Figure 8. The clinical utility of intracoronary propranolol administration in allowing for prolonged balloon inflation. An initial inflation produced marked ST elevation which was accompanied by severe chest pain. These changes necessitated early balloon deflation; the clinical result at this point was unsatisfactory. After intracoronary propranolol, there was a considerable time delay in onset of ischemia, allowing for a more prolonged inflation and a satisfactory angiographic and clinical result.
From Zalewski et al, *Am J Cardiol* 61:54G, 1988. Reprinted with permission.

Oxygenated fluorocarbons

The oxygenated fluorocarbons such as fluosol DA-20% have the advantages of delivering relatively high concentrations of oxygen, while reducing the potential clinical problems attendant with blood perfusion of the myocardium (viscosity, hemolysis). Experimental studies have suggested a significant anti-ischemic effect during coronary artery occlusion when the agents are given both via the intravenous [17] and intracoronary [18] routes. In a clinical study by Anderson, fluosol DA-20% was infused through the dilatation catheter at a rate of 60 ml/min in patients undergoing PTCA [19]. A relatively modest protective effect was demonstrated by a minor prolongation in time to onset of angina (33 to 41 sec) when fluosol was compared to lactated Ringers solution. There was also a moderate increase in the time to development of ST segment elevation; however, a relatively high incidence of ventricular fibrillation in patients treated with intracoronary fluosol infusion limited the efficacy of this approach. More promising results were reported by Cleman et al, [20] who in a controlled study demonstrated preservation of left ventricular function in a group of patients treated with intracoronary oxygenated fluosol during balloon coronary occlusion. In patients treated with similar infusion rates of solutions not as oxygen rich, left ventricular regional function declined during balloon occlusion [20]. Importantly, there were no serious adverse effects of intracoronary fluosol infusion in the latter study.

Mechanical devices used to limit ischemia during balloon angioplasty

The rationale for using a mechanical method of reducing myocardial ischemia during PTCA would be to: (a) extend the use of PTCA to higher risk patients, (b) provide for very prolonged balloon inflations in the 5–15 min range. The purpose of prolonged balloon inflation would be to improve the primary result of PTCA by stabilizing a coronary dissection. In addition, very prolonged inflations conceivably could (c) reduce the current, substantial 35% restenosis rate, and (d) limit ischemic necrosis following failed PTCA.

In order for a mechanical device to have wide applicability in patients undergoing PTCA:
1. It must be practical and easy to deploy. The device should not be more cumbersome or difficult to use than the PTCA procedure itself.
2. The device should provide uniformly reliable myocardial protection in a variety of anatomic circumstances.
3. The device should have a low incidence of complications.

In this section we will review several devices with different mechanisms of action.

Intraaortic balloon counterpulsation

The percutaneous intraaortic balloon is a potentially useful tool to control ischemic injury in high risk patients undergoing balloon angioplasty. It is simple to insert in the catheterization laboratory setting, taking only a few minutes to achieve effective counterpulsation. Previous experimental [21] as well as clinical studies [22] suggest that the intraaortic balloon would be most efficacious in controlling ischemic injury in patients with some residual flow to the hypoperfused myocardial bed. It would be expected that patients with complete interruption of antegrade flow without collateral circulation would experience the least benefit.

In addition, because of the potential significant incidence of local vascular complications, we have limited the use of the intraaortic balloon as an adjunct to PTCA to two circumstances: (a) as a prophylactic measure in very high risk unstable patients with large amounts of myocardium at risk and (b) as a stabilizing device after failed PTCA in patients with hemodynamic compromise on their way to the operating room.

Coronary sinus retroperfusion

The idea of providing oxygen rich blood via an arteriovenous conduit to the coronary circulation was first conceived of as a surgical procedure [23]. More recently, this idea was revived and reapplied as a transcatheter device in which blood is directed from a systemic artery (such as the femoral), through a catheter system which is inserted into the great cardiac vein [24–27]. We studied the effects of arterialization of the coronary sinus in an experimental preparation of coronary artery occlusion designed to assess the degree of myocardial necrosis as a function of the hypoperfused zone (risk area). The findings are demonstrated in Fig. 9, which shows that arterialization of the coronary venous system resulted in a 34% reduction of infarct size as a function of risk area. It should be emphasized that this represents a relatively moderate degree of myocardial protection for this experimental model. Preliminary clinical trials show some potential promise, especially with a newer system of diastolic synchronized retroperfusion. However, the systems are relatively cumbersome, are somewhat time consuming, and involve placement of substantial hardware. Furthermore, the potential adverse consequences of even short term arterialization of the coronary venous system

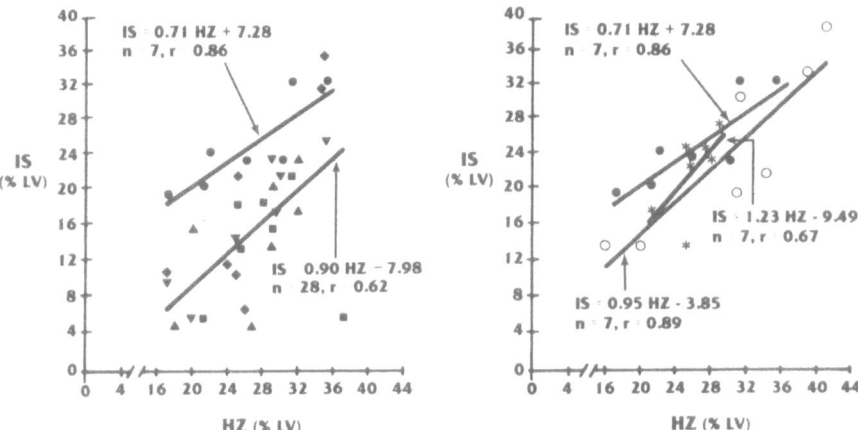

Figure 9. The effects of arterialization of the coronary venous system on reducing exprimental infarct size. The extent of myocardial necrosis, i.e. infarct size (IS) is plotted as a function of the hypoperfused zone (HZ). In the left panel, the upper line represents control animals subject to 6 hour coronary artery occlusion; the lower line represents the animals who underwent coronary artery occlusion plus arterialization of the coronary nervous system. Note the reduction of IS for each given HZ. In the right panel, the upper line shows control animals and the lower 2 lines show the lack of significant IS reduction for venous blood and pressure controlled intermittent occlusion of the great cardiac vein.

From Zalewski et al, *Circulation* 71:1215, 1985. Reprinted with permission.

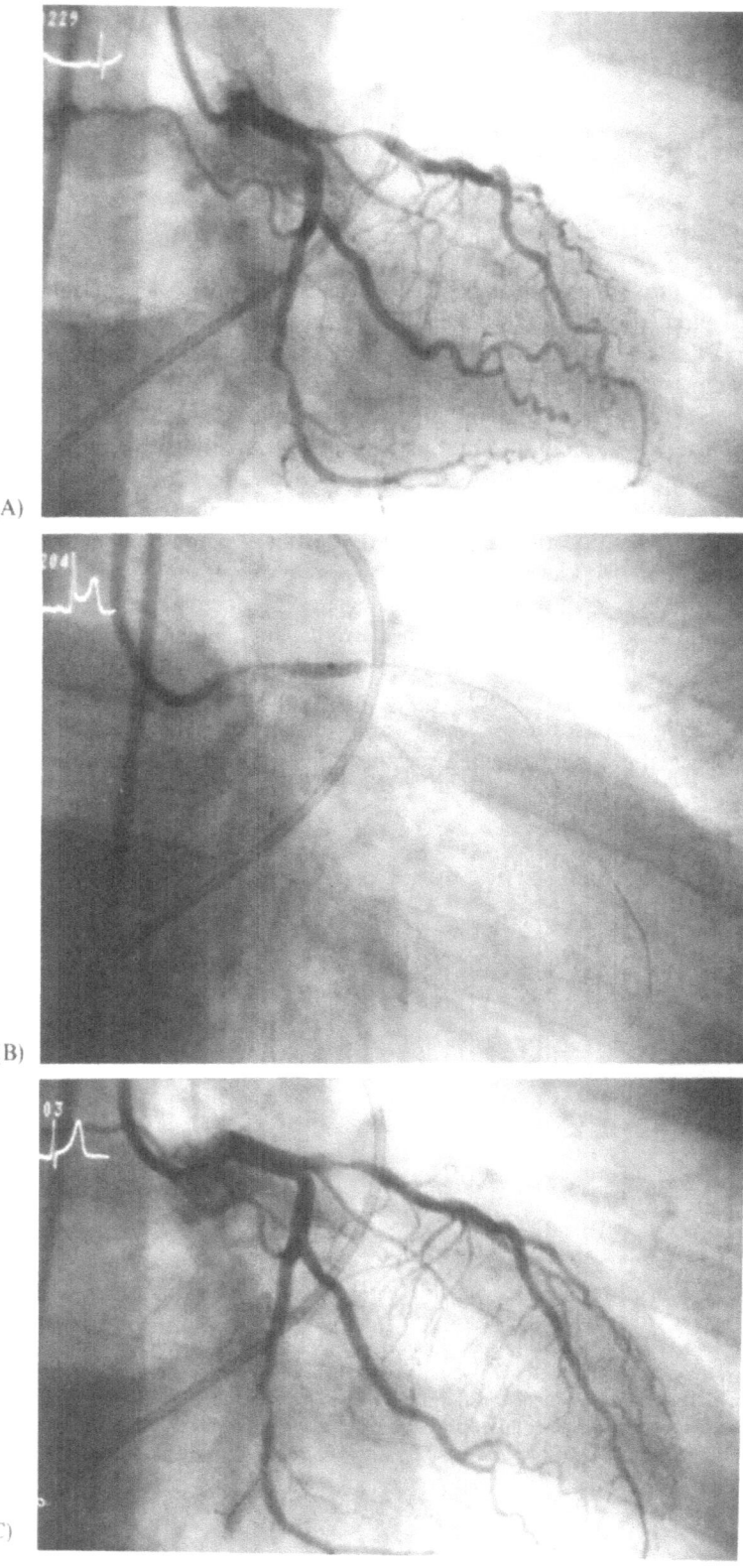

(A)

(B)

(C)

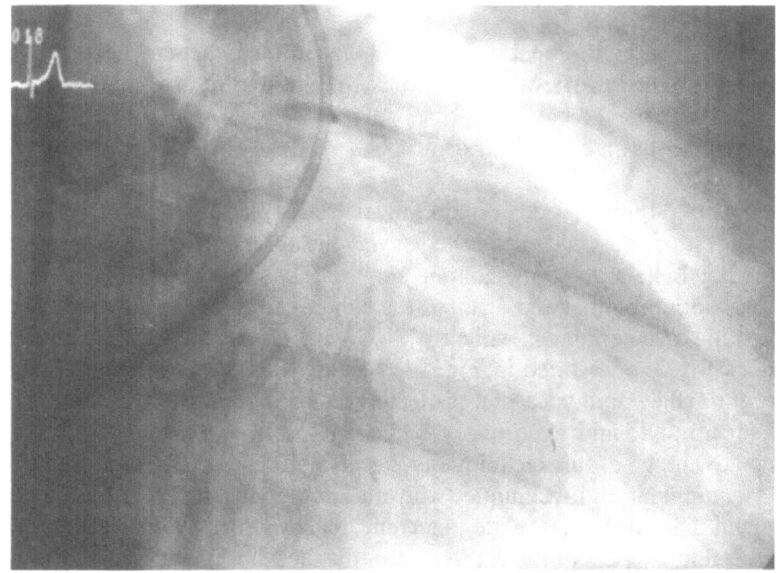

(D)

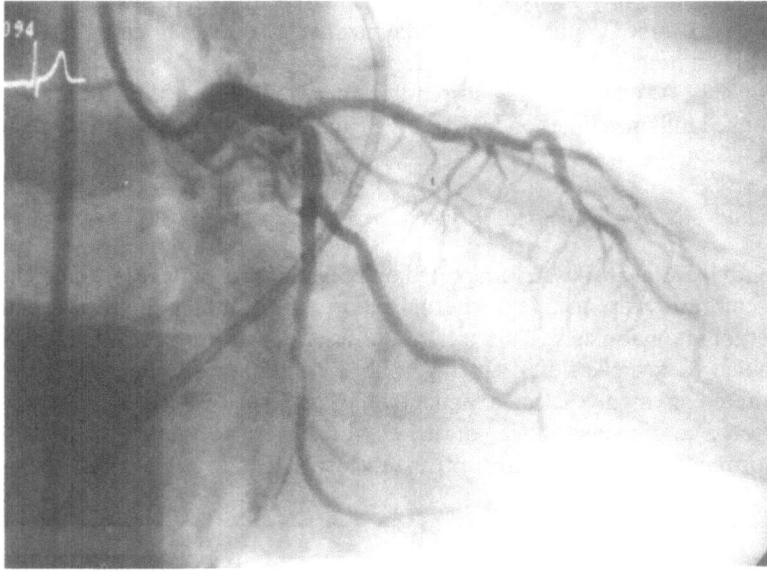

(E)

Figure 10. Efficacy of the autoperfusion balloon in allowing for a prolonged inflation and improvement in angiographic and clinical result.

(A) Baseline left coronary angiogram demonstrating severe proximal left anterior descending stenosis.

(B) Standard short balloon inflation resulted in severe ST elevation and chest pain (note electrocardiogram inset).

(C) Angiographic result after standard balloon inflation shows intimal disruption in area of lesion.

(D) Prolonged inflation of 10 min with autoperfusion balloon; only mild chest discomfort occurred and there is minimal ST segment change.

(E) Angiographic result after prolonged inflation showing marked improvement compared to result obtained with short inflation.

(excess pressure in the venous system, myocardial ischemia) have not been completely studied. Current clinical trials should help resolve these issues.

Distal hemoperfusion catheter devices

Experimental studies [28, 29] and clinical trials [30] have demonstrated the efficacy of autoperfusion catheters in delaying the onset and reducing the extent of myocardial ischemia during balloon angioplasty. The basic concept is that sideholes both proximal and distal to the balloon allow for aortic blood to flow through the catheter lumen, while the PTCA balloon is inflated. The efficacy of this device is demonstrated in Fig. 10. To date, this seems the most practical choice for achieving myocardial protection, allowing for safe balloon inflation times for up to 15 min of coronary occlusion.

The advantage of this technique is that it requires nothing more than basic PTCA equipment and techniques with no additional time required for device placement. Disadvantages relate to technical factors such as the relatively large shaft size and stiffness of the catheter, and the fact that the guidewire has to be withdrawn for effective distal hemoperfusion. In addition, the device would have limited applicability in hypotensive patients due to the reduced aortic-distal coronary pressure gradient in this circumstance. However, to date this seems to be the most practical, reliable, and safe means of achieving myocardial protection during PTCA. Clinical trials currently underway will test the efficacy of very prolonged inflation times on increasing primary success and reducing restenoses rates.

Percutaneous cardiopulmonary bypass support

Recently, several groups have reported on preliminary experience with percutaneous femoral bypass using an external pump oxygenator in 'high risk' patients undergoing angioplasty. This technique requires the use of large (20 French) cannulae to achieve flows ranging from 2.8–5 l/min. This approach may be warranted in highly selected patients such as those with very low ejection fractions, cardiogenic shock, or those who experience severe hemodynamic compromise as a result of abrupt vessel closure [31–33].

References

1. Zalewski A, Savage M, Goldberg S (1988) Protection of the ischemic myocardium during coronary angioplasty. *Am J Cardiol* 61:54G
2. Zalewski A, Goldberg S (1988) Protection of the ischemic myocardium during coronary angioplasty. In: Goldberg S; Brest AN (eds) *Coronary Angioplasty*. Philadelphia: FA Davis Company (Cardiovascular Clinics)
3. Cohen M, Rentrop KP (1986) Limitation of myocardial ischemia by collateral circulation during sudden controlled coronary artery occlusion in human subjects: A prospective study. *Circulation* 74:469
4. Rentrop KP, Cohen M, Blanke H, Phillips RA (1985) Changes in collateral channel filling immediately after controlled coronary artery occlusion by an angioplasty balloon in human subjects. *J. Am Coll Cardiol* 5:587

5. Berry C, Zalewski A, Kovach R, Savage M, Goldberg S (1989) Surface electrocardiogram in the detection of transmural myocardial ischemia during percutaneous transluminal coronary angioplasty. *Am J Cardiol* 63:21
6. Serruys PW, Wijns W, van den Brand M, Meij S, Slager C, Schuurbiers JCH, Hugenholtz PG, Brower RW (1984) Left ventricular performance, regional blood flow, wall motion, and lactate metabolism during transluminal angioplasty. *Circulation* 70:25
7. Wohlgelernter D, Cleman M, Highman HA, Fetterman RC, Duncan JS, Zaret BL, Jaffe CC (1986) Regional myocardial dysfunction during coronary angioplasty: Evaluation by two-dimensional echocardiography and 12 lead electrocardiography. *J Am Coll Cardiol* 7:1245
8. Serruys PW, van den Brand M, Brower RW, Hugenholtz PG (1983) Regional cardioplegia and cardioprotection during transluminal angioplasty, which role for nifedipine? *Eur Heart J* 4(Suppl C): 115
9. Rothman MT, Baim DS, Simpson JB, Harrison DC (1982) Coronary hemodynamics during percutaneous transluminal coronary angioplasty. *Am J Cardiol* 49:1615
10. Feldman RL, Conti CR, Pepine CJ (1983) Regional coronary venous flow responses to transient coronary artery occlusion in human beings. *J Am Coll Cardiol* 2:1
11. Doorey AJ, Mehmel HC, Schwarz FX, Kubler W (1985) Amelioration by nitroglycerin of left ventricular ischemia induced by percutaneous transluminal coronary angioplasty: Assessment by hemodynamic variables and left ventriculography. *J Am Coll Cardiol* 6:267
12. Feldman RL, Joyal M, Conti R, Pepine CJ (1984) Effect of nitroglycerin on coronary collateral flow and pressure during acute coronary occlusion. *Am J Cardiol* 54:958
13. Kern MJ, Deligonul U, Labovitz A, Gabliani G, Vandormael M, Kennedy HL (1988) Effects of nitroglycerin and nifedipine on coronary and systemic hemodynamics during transient coronary artery occlusion. *Am Heart J* 115:1164
14. Gold HK, Leinbach RC, Maroko PR (1976) Propranolol-induced reduction of signs of ischemic injury during acute myocardial infarction. *Am J Cardiol* 38:689
15. Feldman RL, MacDonald RG, Hill JA, Limacher MC, Conti CR, Pepine CJ (1986) Effect of propranolol on myocardial ischemia occurring during acute coronary occlusion. *Circulation* 73:727
16. Zalewski A, Goldberg S, Dervan JP, Slysh S, Maroko PR (1986) Myocardial protection during transient coronary artery occlusion in man: Beneficial effects of regional beta-adrenergic blockade. *Circulation* 73:734
17. Rude RE, Glogar D, Khuri SF, Kloner RA, Karaffa S, Muller JE, Clark Jr LC, Braunwald E (1982) Effects of intravenous fluorocarbons during and without oxygen enhancement on acute myocardial ischemic injury assessed by measurement of intramyocardial gas tensions. *Am Heart J* 103:986
18. Flaherty JT, Jaffin JH, Magovern GJ, Kanter KR, Gardner TJ, Miceli MV, Jacobus WE (1984) Maintenance of aerobic metabolism during global ischemia with perfluorocarbon cardioplegia improves myocardial preservation. *Circulation* 69:585
19. Anderson HV, Leimgruber PP, Roubin GS, Nelson DL, Gruentzig AR (1985) Distal coronary artery perfusion during percutaneous transluminal coronary angioplasty. *Am Heart J* 110:720
20. Cleman M, Jaffee CC, Wohlgelernter D (1986) Prevention of ischemia during percutaneous transluminal coronary angioplasty by transcatheter infusion of oxygenated Fluosol DA 20%. *Circulation* 74:555
21. Maroko PR, Bernstein EF, Libby P, DeLaria GA, Covell JW, Ross J, Braunwald E (1972) Effects of intraaortic balloon counterpulsation on the severity of myocardial ischemic injury following acute coronary occlusion. *Circulation* 45:1150
22. Leinbach RC, Gold HK, Harper RW, Buckley MJ, Austen WG (1978) Early intraaortic balloon pumping for anterior myocardial infarction without shock. *Circulation* 58:204
23. Beck CS, Makao AE (1948) Revascularization of the heart. *Am Surg* 128:854
24. Meerbaum S, Lang TW, Osher JV, Hashimoto K, Lewis GW, Feldstein C, Corday E (1976) Diastolic retroperfusion of acutely ischemic myocardium. *Am J Cardiol* 37:588
25. Zalewski A, Goldberg S, Slysh S, Maroko PR (1985) Myocardial protection via coronary sinus interventions: Superior effects of arterialization compared with intermittent occlusion. *Circulation* 71:1215

26. Farcot JC, Berland J, Cribier A, Letac B, Bourdarias JP (1985) Diastolic synchronized retroperfusion in the coronary sinus during percutaneous transluminal angioplasty: Preliminary experience (abstr). *Circulation* (Suppl III) 72:III–470

27. Gore JM, Weiner BH, Benotti JR, Sloan KM, Okike ON, Cuenoud HF, Gaca JMJ, Alpert JS, Dalen JE (1986) Preliminary experience with synchronized coronary sinus retroperfusion in humans. *Circulation* 74:381

28. Turi Z, Campbell CA, Kloner RA (1987) The autoperfusion balloon angioplasty catheter prevents ischemia during prolonged balloon inflation (abstr). *J Am Coll Cardiol* 9:106A

29. Zalewski A, Berry C, Kosman ZK, Shi Y, Goldberg S (Jan 1990) Myocardial protection with autoperfusion during prolonged coronary artery occlusion. *Am Heart J* (In press)

30. Turi ZG, Rezkalla S, Campbell CA, Kloner RA (1988) Amelioration of ischemia during angioplasty of the left anterior descending coronary artery with an autoperfusion catheter. *Am J Cardiol* 61:1513

31. Tommaso CL, Gundry SR, Zoda AR, Stafford JL, Johnson RA, Vogel RA (1989) Supported angioplasty: Initial experience with high risk patients (abstr). *J Am Coll Cardiol* (Suppl A) 13:159A

32. Shawl FA, Domanski MJ, Punja S, Hernandez TJ (1989) Percutaneous institution of cardiopulmonary (bypass) support: Technique and complications (abstr). *J Am Coll Cardiol* (Suppl A) 13:159A

33. Shawl FA, Domanski MJ, Punja S, Hernandez TJ (1989) Percutaneous cardiopulmonary bypass to support high risk elective coronary angioplasty. *J Am Coll Cardiol* (Suppl A) 13:160A

20. Does Diltiazem protect the ischemic myocardium during PTCA?

M. HALPERN and U. SIGWART

Introduction

Calcium antagonists are currently considered important in the treatment of coronary heart disease. Calcium antagonists have proven their effectiveness in the treatment of classic exertional angina, vasospastic angina, unstable angina, and they may reduce the size of an acute myocardial infarction [1, 2, 3, 4]. It has been postulated that Nifedipine can protect the myocardium during percutaneous transluminal coronary angioplasty (PTCA) by preventing the myocardial cells from becoming anaerobic [4, 5]. Calcium antagonists seem to have a protective effect on the myocardium during coronary bypass operations as well [13]. The hemodynamic effects of an oral and intravenous application of calcium antagonists have frequently been studied in man and animals. However, the hemodynamic and cardioprotective effects of an intra-coronary injection of calcium antagonists have not been frequently studied in man. Our aim was to know whether a super-selective intra-coronary injection of the calcium antagonist Diltiazem can protect the myocardium during acute ischemia of short duration in man.

Methods and material

The study was approved by the Hospital Ethics Committee. Five patients scheduled for PTCA were included. All were males, their age ranging from 49 to 73 years (mean 59). None of the patients had had a previous myocardial infarction and their left ventricular ejection fraction was always superior to 60%. The stenoses which we dilated were always superior to 75% and located proximally in two cases on the LAD, in one case on the circumflex coronary artery, in one case on the RCA, and in one case on a by-pass graft of the circumflex coronary artery. Among the patients three had single vessel disease and two had three vessel disease but in these cases only one vessel was dilated, as the stenoses on the remaining diseased vessels were not considered severe enough to be dilated. All

P.W. Serruys, R. Simon & K.J. Beatt (eds), Percutaneous Transluminal Coronary Angioplasty. ISBN 0-7923-0346-6.
© 1990 Kluwer Academic Publishers, Dordrecht

stenoses were successfully dilated, and there were no complication during of after the procedure.

Twenty-four hours before the procedure, anti-anginal drugs like nitrates and beta-blockers were discontinued and all patients were given aspirin 1000 mg per os. One hour prior to the procedure, the patients were premedicated with Valium 10 mg per os. The procedure was carried out under local anesthesia using the femoral approach. A Zucker F 7 bipolar pacing catheter was placed for pulmonary pressure monitoring and emergency pacing. A Millar PC-770 micro-tip pressure transducer was placed transeptally through a Cordis F 8 long transeptal sheath into the left ventricle and the left atrium. The patients were then given 10'000 U of heparin and left ventricular angiograms were obtained with biplane technique in two perpendicular oblique projections at 50/frames/sec employing a Philips Polydiagnost C with LARC with 9 and 6 inch zoom amplifyer tubes.

Selective coronary angiography was performed before the balloon catheter (Schneider Medintag AG or Advanced Cardiovascular Systems) was introduced into the coronary artery via a USCI F 9 guiding catheter. We have selected different oblique and hemiaxial projections to optimize the visualization of the target lesion. Electrocardiograms, arterial, left auricular and left ventricular pressure, as well as pressure derivatives were monitored continuously by a Mennen System 9000 cath. lab computer and recorded on a photographic recorder (Honeywell LS 8); simultaneously all data were stored on a 16 channel video-PCM digital recorder (Heim KG Elektronische Messgeräte, West Germany). Isovolumetric relaxation time (IVRT) was measured from the closure of the aortic valve (recognized by a small notch on the LA curve, and confirmed by intermittent control on the aortic pressure curve), to the opening of the mitral valve, identified at the point of LV and LA pressure curves cross-over. Total relaxation time (TRT) was measured from the closure of the aortic valve to the lowest pressure point (0 point).

All parameters were monitored and recorded before and during the passage of the balloon catheter, during and between the dilatations, as well as during and after intra-coronary injection of Diltiazem. The moment of coronary occlusion was identified by a sudden pressure drop at the distal end of the balloon catheter which was filled with 30% Urographin 76 and 70% of normal saline at 4 to 14 bars inflation pressure. The patients were asked to avoid deep inspiration during occlusion and to describe all subjective sensation at the time of occurence.

We proceeded to a first therapeutic occlusion (control occlusion), lasting from 15 to 45 sec (according to the degree of the stenosis, the hemodynamic variables as well as the patient's symptoms and ECG changes). After a recovery time of 3 min, after which all variables had returned to baseline, a dose of 0.05 mg/kg Diltiazem was injected super-selectively into the coronary artery undergoing dilatation, distally to the stenosis via the distal orifice of the balloon catheter. One to two minutes after Diltiazem injection, we proceeded to a second therapeutic occlusion, again lasting 15 to 45 sec. The results are expressed as the mean of values ± the standard deviation. Statistical analyses were obtained by a Student's paired T test. A p < 0.05 was considered significant.

Results

(1) *Myocardial ischemia during control occlusion.* Already within the first few seconds of occlusion, we have observed a dramatic disturbance of relaxation, which manifests as a modification of the shape and amplitude of the neg dP/dt; as demonstrated in Fig. 1 and 1 bis, the first signs are: (1) a notch in the ascending portion of the neg dP/dt, due to inhomogenous and asynchronous relaxation; (2) a diminution of the total amplitude of neg dP/dt. The notch in neg dP/dt levels out after about 20 sec of occlusion; at the same time, a modification appears in the diastolic pressure curve of the left ventricle, after the opening of the mitral valve: indeed, the 0 point moves to the right, and the rapid filling wave is flattened; this phenomenon signals a severe disturbance of relaxation. Similar changes are evident on the pos dP/dt curve, but they appear later, are more linear and less pronounced than the changes of neg dP/dt. The LV filling pressure, the LA a-wave and v-wave start to increase after 10 to 13 sec of occlusion, and will progressively increase until the end of the occlusion period. There are no changes in LVSP or heart rate during a 25 to 40 sec occlusion time; after longer coronary occlusions, LVSP starts to decrease progressively and heart rate increases consequently.

(2) *Super-selective intra-coronary Diltiazem injection.* Table 1 shows the values of all parameters before and 1 min after Diltiazem injection. Heart rate did not vary significantly, and there were no rythm disturbance after Diltiazem injection. Peak systolic pressure, end-diastolic pressure, LA a-wave and LA v-wave did not vary significantly. However, all relaxation parameters varied significantly (p < 0.001): neg dP/dt decreased of 10.1%, IVRT increased of 8.4% and TRT increased of 6.7%. In a similar way, contraction was decreased, as shows the drop of pos dP/dt of 9.9%. These events point out a drop of myocardial contractility after intra-coronary Diltiazem injection. Figure 2 shows an original recording before and one minute after intra-coronary Diltiazem injection. One minute after Diltiazem injection, we notice a drop of pos dP/dt and neg dP/dt, and a change in the LV pressure curve which shows a shifting of the 0 point towards the right and the disappearance of the rapid filling wave. This is identical to what we see during coronary occlusion.

(3) *Myocardial ischemia during occlusion following Diltiazem injection.* Figure 3 shows an original recording of the coronary occlusion following i.c. Diltiazem injection. As mentioned above, 1 min after intra-coronary Dilitiazem injection, dP/dt pos and neg are lessened, and there are changes in the LV pressure curve with disappearance of the rapid filling wave, all secondary to diminished

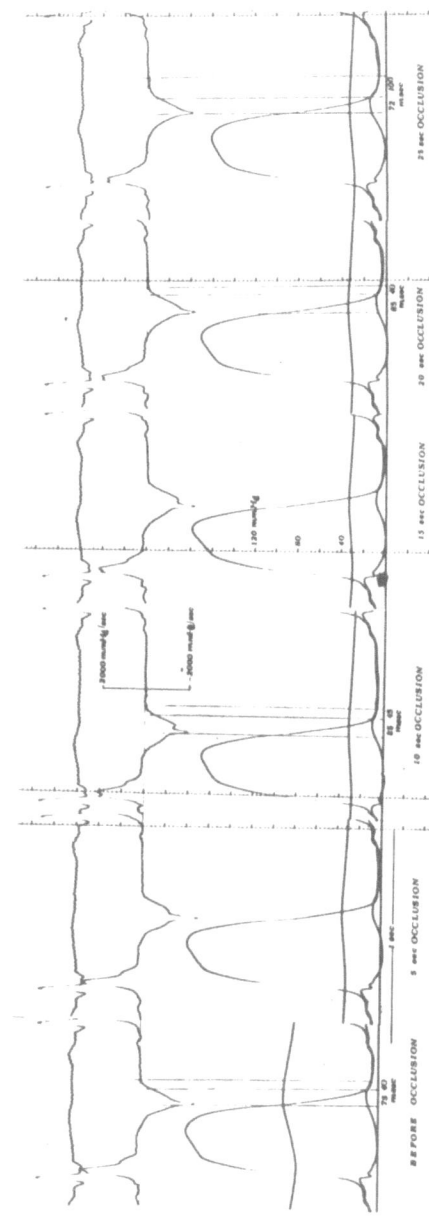

Figure 1. Original recording of cardiac activity before and during LAD occlusion: Parameters are from top to bottom, EKG, dP/dt, LV pressure curve, intra-coronary pressure curve, LA-pressure curve. The recording points out disturbances of relaxation manifested as modification in shape and amplitude of neg dP/dt, and shift of the 0 point of the LV pressure wave to the right, inducing tapering of the rapid filling wave. The typical notch on neg dP/dt curve observed within 5 sec of occlusion, and consequent of asynchronous relaxation of the ventricle, tapers after 15 sec of occlusion, indicating stiffness of the ventricle.

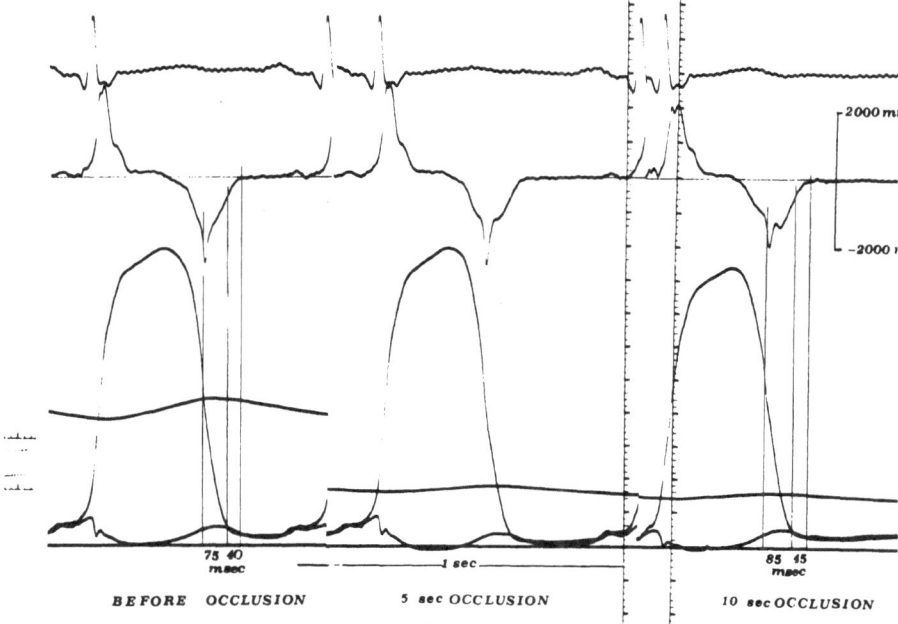

Figure 1 bis. Detail of a recording of LAD occlusion, outlining the changes in contraction and relaxation described in Fig. 1. Parameters are identical as in Fig. 1. Isovolumetric relaxation time is measured from the closure of the aortic valve to the opening of the mitral valve. Total relaxation time is measured from the closure of the aortic valve to the lowest LV pressure point – the 0 point.

Table 1. Comparing parameters before and one minute after 0.05 mg/kg intra-coronary Diltiazem injection. Parameters are heart rate (hr), left ventricular systolic pressure (LVSP), left ventricular end-diastolic pressure (LVEDP), pos dP/Dt, min dP/dt, isovolumic relaxation time (IVRT), total relaxation time (TRT), left atrium a-wave maximal pressure (LA a), left atrium v-wave maximal pressure (LA v). Pos dP/dt, neg dP/dt are significantly decreased; IVRT and TRT are significantly increased after Diltiazem injection demonstrating a drug induced drop in myocardial contractility; HR, LVSP, LA and LV pressure did not vary significantly.

	Before Diltiazem I.C	After Diltiazem I.C 0.05 mg/kg	△ in %
HR (BPM)	71.2 ± 8.7	71.8 ± 7.8	↑ 1.64%
LVSP (mmHg)	138.8 ± 26.6	131.3 ± 19.4	↓ 4.6%
LVEDP (mmHg)	11.6 ± 4.3	12.2 ± 4.9	↓ 5.4%
Max dP/dT (mmHg/sec)	1880 ± 505.7	1669 ± 368.5	↓ 9.9%
Min dP/dT (mmHg/sec)	− 2000 ± 570.1	− 1774 ± 430.9	↓ 10.1%
IVRT (msec)	81 ± 29.9	86.2 ± 24.9	↓ 8.4%
TRT (msec)	145.4 ± 31.7	150.8 ± 25.4	↓ 6.7%
LA-a (mmHg)	13.2 ± 2.4	13.6 ± 4.4	↓ 1.3%
LA-v (msec)	12.2 ± 4.5	13.1 ± 5.9	↓ 5%

myocardial performance. During occlusion which follows i.c. Diltiazem, the dP/dt and LV curves remain almost unchanged, especially within the first 15 sec of occlusion. There is no notch in the dP/dt curve; beyond 15 sec of occlusion, there is more pronounced disappearance of the rapid filling wave and increase in the height of the LA a-wave and LA v-wave.

(4) *Comparing the effects of coronary occlusion on cardiac hemodynamics, before and after Diltiazem injection.* Table 2 and Figs 4 to 12 show how the different parameters of cardiac function evolve during the first 16 sec of occlusion, before and after i.c. Diltiazem injection.

1. Heart rate: there is no significant change in heart rate during neither occlusion.

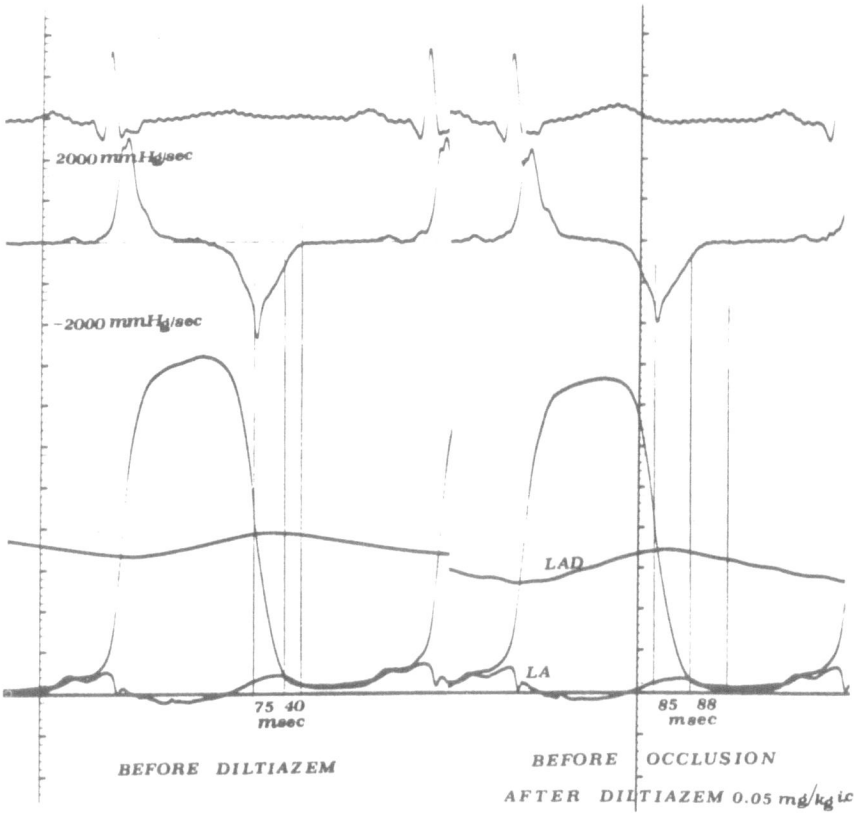

Figure 2. Original recording of cardiac activity before and one minute after intra-coronary selective Diltiazem injection (parameters are the same as in Fig. 1). One minute after Diltiazem injection, there is a drop in pos dP/dt and neg dP/dt, a change in the LV pressure curve with a shift of the 0 point to the right.

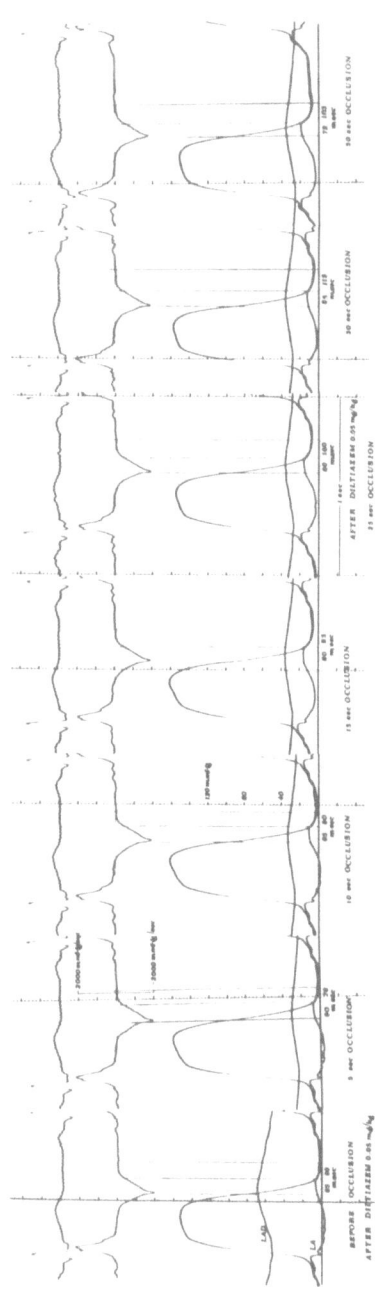

Figure 3. Original recording of cardiac activity, pretreated with intra-coronary Diltiazem, before and during LAD occlusion. Parameters are identical to Fig. 1: the dP/dt and LV curves remain almost unchanged within 15 sec of occlusion, there is no 'notch' in the dP/dt curve; beyond 15 sec, there is disappearance of the ventricular rapid filling wave, and increase in the height of the LA a-wave and v-wave.

2. Peak systolic pressure: LVSP is slightly lower after Diltiazem injection, but the difference is not significant. LVSP does not vary significantly during the first 16 sec of either occlusion.

3. End-diastolic pressure: LVEDP increases slowly with the last seconds of occlusion. Figure 5 shows that when occlusion is prolonged until 42 sec LVEDP continues to increase gradually until the end of occlusion. The difference between the values before and after Diltiazem injection is not significant.

4. Neg dP/dt: typically, occlusion induces within the first seconds a drop in neg dP/dt which is most rapid within the 10 first sec of occlusion, but continues until the end of the observed period of 16 sec of occlusion (see Fig. 6). On different occasions we have also noticed that when occlusion lasts as long as 30 sec, neg dP/dt continues to drop until the end of the occlusion. After i.c. Diltiazem, neg dP/dt starts to drop from a 10.1% lower value ($p < 0.001$); however, during the occlusion following the anti-calcic agent, neg dP/dt drops less than during the control occlusion ($p < 0.001$). In consequence, the curve of neg dP/dt values is flatter for coronary occlusion following i.c. Diltiazem injection than for control occlusion. After 12 sec of occlusion, the two curves have a similar slope.

5. Isovolumetric Relaxation Time: Fig. 7 shows that coronary occlusion induces a prolongation of IVRT as a consequence of the decrease of myocardial contractility. IVRT is 8.4% longer 1 min after i.c. Diltiazem injection, but during the occlusion following the anti-calcic agent, IVRT increases less than

Table 2. Comparing the evolution of 8 parameters (see Table 1 for parameters legends), at 0 and 16 sec of coronary occlusion, prior and after intra-coronary i.c. Diltiazem injection neg dP/dt was significantly less decreased at 16 sec of occlusion after Diltiazem injection; IVRT, TRT and LA a-wave significantly less increased; indicating lesser impairment of myocardial contractility during coronary occlusion when the myocardium is treated with Diltiazem injected selectively into the dilated artery.

	Control coronary balloon occlusion (0–16 sec)		Coronary balloon occlusion (0–16 sec) after Diltiazem 0.05 mg/kg I.C	
		△ in %		△ in %
LVSP (mmHg)	↓ 138.8± 26.6 / 141.8± 20.9	↑ 2.7%	↓ 131.4± 19 / 127 ± 25.7	↓ 3.8%
LVEDP (mmHg)	↓ 11.2± 4.6 / 16.4± 6.7	↑ 50.2%	↓ 10.8± 4 / 16.4± 7.1	↑ 49.8%
Max dP/dT (mmHg/sec)	↓ 1880 ±505.7 / 1720 ±334.7	↓ 7.1%	↓ 1669 ±368.5 / 1530 ±303.3	↓ 7.9%
Min dP/dT (mmHg/sec)	↓ −2000 ±570 / −1610 ±461.5	↓ 19.4%	↓ −1774.5±430.9 / −1470 ±361.6	↓ 16.3%
IVRT (msec)	↓ 80 ± 28.9 / 94 ± 29.4	↑ 18.9%	↓ 85.4± 25.4 / 97.7± 25.3	↑ 15.1%
TRT (msec)	↓ 143 ± 31.9 / 160.6± 33.2	↑ 14.1%	↓ 148.4± 22.9 / 165 ± 17.7	↑ 11.9%
LA-a (mmHg)	↓ 12.6± 2.6 / 17.6± 4.8	↑ 38.9%	↓ 12.8± 3.8 / 17.4± 5.4	↑ 35.4%
LA-v (mmHg)	↓ 12 ± 4.7 / 18.2± 8.4	↑ 50.1%	↓ 11.6± 4.7 / 17.4± 5.8	↑ 40.1%

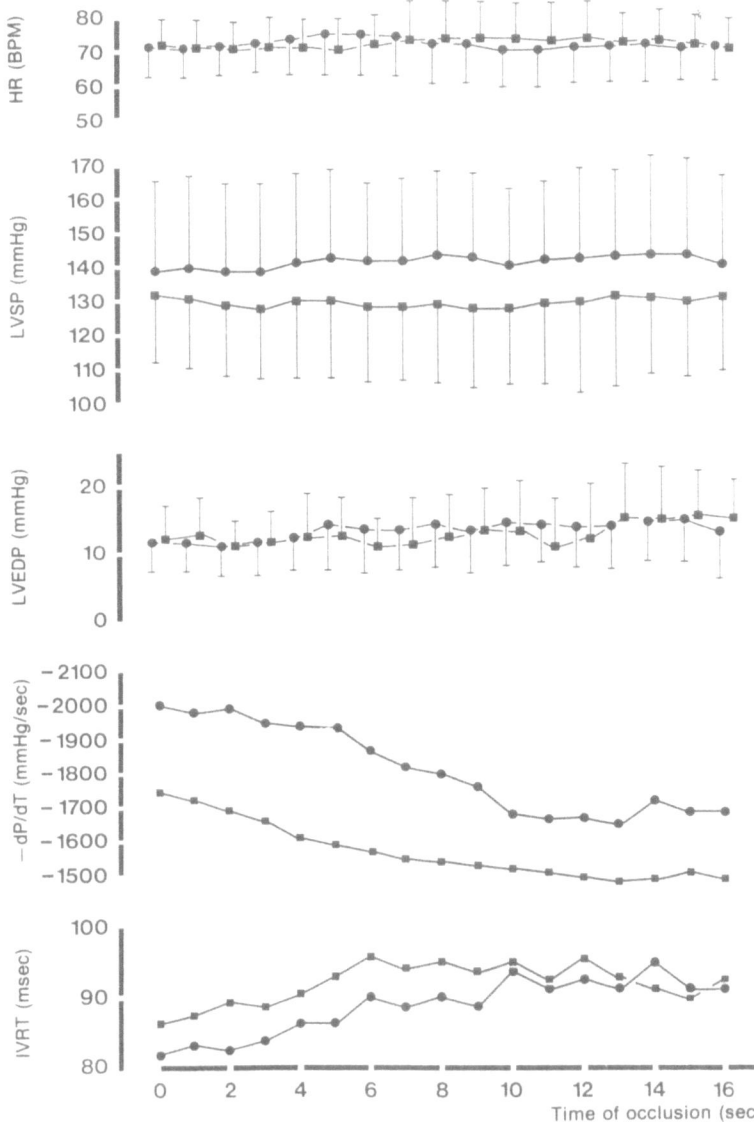

Figure 4. Evolution of cardiac parameters during 16 sec of coronary occlusion, before and after intra-coronary injection of Diltiazem 0.05 mg/kg. Y-axis parameters are, from top to bottom: heart rate (beats per min), left ventricular systolic pressure (LVSP, in mmHg), left ventricular end-diastolic pressure (LVEDP, in mmHg), neg dP/dt (mmHg per sec) and isovolumetric relaxation time (milliseconds msec). The X-axis is time of occlusion in seconds. The ● round points represent values during control occlusion; the ■ square points represent values during occlusion after i.c. injection of Diltiazem. Heart rate and LVSP do not vary significantly, LVEDP increases slowly in the last seconds of occlusion. For hr, LVSP and LVEP, the difference of the values before and after i.c. Diltiazem is not significant.

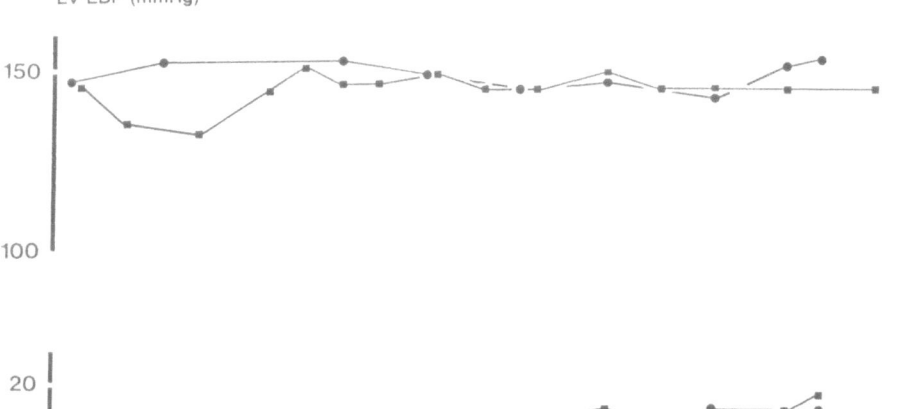

Figure 5. Evolution of left ventricular end-diastolic pressure (LVEDP) and left systolic pressure (LVSP) during a 40 sec coronary occlusion before (●) and after (■) intra-coronary injection of 0.05 mg/kg Diltiazem in one patient. LVEDP increases slowly after the 10th second of occlusion, until the end of occlusion, as the ventricle looses compliance. The difference between the values before and after Diltiazem injection is not significant. LVSP did not change significantly at either occlusion.

during control occlusion (p < 0.001). The two curves meet at the end of the 16 sec occlusion period.

6. Total Relaxation Time: Fig. 8 shows that TRT increases during coronary occlusion, as a consequence of ischemia. TRT is prolonged by 6.7% 1 min after i.c. Diltiazem injection, but increases less during the occlusion following Diltiazem injection than during control occlusion (p < 0.001). However, at the end of the observed period, there is again a superposition of both curves of values preceding and following Diltiazem treatment.

7. Pos dP/dt: as shown in Fig. 9, occlusion induces a drop of pos dP/dt as it did for neg dP/dt, but less pronounced. The drop is even less pronounced after Diltiazem injection. Figure 10 shows that pos dP/dt continues to drop when occlusion is prolonged to 30 sec.

8. LA v-wave: occlusion induces a rise of LA v-wave, most importantly after 10 sec (see Fig. 11). Comparing the curves of values of occlusion before and after i.c. Diltiazem injection, we notice a separation after 5 sec of occlusion, followed by a superimposition of the curves after 13 sec of occlusion. Similar

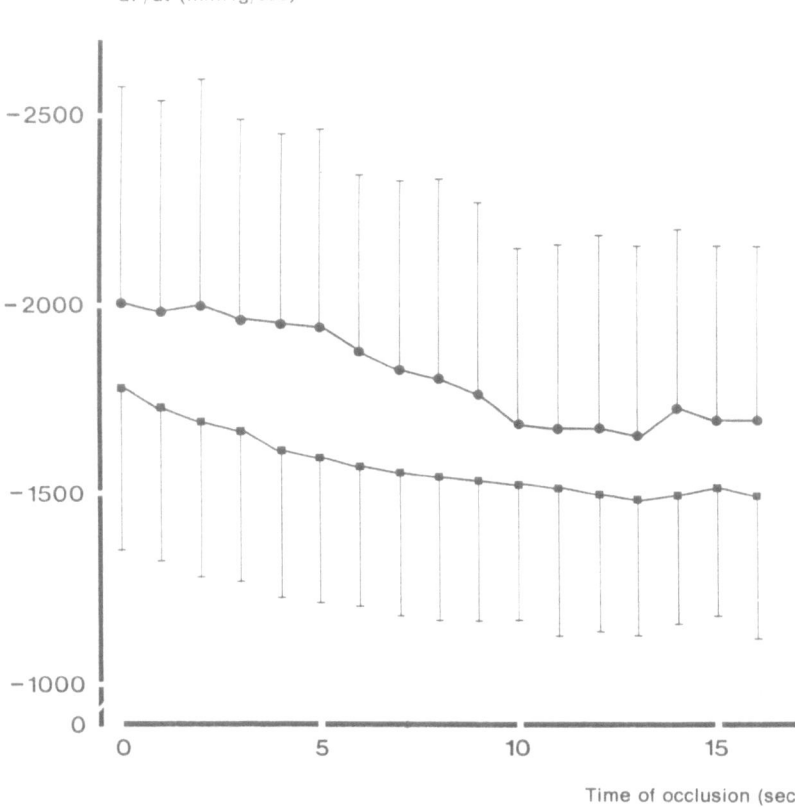

Figure 6. Evolution of the negative left ventricular dP/dt min during coronary occlusion before (●) and after (■) intra-coronary injection of 0.05 mg/kg of Diltiazem. Coronary occlusion induces within the first seconds a significant drop in min dP/dt which is maximal in the first 10 sec of occlusion. The occlusion following Diltiazem injection induces less of a drop and a flatter curve than control occlusion; after 12 sec of occlusion, however, the two curves have a similar slope; before the onset of occlusion at time 0, the initial values of min dP/dt are 10.1% less for the group pretreated with Diltiazem.

events are apparent for the evolution of LA a-wave during occlusion (see Fig. 12).

Discussion

At least three mechanisms are involved in myocardial protection with calcium antagonists:
1. Potent dilation of large conductance coronary arteries and of coronary

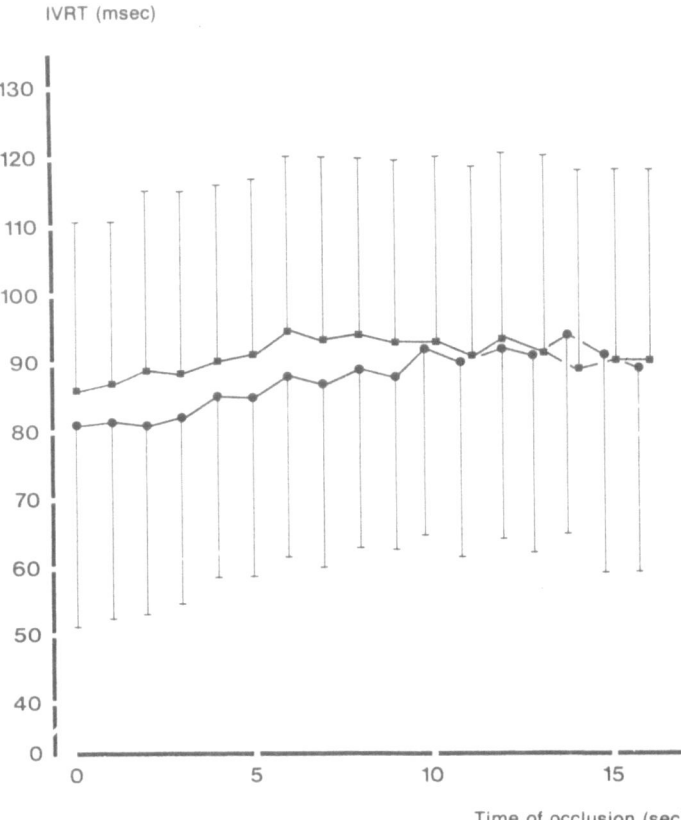

Figure 7. Evolution of Isovolumetric relaxation time (IVRT) in milliseconds during 16 seconds of coronary occlusion before (●) and after (■) intra-coronary injection of Diltiazem (0.05 mg/kg). Prior to occlusion at time 0, IVRT is 8.4% longer in patients pretreated with i.c. Diltiazem (p < 0.001). During coronary occlusion, IVRT increases as a consequence of impaired myocardial contractility, but increases less in patients pretreated with i.c. Diltiazem than in non treated patients. The two curves of values meet at 12 sec of occlusion.

collaterals, due to selective and specific inhibition of calcium influx into the smooth muscle cells of coronary arteries; this has been demonstrated in man [14–16], on normal prestenotic and poststenotic segments of large coronary arteries [17–19], and on collateral coronary arteries [4, 20–27]. The effect seems to be dose dependant [16, 19] and induced by calcium antagonists injected intravenously [14, 4] as well as into the coronary arteries. Effects on collaterals has been shown to favour a beneficial redistribution of subendocardial blood flow (increased endocardium/epicardial ratio) [21, 20, 28, 29], and allows a decrease in myocardial oxygen consumption, an increased blood flow

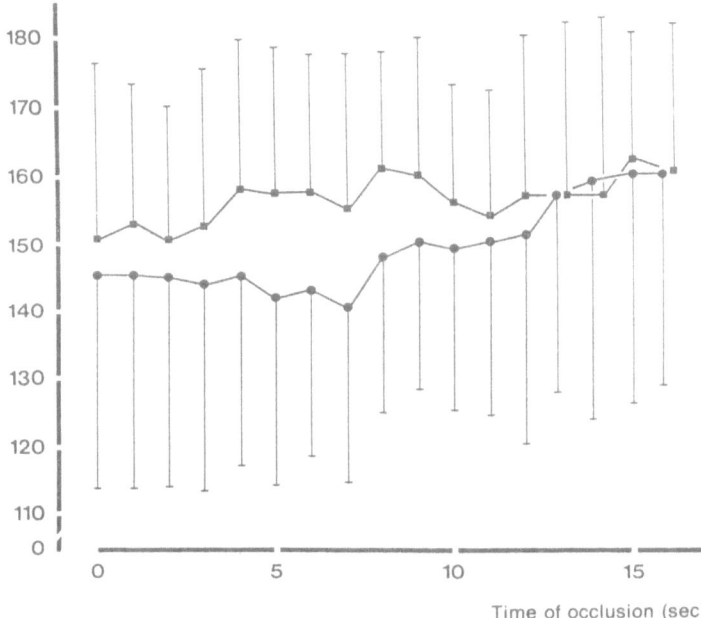

Figure 8. The effects of coronary occlusion on total relaxation time (TRT) before (●) and after (■) intra-coronary Diltiazem injection (0.05 mg/kg) are similar to the ones described for IVRT. At time 0, TRT is 6.7% longer (p < 0.001) after i.c. Diltiazem injection but increases less during coronary occlusion than during control occlusion. After 13 sec of occlusion, the two curves of values meet.

at the perimeter of transmurally ischemic myocardium [18, 20, 30], improved function of ischemic myocardium [21–23] and a reduction of myocardial infarction size in man and animal [4, 31, 20].

2. A peripheral vasodilating effect, when used i.v. or per os, inducing a drop in afterload and blood pressure [14, 31, 32, 1].

3. A cardioplegic effect: organic calcium channel blockers can produce a selective blockade of the slow inward current of calcium ions into the myocardial cells [33]. In consequence less calcium will be available to interact with troponin, and therefore muscular contraction will be inhibited; this defines the cardioplegic effect of calcium channel blockers.

Electromechanical uncoupling will prevent depletion in ATP stores of myocardial cells. It has been shown that myocardial ischemia is characterized by a reduction of myocardial ATP stores, which raises myoplasmic calcium; this triggers a vicious cycle by further depleting ATP stores, as calcium will interfere with the cell's capacity to generate ATP. This mechanism appears to be responsible at least in part for the death of ischemic cells [1]. Therefore electromechanical uncoupling by calcium blockers might be beneficial to the ischemic myocardial

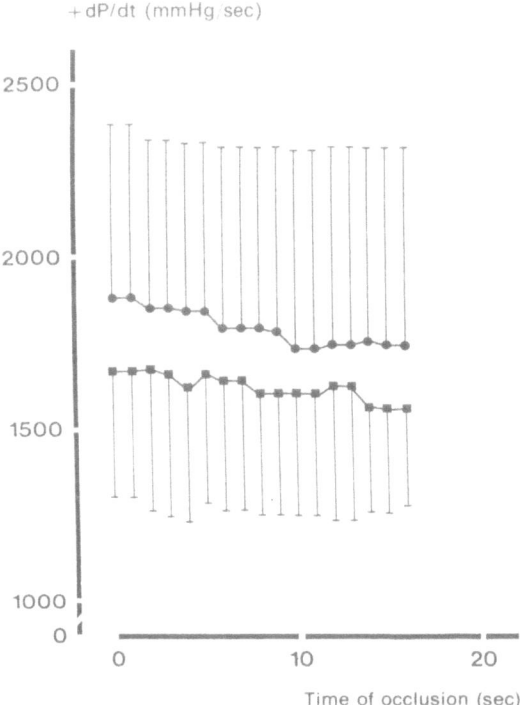

Figure 9. The effects of coronary occlusion before (●) and after (■) intra-coronary injection of 0.05 mg/kg of Diltiazem are similar to the ones described for min dP/dt (Fig. 6), although less pronounced.

cell. It has been demonstrated [9] that 1 hr of severe ischemia induces a four-fold rise in mitochondrial calcium which was concomittent with ischemic ventricular contracture and an elevated ventricular diastolic pressure; administration of Nifedipine prevented ischemic contracture and permitted recovery of myocardial relaxation and contraction; these effects were associated with a marked reduction of the accumulation of calcium in the mitochondria. In vitro experiments, in which reflex activity does not occur, show that all calcium channels blockers exert a dose-dependent inhibition of myocardial contractility that can be reversed by increasing the extracellular calcium concentration [34]; on a weight basis, relative potency of this direct negative inotropic effect is in descending order Nifedipine, Verapamil, Diltiazem and Perhexilline [5]. In vivo studies in man and animal have also demonstrated a cardioplegic, direct negative inotropic effect [40, 4, 17, 35], represented by decreased pos and neg dP/dt [4, 15, 35, 17], increased time constant of isovolumic pressure decay (T) [35, 15, 17], decreased mean wall velocity [17] and maximal velocity of shortening (V max) [4]. Serruys et al have demonstrated depressed, delayed and prolonged segmental

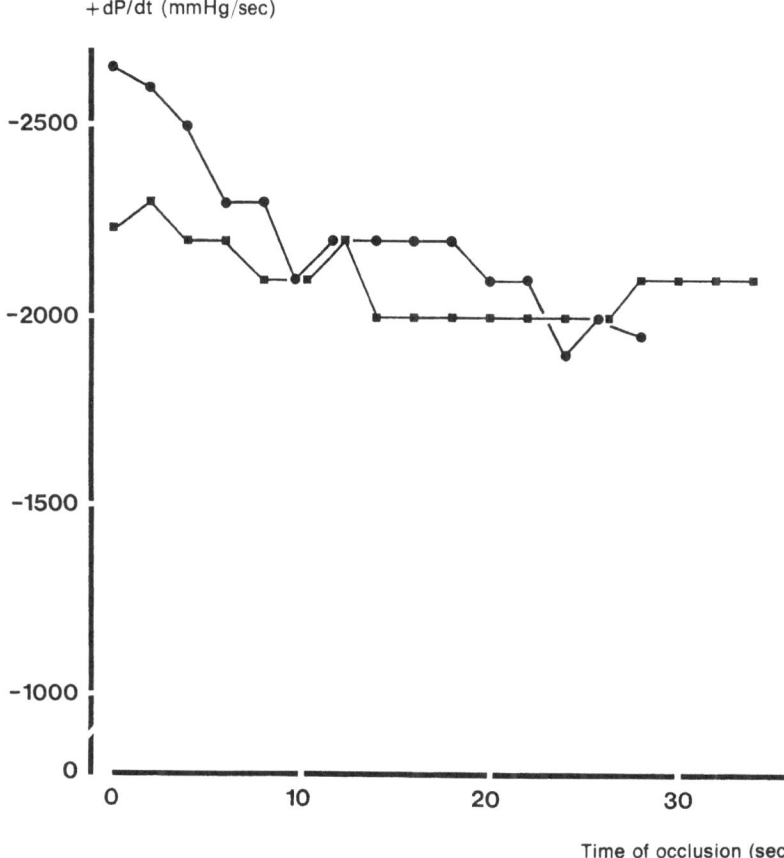

Figure 10. Evolution of pos dP/dt (mmHg/sec) during LAD occlusion before (●) and after (■) i.c. Diltiazem 0.05 mg/kg injection in one patient. During occlusion, pos dP/dt drops as a consequence of impaired myocardial contractility. When the occlusion is prolonged to 30 sec, pos dP/dt continues to drop, but the drop is far less pronounced when the myocardium is pretreated selectively with i.c. Diltiazem (0.05 mg/kg).

contraction and relaxation of the ventricular wall after intra-coronary Nifedipine injection in normal human hearts [17]. Several groups [17, 15] have noted that systolic and diastolic function are depressed by intra-coronary Nifedipine in humans, while coronary sinus blood flow was augmented through the vasodilating effect on coronary arteries of intra-coronary Nifedipine: interestingly coronary sinus blood flow remained increased long after changes in left ventricular function has subsided. These temporal differences are consistent with a differential depressant effect of Nifedipine on calcium uptake in smooth muscle and cardiac muscle. Associated with a negative inotropic effect of calcium channel blockers is a dose-dependent decrease in myocardial oxygen consumption [4, 17, 22, 23, 36], which allowed favourable use of aerobic pathways and near

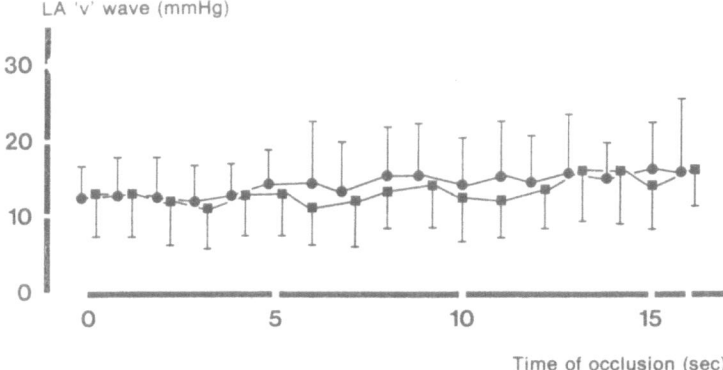

Figure 11. Progression of left atrium v-wave maximal pressure in mmHg during coronary occlusion in seconds before (●) and after (■) i.c. Diltiazem injection (0.05 mg/kg). Coronary occlusion induces a rise in LA v-wave pressure, most importantly after 10 sec of occlusion. Between the 5th and 13th sec, LA v-wave pressure increases less during the occlusion following i.c. Diltiazem injection.

suppression of lactate production by ischemic myocardial cells. In clinical use of calcium antagonists, such as for classic angina, Prinzmetal angina or hypertension, peripheral arterial vasodilatation will induce a baroreceptor mediated reflex positive inotropic response and tachycardia, which will offset their direct negative inotropic effect [36, 17]. However, clinical situations such as PTCA allow selective intra-coronary application of calcium channel blockers and provide means of not only treating coronary artery disease, but also of studying during exactly timed coronary occlusion the effect of ischemia on left ventricular performance. Ischemia has been studied extensively in dogs during coronary occlusion [37, 40, 47]. In the rat, substantial myocardial ATP decrease has been shown to occur before the onset of myocardial contraction failure [12]. In humans, however, the study of myocardial ischemia is rather complex since coronary occlusion similar to the dog model could not be applied until recently. Up to now, ischemia had to be generated by increase of myocardial oxygen consumption with pacing or dynamic exercise [41, 43], or cathecholamines [46], thus rendering fixed coronary artery stenoses sufficiently important to produce ischemia. Provocative testing has provided a large amount of knowledge on ischemia. It is evident however, that slight and intermediate cases of myocardial ischemia escaped from observation, and it had not been possible to study the sequence of events in the development of myocardial ischemia. In severe ischemia during exercise, left ventricular ejection fraction decreases significantly [43], left ventricular end- diastolic pressure is augmented together with pulmonary artery pressure and pulmonary capillary wedge pressure; more recently, diastolic changes have also been recognized during ischemia [37, 47, 50].

Our first observations of impaired myocardial activity during localized ischemia induced by PTCA date back to 1981, when we observed a rapid fall of

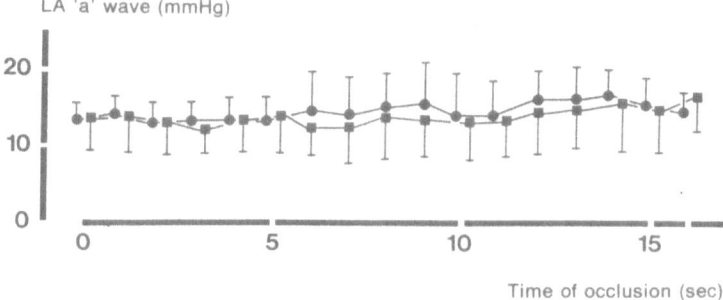

Figure 12. The effects of coronary occlusion on LA-a wave pressure before (●) and after (■) i.c. Diltiazem injection (0.05 mg/kg) are similar to what was described for LA-v wave (Fig. 11), although less marked.

positive and negative dP/dt during the first seconds of coronary artery occlusion at the time of angioplasty [6]. We were struck by the observation that the negative dP/dt was the first parameter to change during coronary artery occlusion followed after few seconds by a drop of the dP/dt max. Thus it seemed that myocardial diastole is more sensitive to ischemia than systole. We therefore have continued to study different parameters of myocardial performance during short intermittent coronary occlusion at the time of angioplasty e.g. systolic performance as well as the global pump function [6, 51, 53]. Echocardiography has not been found to be sufficiently reproducable in this experimental setting. Radioisotope tests do not provide sufficient accuracy in delimitating small segmental wall motion changes. We therefore used biplan left ventricular angiography to study systolic events during ischemia [6, 52]. It became evident that systolic wall motion diminishes rapidly during acute coronary occlusion, thus depressing left ventricular ejection fraction after some 7 sec of interruption of the left anterior descending coronary artery flow. This phenomenon is preceeded by diastolic abnormalities however [6].

Relaxation of the heart represents a change in the material properties of the myocardium and means the return to its initial presystolic length and tension. Relaxation is an energy dependent process. It is modulated by the myocardium's prevailing load (forces affecting myocardial fiber length), deactivation (decay of active force generating capacity), and the regional and temporal non-uniform distribution of the mentioned load and deactivation [49, 50, 57]. The exact quantification process of myocardial relaxation is difficult [49, 55]. The peak negative dP/dt is influenced by heart rate, systolic pressure, endsystolic volume and other factors. The time constant T of the left ventricular pressure fall during isovolumic relaxation seems relatively independent of other determinents of cardiac performance and has been proposed as an index of left ventricular relaxation. This parameter, however, has been criticized, since it constitutes a mere mathematic approximation of the pressure decay which is now considered to be a complex function of time, sometimes influenced in the opposite way, even by minor alterations of different factors [56]. It has been suggested that, in the diseased heart, as in experimental ischemia, left ventricular pressure fall during the isovolumic relaxation period looses its exponential nature [47, 56].

None of the as yet above described parameters provides a true description of the left ventricular relaxation process. In this study, we have used left ventricular isovolumic relaxation time, as well as the time from the beginning of relaxation to the lowest point of left ventricular pressure (which we called total relaxation time), the height of the a-wave and v-wave, and the maximal speed of left ventricular pressure drop during diastole (neg dP/dt). Beat-to-beat analysis of myocardial function rendered ischemic via PTCA confirmed previous observations; neg dP/dt drops earlier and faster than pos dP/dt during ischemia, ventricular relaxation being more sensitive to ischemia than contraction. Striking is the early appearance of a notch in the ascending portion of the neg dP/dt curve, probably due to inhomogeneous and asynchronous relaxation of the locally ischemic myocardium, which levels out after about 20 sec of ischemia, when the myocardium becomes totally anoxic and therefore stiff. Simultaneously, modifications of the left ventricular pressure curve shows disappearance of the rapid systolic filling wave-causing a 'hamac' appearance of the left ventricular diastolic pressure curve, which coincides with the prolongation of our measured relaxation parameters IVRT and TRT. Left ventricular filling pressure and left atrial pressures increase within 20 sec of ischemia, and can easily double or triple in value during ischemia, but this occurs later than any of the dramatic relaxation disturbance described above.

Even if one admits that none of these parameters nor the sum of all the different parameters studied represents true left ventricular relaxation, it is legitimate to compare the left ventricular relaxation behaviour before and after application of calcium antagonists. By injecting Diltiazem super-selectively in coronary arteries beyond the stenosis to be dilated during PTCA, we were providing selective and direct effect of this *calcium antagonist*, and could monitor its cardioplegic effect Diltiazem injection induced a significant change in all relaxation parameters, in particular a drop in neg dP/dt, a prolongation of IVRT and TRT, and a 'hamac' appearance of the left ventricular diastolic pressure curve. These observations are identical to the ones we described during myocardial ischemia induced by in coronary occlusion.

After Diltiazem, within 15 sec of occlusion, relaxation and contraction parameters and the left ventricular pressure curve configuration do not behave as during control coronary occlusion: there is no notch in the neg or pos dP/dt curves therefore no evidence of ischemic asynchronous relaxation or contraction; during coronary occlusion after Diltiazem pretreatment the left ventricular pressure curve configuration remains almost unchanged. In other words the cardioplegic effect observed after intra-coronary Diltiazem injection seems to modify the initial period of occlusion induced ischemia.

Ischemic changes in patients treated with intra-coronary Diltiazem prior to PTCA seem to be less pronounced during the observation period as compared with the non-treated patients. In particular, the duration of isovolumic relaxation and of total relaxation depicts a tendency towards normality during PTCA following application of the calcium antagonist. However, this tendency towards normal behaviour was not maintained longer than some 15 sec. One can possibly explain this phenomenon by the fact that ischemia reaches an end point after some 15 sec of total coronary occlusion, where the myocardium becomes stiff and its material properties would not seem to change any further, no matter what treatment had been installed beforehand. It appears as if only the transition period from the normal performance until the development of total anoxia is susceptible to be altered with calcium channel blockers, and that this critical period lasts only 15 sec in the case of total coronary artery occlusion. In contrast to what used to be believed, myocardial failure occurs before the appearance of angina [6]. The appearance of angina pectoris can further be delayed after intra-coronary injection of very small amounts of calcium antagonists [58]. The latter observation points towards a mechanism which is not entirely dependent on pure diminution of myocardial oxygen demand, since the amplitude of changes after treatment with calcium channel blockers is larger than could be expected from pure oxygen consumption reduction.

In conclusion, calcium antagonists injected into the coronary arteries in small enough amounts not to produce systemic effects may prolong the myocardial tolerance to ischemia during the time of coronary balloon occlusion. Whether it might be beneficial to locally treat the myocardium with a calcium antagonist immediately before PTCA needs to be demonstrated.

References

1. Braunwald E (1982) Mechanism of action of calcium-channel-blocking agents. N Eng 307 (26):1618–1628
2. De Boer LMV, Strauss HW, Kloner RA et al (1980) Autoradiographic method for measuring the ischemic myocardium at risk: Effects of Verapamil on infarct size after experimental coronary artery occlusion. *Proc Natl Acad Sci USA* 77:6119–6123
3. Bussman WD (1982) Use of vasodilators in acute myocardial infarction. *Proc Intern Symp on Limiting Infarct Size. Tagung der Deutschen Gezellshaft für Inners Medizin* 129 Abstract
4. Nakamura M, Kikuchi Y, Senda Y, Yamada A, Koiwaya Y (1980) Myocardial blood following experimental coronary occlusion: Effects of Diltiazem. *Chest* 78:1 (Suppl) 205–209
5. Serruys PW, Van den Brand M, Brower RW, Hugenholtz PG (1983) Regional cardioplegia and cardioprotection during transluminal angioplasty, which role for Nifedipine? *Eur Heart J* 4 (Suppl C): 115–121
6. Sigwart U, Grbic M, Payot M, Goy J-J, Essinger A, Fischer A (1984) Ischemic events during coronary artery balloon obstruction. In: *Silent Myocardial Ischemia*, pp 29–36 W Rutushauser and H Rostramm (eds) Berlin, Heidelberg, New-York, Tokyo: Springer Verlag
7. Tennant R, Wiggers CJ (1935) The effect of coronary occlusion on myocardial contraction. *Am J Physiol* 112:351–361
8. Sigwart U, Grbic M, Essinger A, Rivier J-L (1982) L'effet aigu d'une occlusion coronarienne lors de la dilatation transluminale. *Schweiz Med Schr* 1631:45 Abstract
9. Sigwart U, Grbic M, Essinger A, Fischer A, Morin D, Sadeghi H (1982) Myocardial function in man during acute coronary balloon occlusion. *Circulation* 66, Supp II–86 Abstract

10. Serruys PW, Van den Brand M, Mey S, De Ruiter R, Hugenholtz PP (1983) Left ventricular function, coronary blood flow and lactate metabolism during PTCA of the left anterior descending artery (LAD). In: *Transluminal angioplasty* (Toulouse) VIII–65

11. Bertrand ME, Lablanche JM, Tilmant PY, Thieuleux FA (1983) Left ventricular hemodynamic changes during percutaneous transluminal angioplasty (PTCA). In: *transluminal angioplasty* (Toulouse) C-20

12. Hearse DJ (1979) Oxygen deprivation and early myocardial contractile failure: a reassessment of the possible role of adenosine triphosphate. *Am J of Cardiol* 44:1115–1121

13. Clark RE, Ferguson TB, West PN, Sherchleib RC, Henry PD (1977) Pharmacological preservation of the ischemic heart. *Ann of Thoracic Surg* 24(4):307–314

14. Bourassa MG, Cote P, Theroux P, Tuban JF, Genain C, Waters DD (1980) Hemodynamics and coronary flow following Diltiazem administration in anesthetized dogs and in humans. *Chest* 78:1 Suppl: 224–230

15. Amende I, Simon R, Hood P Jr, Hetzer R, Lichtlen PR (1983) Intracoronary Nifedipine in human beings: magnitude and time course of changes in left ventricular contraction/relaxation and coronary sinus flow. *JACC* Vol 2(6):1141–1145

16. Bertrand ME, Dupuis BA, Lablanche JM, Timant PY, Thieuleux FA (1982) Coronary hemodynamics following intravenous or intracoronary injection of Diltiazem in man. *J Cardio-Vascular Pharm* 4(5):695–699

17. Serruys PW, Hooghoudt TEH, Reiber JHC, Slager C, Brower RW, Hugenholtz PG (1983) Influence of intracoronary Nifedipine on left ventricular function, coronary vasomotility, and myocardial oxygen consumption. *British Heart J* 49:427–441

18. Millard RW, Lathrop DA, Grapp G, Ashraf M, Grupp I, Schwartz A (1982) Differential cardio-vascular effects of calcium-channel blocking agents: Potential mechanisms. *Am J Cardiol* 49:499–505

19. Engle HJ, Lichtlen PR (1981) Beneficial enhancement of coronary blood flow by Nifedipine: Comparison with nitroglycerin and beta blocking agents. *Am J Med* 71:658–666

20. Warltier DC, Meils CM, Gross GJ, Brook HL (1981) Blood flow in normal and acutely ischemic myocardium after Verapamil, Diltiazem and Nisoldirine (Bay K 5552): A new dihydropyridine calcium antagonist. *J Pharmacol & experim Therap* 218(1):296–302

21. Clozel JP, Theroux P, Bourassa M (1983) Effects of Diltiazem on experimental myocardial ischemia and on left ventricular performance. *Circ Res* 52(Suppl I):I-120–128

22. Henry PD, Shuchleib R, Clark RE, Perez JE (1979) Effects of Nifedipine on myocardial ischemia: analysis of collateral flow, pulsatile heat and regional muscle shortening. *Am J Cardiol* 44:817–824

23. Henry PD, Shuchlieb R, Bordal LJ, Roberts R, Williamson JR, Sobel BE (1978) Effects of Nifedipine on myocardial perfusion and ischemic injury in dogs. *Cir Res* 43:372–380

24. Nakamura M, Kojwaya Y, Yamada A et al (1979) Effects of Diltiazem: A new antianginal drug on myocardial blood flow following experimental coronary occlusion. In: Winbury MM, Abiko Y (eds) *Ischemic Myocardium and Antianginal Drugs*, pp 129–142. New-York: Raven Press

25. Schmier J, Van Ackern K, Bruckner U (1975) Investigations on tachyphylaxis and collateral formation after Nifedipine whilst taking into consideration the direction of flow and the mortality rate due to infarction. In: Hashimoto K, Kimura E, Kobayashi T (eds) The First Nifedipine Symposium, pp 45–52. Tokyo: Tokyo Press

26. Van Ackern K, Braasch W, Bruckner UB, Heger W, Schmier J (1974) Development of coronary collaterals following oral long term therapy with Nifedipine: increased survival rate after experimental coronary occlusion. *Arzneim Forsch* 24:1577–1581

27. Da Luz PL, De Barros LFM, Leite JJ, Pileggi F, Decourt LV (1980) Effect of Verapamil on regional coronary and myocardial perfusion during acute coronary occlusion. *Am J Cardiol* 45:269–275

28. Zyvoloski MG, Brooks HL, Gross GJ, Warltier DC (1982) Myocardial perfusion distal to an acute or chronic coronary artery occlusion: effects of Diltiazem and Nifedipine. *J Pharm & Experim Therap* 222(2):494–500

29. Franklin D, Millard RW, Nagao T (1980) Responses to coronary collateral flow and dependent myocardial mechanical function to the calcium antagonist Diltiazem. *Chest* 78:1 Suppl 200–204
30. Millard RW (1980) Changes in cardiac mechanisms and coronary blood flow of regionally ischemic porcine myocardium induced by Diltiazem. *Chest* 78:193–199
31. Ferlintz J, Turbow ME (1980) Antianginal and myocardial metabolic properties of Verapamil in coronary artery disease. *Am J Cardiol* 46:1019–1026
32. Kaltenbach M, Schulz W, Kober J (1979) Effects of Nifedipine after intravenous and intracoronary administration. *Am J Cardiol* 44:832–838
33. Fleckenstein A (1977) Specific pharmacology of calcium in myocardium, cardiac pacemakers, and vascular smooth muscle. *Ann Rev Pharm Toxicol* 17:149–166
34. Stone PH, Antman EM, Muller JE, Braunwald E (1980) Calcium channel blocking agents in the treatment of cardiovascular disorders, Part II: Hemodynamic effects and clinical application. *Annals of Int Med* 93:886–904
35. Rousseau MF, Veriter C, Detry J-M, R, Brasseur L, Pouleur H (1980) Impaired early left ventricular relaxation in coronary artery disease: effects of intracoronary Nifedipine *Circulation* 62, 4:764–772
36. Vater W, Schlosmann K (1976) Effects of Nifedipine on the haemodynamics and oxygen consumption of the heart in animal experiments. In: Jatene AD, Lichtlen PR (eds) *The Third International Adalat Symposium*, pp 33–41. Amsterdam: Excerpta Medica
37. Smalling RW, Kelley KO, Kirkeeide RL, Gould KL (1983) Comparison of early systolic and early diastolic regional function during regional ischemia in a chronically instrumented canine model. *JACC* 2(2):263–269
38. Koiwa Y, Nunokawa T, Ishide N, Isoyama S, Kitao S, Tamaki K, Satoh S, Suzuki H, Shimizu Y, Kakuta Y, Ino-Oka E, Takishima T (1980) The effect of graded coronary flow reduction in the left anterior descending and septal arteries on left ventricular function in the canine heart. *Circulation* 62(4):745–755
39. Heyndrick GR, Millard RW, McRitchie RJ, Maroko PR, Vatner SF (1975) Regional myocardial functional and electrophysiological alterations after brief coronary artery occlusion in conscious dogs. *J Clin Investig* 56:978–985
40. Hess OM, Koch R, Bonnert C, Krayenbuehl HP (1980) Regional wall stiffness during acute myocardial ischemia in the canine left ventricle. *Eur Heart J* 1:435–443
41. Carroll JD, Hess OM, Hirzel HO, Krayenbuehl HP (1983) Dynamics of left ventricular filling at rest and during exercise. *Circulation* 68(1):59–67
42. Carroll JD, Hess OM, Hirzel HO, Krayenbuehl HP (1983) Exercise-induced ischemia: the influence of altered relaxation on early diastolic pressures. *Circulation* 67(3):521–528
43. Rutishauser W, Amende J, Mehmel H (1972) Comparison of left ventricular dynamics in normal and patients with ischemic heart disease at rest, during pacing and exercise. *Eur J Clin Investig* 2:304
44 Bahler RC, Martin P (1985) Effects of loading conditions and inotropic state on rapid filling phase of left ventricle. *Am Physiology Soc* H523–H533
45. McLaurin LP, Rolett EL, Grossman W (1973) Impaired left ventricular relaxation during pacing-induced ischemia. *Am J Cardiol* 32:751–757
46. Vatner SF, Millard RV, Patrick TA, Heymdrick FR (1976) Effect of Isoprorenol on regional myocardial function, electrocardiogram and blood flow in conscious dogs with myocardial ischemia. *J Clin Investig* 57:1261
47. Kumada T, Karliner JS, Pouleur H, Gallacher KP, Shirato K, Ross J, Jr (1979) Effects of coronary occlusion on early ventricular diastolic events in conscious dogs. *Am Physiological Soc* H542–H549
48. Van Houten FX, Serur JR, Borkenhagen DM, Adams DF, Abrams HL (1980) Experimental myocardial ischemia, IV: Shape and volume changes during 'isovolumetric relaxation' in normal and ischemic ventricles. *Circulation* 62(2):350–356
49. Brutsaert DL, Rademakers FE, Sys SU (1984) Triple control of relaxation: implications in cardiac disease. *Circulation* 69(1):190–196

50. Brutsaert DL, Rademakers FE, Sys SU, Gillebert TC, Housmans PR (1985) Ventricular relaxation. In: Levine HJ, Gaasch WH (eds) *The Ventricle. Basic and Clinical Aspects.* Dordrecht – Boston – Lancaster: Martinus Nijhoff Publishers

51. Gibson DG, Prewitt TA, Brown DJ (1976) Analysis of left ventricular wall movement during isovolumic relaxation and its relation to coronary artery disease. *British Heart J* 38:1010–1019

52. Grbic M, Sigwart U (1986) Left ventricular filling during acute ischemia. In: PW Serruys, GT Meester (eds) *Coronary angioplasty: A controlled model for ischemia*, pp 141–149. Dordrecht – Boston – Lancaster: Martinus Nijhoff Publishers (DICM 58); reprinted in this volume, Chapter 13, pp 167–174

53. Shimizu G, Zile MR, Blaustein AS, Gaasch WH (1985) Left ventricular chamber filling and midwall fiber lengthening in patients with left ventricular hypertrophy: Overestimation of fiber velocities by conventional midwall measurements (echography), *Circulation* 71(2):266–272

54. Gruntzig AR, Senning A, Siegenthaler WE (1979) Nonoperative dilatation of coronary artery stenosis: percutaneous transluminal coronary angioplasty. *N Eng J Med* 301(2):61–68

55. Mirsky I (1984) Assessment of diastolic function: suggested methods and future considerations. *Circulation* 69(4):836–841

56. Katayama K, Kumada T, Fujii T, Moritani K, Miura T, Toma Y, Kohno M, Yoshino F, Ogawa H, Ozaki M, Matsuzaki M, Matsuda Y, Kusukawa R (1984) Clinical characteristics of left ventricular pressure decline during isovolumic relaxation in normal and diseased hearts. *Am Heart J* 332–338

57. Gaasch WH, Apstein CS, Levine HJ (1983) Diastolic properties of the left ventricle

58. Sekoranja L, Grbic M, Halpern M, Sigwart U (1985) Effect of Verapamil on the ischemic myocardium. *In:* Hypertension – the next decade; Verapamil in focus. Fleckenstein A, Laragh JH (eds)

21. Influence of anti-ischemic drug treatment on the ischemic response to acute coronary occlusion in man

RÜDIGER SIMON, GUNHILD HERRMANN, IVO AMENDE, GERT H. REIL and PAUL R. LICHTLEN

Introduction

Percutaneous transluminal coronary angioplasty offers a unique opportunity to study the human cardiac response to acute ischemia in conscious man. Numerous studies have confirmed a typical sequence of events following the abrupt total occlusion of a major coronary artery. Blood flow in the dependent myocardial area drops within 10 to 15 sec to a level that is defined by the presence or absence of collaterals [1, 2, 3]. This is associated with a very early impairment in the regional myocardial action potential (see Rickards et al this volume) and in ventricular relaxation, followed by a depression of systolic contractility, a progressive increase in left ventricular filling pressure, typical alterations in the surface electrocardiogram and finally angina pectoris [4]. Despite a long-standing use of antianginal and anti-ischemic drug treatment, it is not completely understood by which mechanisms and to which extent these drugs interfere with the chain of events in the situation of acute coronary occlusion. The present article summarizes some of the results that we have gained over the last years on the effects of nitrates and calciumantagonists on hemodynamics and angiographic parameters of left ventricular function during balloon occlusion of major coronary arteries in patients undergoing coronary angioplasty.

Patients and methods

In total 155 patients aged 31 to 70 yrs have been included in a series of studies, the results of which are presented in this article. All patients underwent balloon dilatation of a proximal stenosis in the left anterior descending coronary artery (LAD). Standard lead ECG (lead I or avF), the epicardial i.e. intracoronary ECG in the LAD area (from the guide wire), aortic and pulmonary pressures were recorded continuously throughout the procedure. To determine left ventricular volumes, pump function, and regional contraction, digital angiography was performed before and after drug administration in subgroups of patients.

P.W. Serruys, R. Simon & K.J. Beatt (eds), Percutaneous Transluminal Coronary Angioplasty. ISBN 0-7923-0346-6.
© *1990 Kluwer Academic Publishers, Dordrecht*

Thirty-five ml of a non-ionic contrast agent (Ultravist[R] 370) were injected into the pulmonary artery via an especially designed balloon-tipped catheter, and angiograms were recorded on a digital disk at a frame rate of 25/sec, using a matrix of 512 times 512 pixel and a grey resolution of 8 bit. To obtain an optimal contrast, these raw angiograms were processed by R-wave-gated cyclic mask mode subtraction (ADAC 4100). A typical result is demonstrated in Fig. 1. Left ventricular borders were then outlined in the video frame and volumes were calculated according to the area-length-method. Local contraction was assessed in 5 left ventricular regions (Fig. 3) by superimposing the centre of gravity in end-diastole and end-systole and applying a radial method of analysis similar to the technique described previously [6, 7].

For statistical analysis, students paired and unpaired T-test was applied and p-value of < 0.05 was considered to be significant.

Results

Typical examples of hemodynamics and left ventricular silhouettes before and during balloon occlusion of the proximal LAD are given in Figs 2 and 3. At the end of a 60 sec lasting balloon inflation period, pulmonary wedge pressure was increased markedly and there were signs of transmural ischemia in the epicardial

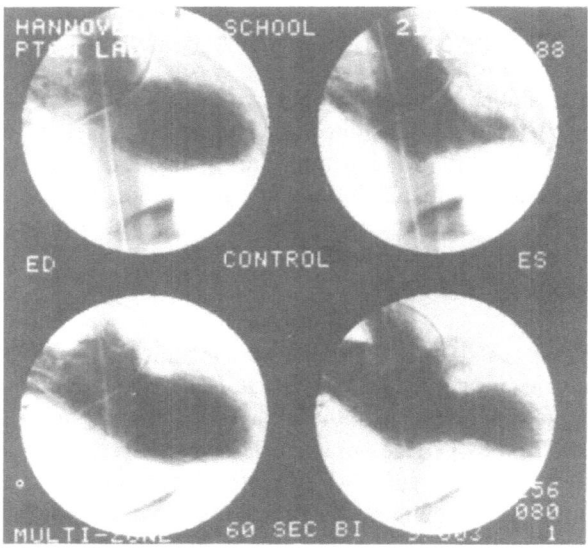

Figure 1. Digital subtraction angiograms of the left ventricle before (control upper part) and at the end of a 60 sec lasting balloon occlusion (60 sec BI, lower part) of the proximal LAD. ED = end-diastole; ES = end-systole.

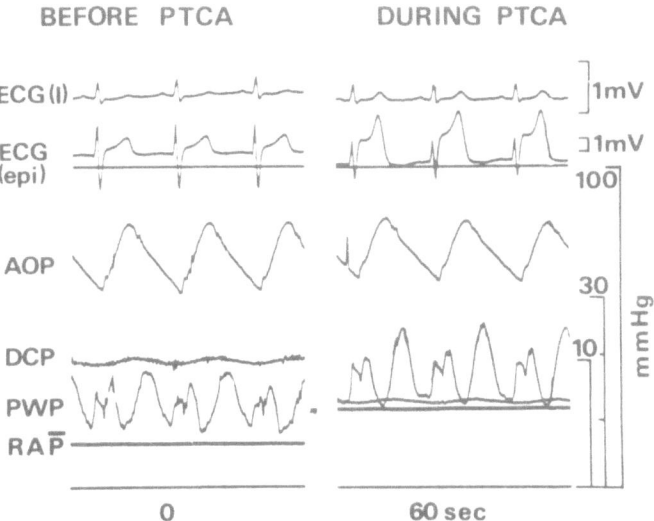

Figure 2. Hemodynamics before (left side) and at the end of a 60 sec lasting period of balloon inflation in the proximal LAD (right side).
ECG (I) = lead I; ECG (epi) = epicardial (intracoronary) ECG recorded from guide wire; AOP = aortic pressure (guiding catheter); DCP = distal coronary pressure (balloon catheter); PWP = pulmonary wedge pressure; RAP = mean right atrial pressure.

ECG, whereas the aortic pressure remained unchanged (Fig. 2). This was associated with a profound anterior and apical hypokinesis of the left ventricle in the digital angiogram (Fig. 3).

Nitroglycerin, hemodynamics and electrocardiogram

In 21 patients the effect of intracoronary nitroglycerin on hemodynamic parameters of ischemia was investigated. In order to avoid a possible interference with the impact of balloon dilatation itself on potential ischemia before dilatation, two subsequent balloon inflations were performed each lasting 1 min, before the study was started. Then, 0.2 mg nitroglycerin were injected into the distal LAD via the balloon catheter and 1 min later a third balloon inflation took place. Figure 4 summarizes the effects on pulmonary wedge pressure as an equivalent of left ventricular filling pressure. Nitroglycerin given ic. reduced wedge pressure before as well as during a 60 sec period of balloon occlusion of the LAD significantly.

In a subsequent study on 119 patients, the same protocol was followed, but patients were randomly allocated to 0.2 mg nitroglycerin given directly into the distal LAD or as an intravenous bolus into the left femoral vein. In this study, both intracoronary and intravenous nitroglycerin decreased pulmonary wedge

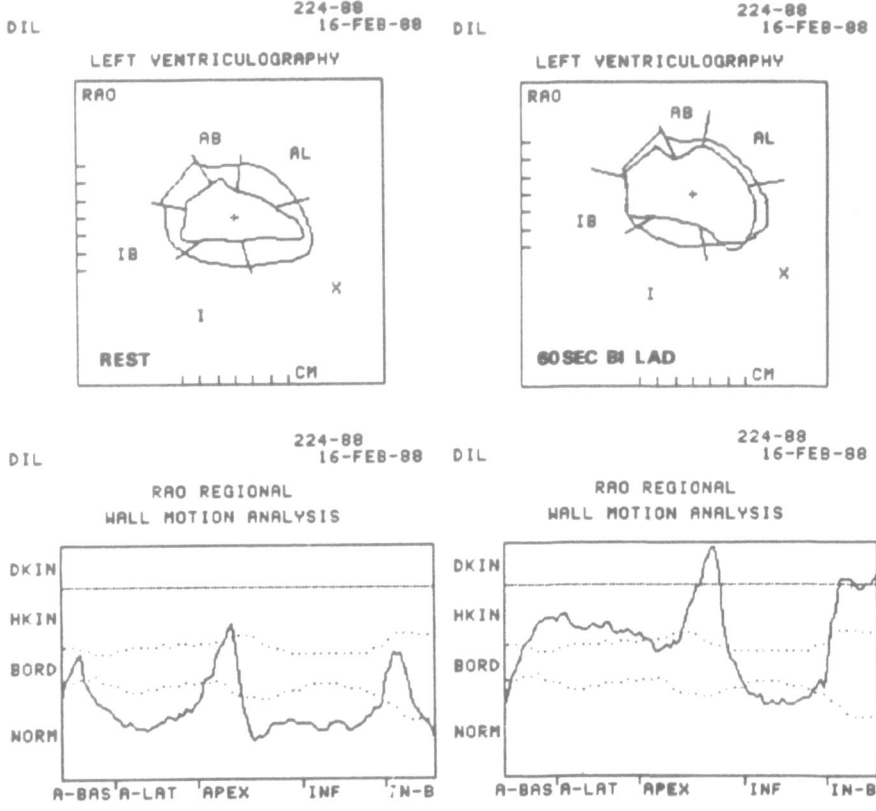

Figure 3. *Upper part:* left ventricular silhouettes in end-diastole and end-systole, traced from digital angiograms and superimposed by the computer program. Note a marked contraction abnormality in the anterior wall and apex at 60 sec balloon inflation time.

Lower part: regional analysis of systolic wall motion (normal range between dotted lines).

pressure and right atrial pressure to a similar extent in the control state before balloon inflation as well as during LAD occlusion by the inflated balloon (Fig. 5). This was associated with a comparable drop in mean aortic pressure by about 5 mmHg one minute after drug administration by either route (Table 1). These results indicate a significant systemic action of intravenous as well as intracoronary nitroglycerin, leading to a decrease in both left and right ventricular preload. There were also significant effects on the ECG during balloon occlusion (Table 2). The average time interval from balloon inflation to the appearance of ST-changes of >0.1 mV in the ECG was prolonged by intracoronary as well as intravenous nitroglycerin to a similar degree.

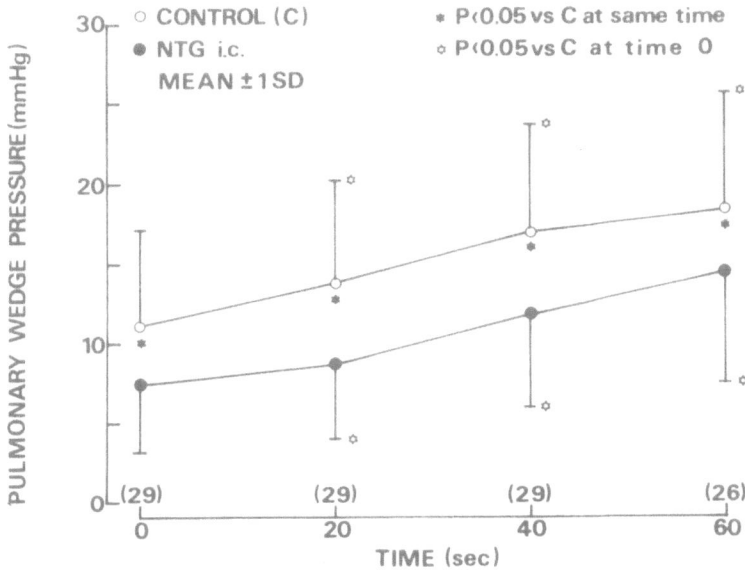

Figure 4. Effect of intracoronary nitroglycerin (0.2 mg) on pulmonary wedge pressure during 60 sec balloon occlusion of the proximal LAD in 29 patients.

Calciumantagonists, hemodynamics and electrocardiogram

The dihydropyridine-type calciumantagonist nifedipine was investigated in 22 patients. After two balloon inflations, each of 60 sec duration, 0.1 mg nifedipine were injected into the distal LAD via the balloon catheter and 2 subsequent balloon inflations were performed starting 2 and 4 min after drug administration. An example of hemodynamics before and 2 min after intracoronary nifedipine is demonstrated in Fig. 6. Figure 7 summarizes the effects on aortic pressure and pulmonary wedge pressure in the entire study group. Neither balloon inflation nor intracoronary nifedipine exerted any significant effect on mean aortic pressure. Pulmonary wedge pressure was comparable at the end of 60 sec balloon occlusions of the LAD before as well as 2 and 4 min after intracoronary nifedipine. It is noteworthy, however, that 2 min after nifedipine wedge pressure before balloon inflation was slightly but significantly elevated when compared to the control value (see Fig. 7), presumably due to the negative inotropic direct action of the drug on the dependent myocardium. Thus, the relative increase to the final wedge pressure at the end of the balloon inflation period was slightly reduced 2 min after drug administration, but this small effect had disappeared at 4 min.

In a group of 7 patients, the same protocol was followed but, 0.1 mg nifedipine were injected as a bolus intravenously. In these patients no effect was detected on

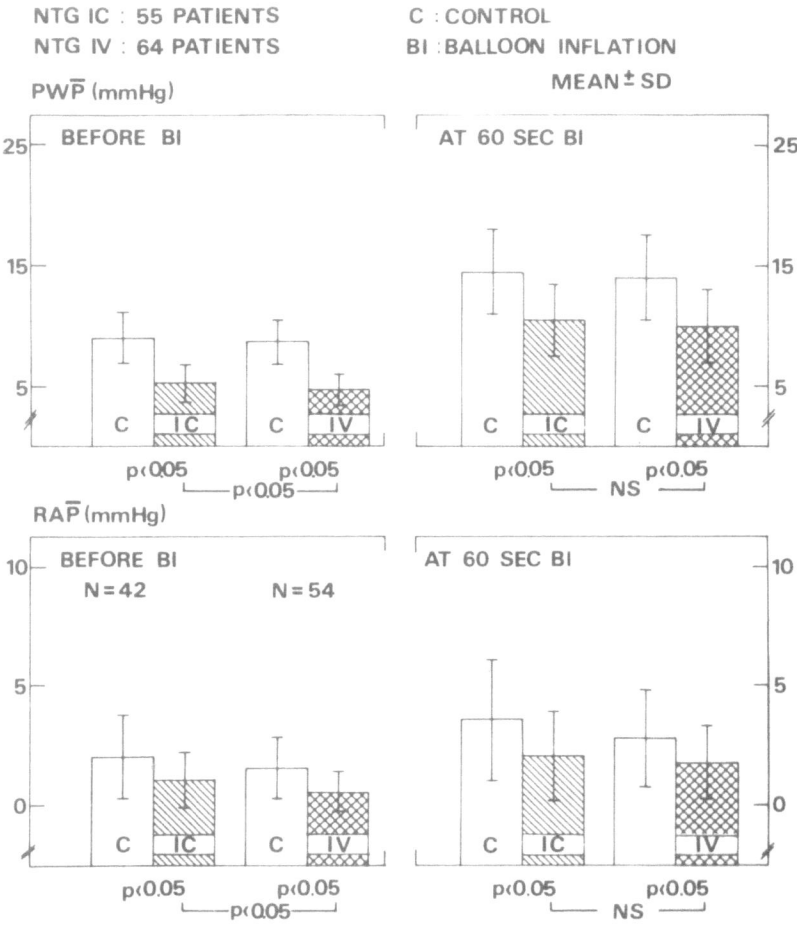

Figure 5. Effect of nitroglycerin on mean pulmonary wedge pressure (PWP) and mean right atrial pressure (RAP) before and during balloon inflation in the proximal LAD.
Left side: effects in the control state before (c) and 1 minute after 0.1 mg intracoronary (ic) or intravenous (iv) nitroglycerin.
Right side: pressures at the end of a 60 sec lasting occlusion of the LAD due to balloon inflation before (c) and after intracoronary or intravenous nitroglycerin.
Mean values ± SD

hemodynamics as well as on the electrocardiograms 2 and 4 min after drug administration as well as during balloon occlusion of the LAD when compared to the same balloon inflation period before nifedipine.

It is of interest, that despite the minor changes in hemodynamics, electrocardiographic signs of ischemia were influenced significantly by intracoronary

Table 1. Intracoronary and intravenous nitroglycerin in PTCA

			Control	60 sec BI	60 sec after NTG	NTG + 60 sec BI
NTG ic						
	HR	(bpm)	84 ± 13	84 ± 13	88 ± 13*	84 ± 13
	AOP	(mmHg)	80 ± 13	78 ± 15	76 ± 13*	77 ± 15
NTG iv						
	HR	(bpm)	86 ± 14	86 ± 15	92 ± 14*	87 ± 15
	AOP	(mmHg)	82 ± 17	83 ± 17	78 ± 14*	80 ± 15**

ic = intracoronary; iv = intravenous; HR = heartrate (beats per min); AOP = mean aortic pressure (mmHg); control = before balloon inflation; 60 sec BI = at 60 sec balloon inflation time.
Mean values ± SD; *p < 0.05 vs control; **p < 0.05 vs 60 sec BI.

Table 2. Nitroglycerin, calcium-antagonists and time to ST-changes during PTCA

Drug tested	n (pat.)	ECG lead	Time before drug (sec)	Time after drug (sec)	p
NTG ic	53	I/avl	26 ± 14	34 ± 15	< 0.05
NTG iv	57	I/avl	22 ± 10	28 ± 13	< 0.05
NIF ic	22	epi	12 ± 4	17 ± 8	< 0.05
NIS ic	14	epi	12 ± 5	21 ± 10	< 0.05

NTG = nitroglycerin (0.2 mg); NIF = nifedipine (0.1 mg); NIS = nisoldipine (0.05 mg); ic = intracoronary; iv = intravenous; epi = epicardial (intracoronary) nECG.

nifedipine (see also Fig. 6). In those patients who exhibited ST-elevations during balloon inflation, the appearance of these ST-changes were delayed from 15 to 31 sec 2 min after nifedipine (p < 0.05). In another study on 14 patients with the dihydropyridine-type calciumantagonist nisoldipine, a similar effect on electrocardiographic parameters of ischemia were observed (Table 2).

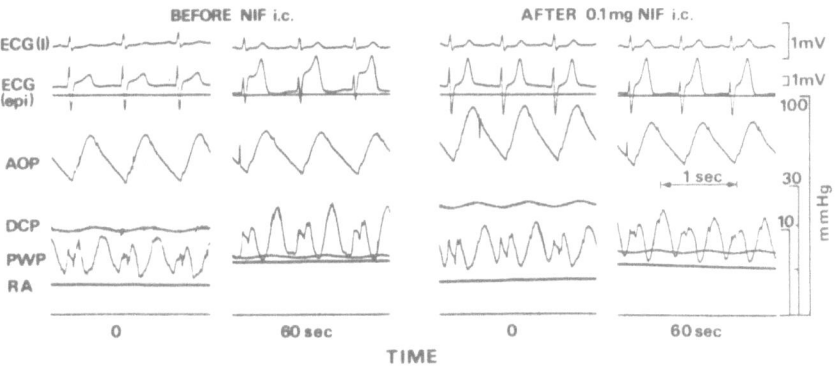

Figure 6. Hemodynamics before (0) and at 60 sec balloon inflation time in the proximal LAD (60 sec) before (left side) and 2 min after 0.1 mg intracoronary nifedipine (right side). Abbreviations as in Fig. 2.

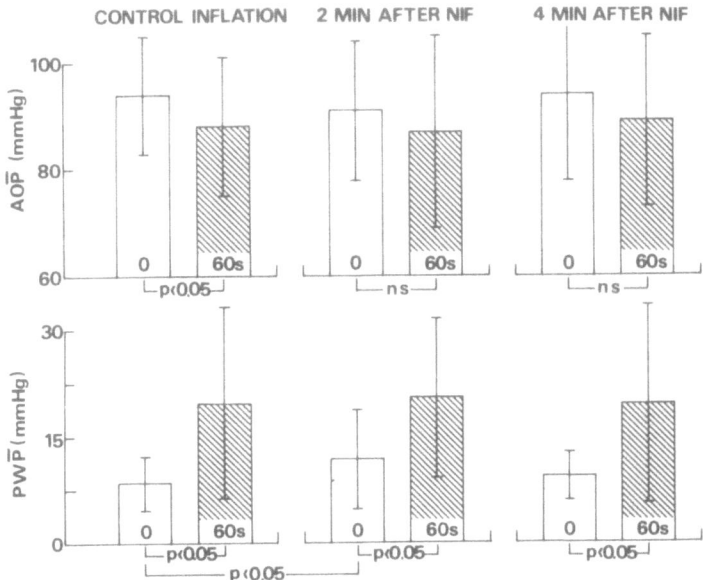

Figure 7. Effect of intracoronary nifedipine on mean aortic and pulmonary wedge pressure in 22 patients.
0 = before inflation; 60 s = at 60 sec balloon inflation.
Mean values ± SD

Digital angiograms

The effects of intracoronary nitroglycerin on left ventricular volumes, ejection fraction and regional wall motion were investigated in 6 patients undergoing dilatation of LAD obstructions (Fig. 8). Digital angiograms were obtained in the control state before dilatation, at the end of a 60 sec lasting second balloon occlusion of the proximal LAD (60 sec BI), and at the end of a third balloon inflation of equal length that started 1 minute after nitroglycerin administration. The acute occlusion of the LAD by the balloon caused a significant increase in end-systolic volume of the left ventricle associated with a drop in ejection fraction, that was due to development of hypokinesia or akinesia in the anterior and apical regions. Intracoronary nitroglycerin almost normalized end-systolic volume and in part reversed the drop in ejection fraction. Interestingly this effect was due to an enhanced contraction of the contralateral inferior wall rather than an improvement in the ischemic anterior and apical regions.

Nisoldipine was used to investigate the effects of dihydropyridine-type calciumantagonists on ventricular pump function in another 7 patients. Digital angiography was performed before and at the end of a 60 sec lasting occlusion period of the LAD. Then, 0.05 mg nisoldipine were injected directly in the left coronary artery and a third digital angiogram was stored at the end of another

6 PTS, MEAN ± SD (←: p < 0.05)

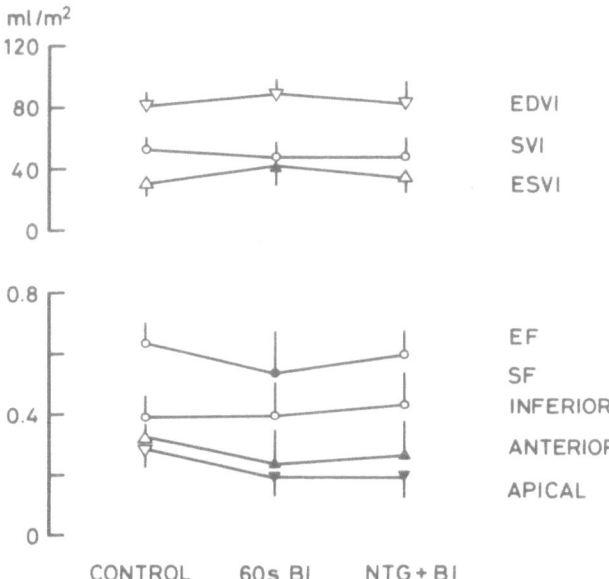

Figure 8. Effect of intracoronary nitroglycerin (0.2 mg) on left ventricular volumes and regional systolic shortening fraction (SF) in the inferior, anterior, and apical area during balloon inflation in the proximal LAD.
Control = before balloon inflation; 60 s BI = at the end of a 60 sec lasting balloon inflation period before NTG; NTG + BI = at 60 sec balloon inflation time, 2 min after nitroglycerin administration; EDVI, ESVI, SVI = end-diastolic, end-systolic, stroke volume indices; EF = ejection fraction.

60 sec lasting balloon inflation that was started 2 min after drug administration. In contrast to nitroglycerin, nisoldipine did not reverse the ischemia-induced changes in end-systolic volume and in ejection fraction in these patients (Fig. 9) and regional wall motion equally remained unaltered in the anterior as well as in the inferior regions of the left ventricle.

Discussion

Nitrates and calciumantagonists are widely used in the treatment of coronary disease. In coronary angioplasty, these drugs are often administrated directly into the coronary arteries in an attempt to prevent ischemia during balloon inflation. In the past, the salutary effects of nitrates have been attributed primarily to peripheral vasodilation and venous pooling that is associated with ventricular unloading and a decrease in myocardial oxygen demand [8, 12]. More recently, a direct dilatory effect on eccentric coronary artery obstructions has been

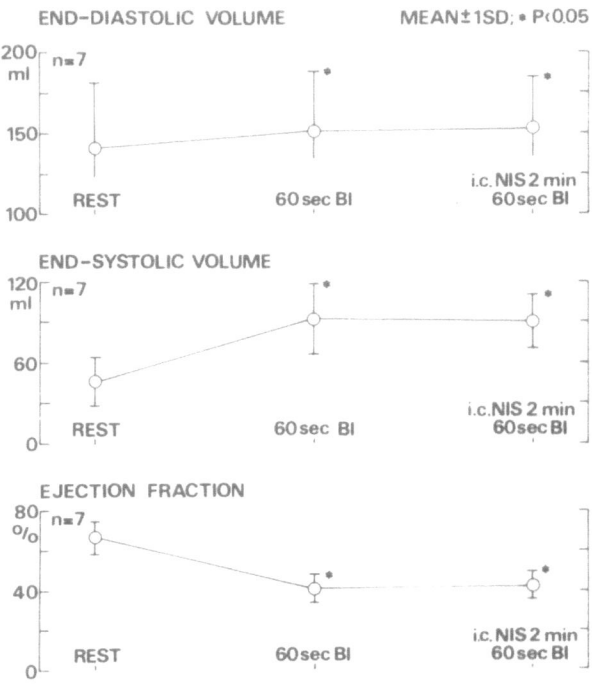

Figure 9. Left ventricular volumes and ejection fraction at rest, at the end of a 60 sec lasting balloon inflation in the proximal LAD (60 sec BI) and at 60 sec balloon inflation performed 2 min after 0.05 mg nisoldipine injected into the left coronary artery (i.c. NIS 2 min; 60 sec BI).

demonstrated after intracoronary administration of nitrates that caused an amelioration of oxygen supply [13]. In the setting of coronary angioplasty, this is an unlikely mechanism for an improvement during ischemia since the vessel under scrutiny is totally occluded during the phase of balloon inflation. Nonetheless, several groups could demonstrate a beneficial effect of intracoronary nitroglycerin during acute coronary occlusion that raises the question of the underlying mechanism [14, 15].

The present study clearly indicates that at least during an acute occlusion of a major coronary artery, all salutary effects of intracoronary nitroglycerin on hemodynamics, on electrocardiographic signs of ischemia and on ventricular pump function and volumes are equivalent to those that can be evoked by an intravenous injection of the same amount of the drug. It is therefore justified to conclude that the observed effects after intracoronary nitroglycerin are primarily due to a peripheral systemic action that occurs when the compound has left the coronary system and reached the systemic circulation. This is confirmed by the fact that after intracoronary nitroglycerin, ventricular pump function is improved by an unloading effect on the non-ischemic contralateral regions of the ventricle whereas wall motion in the occlusion-dependent area stays unimproved, although the drug had been administered directly into this area. Similar observations have been reported by other groups for an intravenous administration of nitroglycerin [16]. Further evidence may come from previous studies, in which we could show a typical vasodilatory effect on the arterial system and a decrease on right and left ventricular filling pressures within 30 sec after intracoronary administration of nitroglycerin [17].

It is well established that orally or intravenously administered dihydropyridine-type calciumantagonists have an anti-ischemic and antianginal effect in subjects with coronary disease that can be attributed to cardial unloading associated with increase in myocardial perfusion [18]. When given directly into the coronary circulation however, any beneficial effects on ischemia seem to have different reasons that are not completely understood. We have found no evidence of any significant peripheral systemic action of nifedipine as well as nisoldipine given in dosages that have been advocated for intracoronary administration. This is in accordance with the findings of Erbel et al [14]. On the other hand, there was a significant reduction in ST-changes in the electrocardiogram after intracoronary administration of calcium-antagonists. Nifedipine as well as nisoldipine given intracoronarily could clearly delay the onset of ischemic ST-changes. So far, there is no established explanation for this phenomenon. The situation is complicated by the fact that calcium-antagonists per se exhibit a negative inotropic effect on the myocardium when administered directly in the coronary circulation [19] and thus can induce alterations in hemodynamics and pump function that are similar to those induced by acute ischemia. In this context, it may be of importance that the relative extent of the increase in pulmonary wedge pressure during acute occlusion of the LAD was slightly reduced by intracoronary nifedipine. The disappearance of ST-alterations despite an increase in left ventricular filling pressure in some cases (see Fig. 5) could potentially be explained by a 'cardioprotective' effect that has been postulated for calciumantagonists. Further studies, however, have to show whether or not the extent of ischemia can definitely be reduced by a direct administration of calciumantagonists into the coronary circulation.

Clinical implications

We have concluded from our study that there is no difference between the intracoronary or intravenous administration of nitrates during acute coronary occlusions. We therefore use the intravenous route when giving nitroglycerin during balloon dilatation, and we perform repeated bolus injections to avoid marked increases in filling pressures when longer periods of balloon inflation or very proximal balloon positions are required.

Calciumantagonists, on the other hand, are preferentially administered orally since their effect on hemodynamics and pump function during ischemia had been of only minor degree after intracoronary and intravenous administration.

References

1. Simon R, Amende I, Herrmann G, Reil GH, Lichtlen PR (1986) Effect of prolonged balloon inflations on hemodynamics and coronary flow with respect to balloon position in patients undergoing coronary angioplasty. In: Serruys PW, Meester GT (eds) *Coronary Angioplasty: A Controlled Model for Ischemia* pp 63–76. Dordrecht – Boston – Lancaster: Martinus Nijhoff Publishers (DICM Volume 58)
2. Rentrop KP, Cohen M, Blanke H, Philipps RA (1985) Changes in collateral channel filling immediately after controlled coronary artery occlusion by an angioplasty balloon in human subjects. *JACC* 5:587
3. Propst P, Zangel W, Pachinger O (1985) Relation of coronary arterial occlusion pressure during percutaneous transluminal coronary angioplasty to presence of collaterals. *AJC* 50:1264
4. Grbic M, Sigwart U (1986) Left ventricular filling during acute ischemia. In: Serruys PW, Meester GT (eds) *Coronary Angioplasty: A Controlled Model for Ischemia*, pp 141–150. Dordrecht – Boston – Lancaster: Martinus Nijhoff Publishers
5. Meyer B, Rutishauser W (1986) Intracoronary electrocardiogram during transluminal angioplasty. In: Serruys PW, Meester GT: *Coronary Angioplasty: A Controlled Model for Ischemia*, pp 33–38, Dordrecht – Boston – Lancaster: Martinus Nijhoff Publishers
6. Rickards A, Seabra-Gomez R, Thuston P (1976) The assessment of regional abnormalities of the left ventricle by angiography. *Eur J Cardiol* 5:167
7. Hood WP, Amende I, Simon R, Lichtlen PR (1979) Relationship between left ventricular geometry and diastolic function: A computer analysis of the effect of nitroglycerin and the β-blocking agent atenolol, *Computers in Cardiology*, p 391f. Longbeach: IEE Computers Society
8. Lichtlen, PR, Halter J, Gattiker K (1974) The effect of isosorbiddinitrate on coronary blood flow, coronary resistance and left ventricular dynamics under exercise in patients with coronary disease. *Basic Research Cardiology* 69:402
9. Bernstein L, Friesinger GC, Lichtlen PR, Ross RS (1966) The effect of nitroglycerin on systemic coronary circulation on man and dogs. *Circulation* 33:107
10. Amende I, Simon R, Hood WP Jr, Lichtlen PR (1979) The effect of the β-blocker atenolol and nitroglycerin on left ventricular function and geometry in man. *Circulation* 60:836
11. Amende I, Simon R, Hood WP Jr, Daniel W, Lichtlen PR (1981) Direct and indirect effects of nitroglycerin on systemic and diastolic left ventricular function. In: Lichtlen PR, Engel HJ, Schrey A, Swan HJL (eds) *Nitrates III*, pp 126f. Berlin: Springer
12. Simon R, Amende I, Engelhard J, Lichtlen PR (1984) The effect of nitroglycerin and isosorbidinitrate on myocardial perfusion and hemodynamics in patients with and without coronary disease. *Scandinavian Journal of clinical and laboratory investigation* 44:47
13. Brown BG, Bolson E, Petersen RB, Piers Ed, Dodge HT (1981) The mechanisms of nitroglycerin action: Stenosis vasodilatation as a major component of the drug response. *Circulation* 64:1089
14. Erbel R, Henkel B, Schreiner G, Clas W, Brennecke R, Kopp K, Meyer J (1986) Clinical, electrocardiographic and hemodynamic changes during coronary angioplasty. Influence of nitroglycerin and nifedipine. In: Serruys PW, Meester GT: *Coronary Angioplasty: A Controlled Model for Ischemia*, pp 39–54. Dordrecht – Boston – Lancaster: Martinus Nijhoff Publishers
15. Hombach V, Höpp HW, Behrenbeck DW, Fuchs HM, Osterspy A, Hilgar HH (1985) Ischämietoleranz unter intrakoronar verabreichtem Nifedipin während transluminaler Koronarangioplastie. In: Meyer J, Erbel R (eds) *Intravenöse und intrakoronare Anwendung von Adalat*, pp 80f. Berlin: Springer
16. Doorey AJ, Mehmel HC, Schwarz FX, Kübler W (1985) Amelioration by nitroglycerin of left ventricular ischemia induced by PTCA: Assessment by hemodynamic variables and left ventriculography. *JACC* 6:267
17. Herrmann G, Simon R, Lichtlen PR (1985) Intracoronary versus intravenous nitroglycerin during coronary angioplasty. *Eur Heart J* 6:24
18. Lichtlen PR (1975) Coronary and left ventricular dynamics under nifedipine in comparison to

nitrates, β-blocking agents and dipyridamole. In: Lochner W, Braasch W, Kroneberg G (eds) *II. International Adalat Symposium*, pp 212f. Berlin: Springer

19. Amende I, Simon R, Hood WP Jr, Hetzer R, Lichtlen PR (1983) Intracoronary nifedipine in human beings: Magnitude and time course of changes in left ventricular contraction/relaxation and coronary sinus blood flow. *JACC* 2:1141

22. Cardioprotective effects of coronary sinus retroperfusion during LAD angioplasty

J. BERLAND and J.E. FARCOT

Introduction

Since the pioneering efforts of Beck and his associates [1] the concept of coronary venous retroperfusion treatment of myocardial ischemia has evolved from largely surgical toward clinically oriented applications [2–4]. In 1976, an ECG synchronized phased retroperfusion was developed featuring diastolic delivery of arterial blood into the coronary sinus veins, along with normal coronary venous drainage during cardiac systole [5]. In a 1978 follow-up study, Farcot et al [6] introduced an autoinflatable balloon at the tip of the retroperfusion catheter in order to enhance the reliability of phasic retroperfusion. Extensive experimental studies have confirmed the beneficial effects of the synchronized retroperfusion system during coronary artery occlusions, indicating significant extension of myocardial viability and improvements in function [7–9]. More recently safety, feasibility and absence of hemodynamic derangements during diastolic retroperfusion were demonstrated in humans [10]. Preliminary clinical system effectiveness studies have also been reported both during unstable angina [2] or PTCA treatment [11]. In view of the persisting PTCA complications, and a trend to seek prolonged intracoronary balloon inflation period, we examined in 17 patients undergoing proximal LAD angioplasty the feasibility, safety and efficacy of a new diastolic coronary venous retroperfusion support. The FDA approved clinical protocol was designed to assess the effects of retroperfusion on incidence of pain, anterior electrocardiographic changes and echographic wall motion of the left ventricle during the PTCA balloon-induced ischemia.

Methods

Patients' selection

Seventeen candidates for PTCA with severe proximal LAD stenosis, and without previous anterior myocardial infarction, were selected for study of the diastolic

P.W. Serruys, R. Simon & K.J. Beatt (eds), Percutaneous Transluminal Coronary Angioplasty. ISBN 0-7923-0346-6.
© 1990 Kluwer Academic Publishers, Dordrecht

retroperfusion system. Patients with multivessel coronary disease and/or with resting anterior left ventricular dysfunction were excluded. Informed consent was obtained from all the patients. Sixteen if whom were males and one female (mean age 58 ± 10).

Retroperfusion system (Fig. 1)

The new synchronized diastolic retroperfusion system (Retroperfusion Systems Inc.*) delivers pulsatile arterial blood via the coronary sinus during diastole and facilitates venous drainage during systole. To ease and enhance the retroperfusion flow delivery the 8 F radio-opaque coronary sinus retroperfusion catheter is equipped wth a special valve at its tip. A side hole near the catheter tip serves to

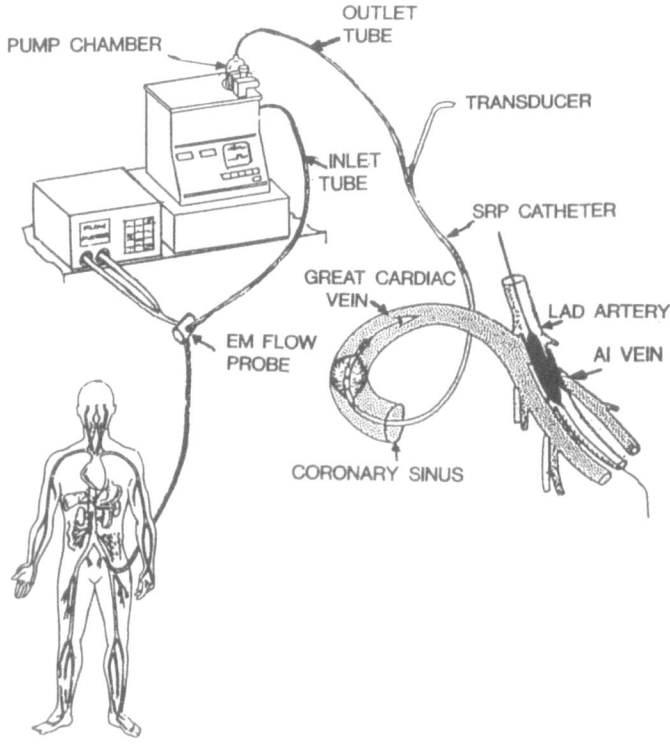

Figure 1. Schematic representation of the diastolic synchronized circuit. SRP = Synchronized retroperfusion; EM = Electromagntic.

*Retroperfusion Systems Inc.: 3178 Pullman Avenue, Costa Mesa, CA 92626, USA

continuously monitor the coronary venous pressure throughout the synchronized retroperfusion.

The system consists of a cardiac monitor, a pump controller, a piston driven pump cassette controlling the retroperfusion flow and an extracorporeal circuit. The monitor is a 3 channel unit capable of monitoring and displaying the electrocardiogram, the coronary vein blood pressure, as well as the pump piston reflecting retroperfusion motion. Information from the patients' ECG is fed and processed by the pump controller, which maintains pump flow and precise pump phasing through a feedback system appropriately compensating for variations in heart rate. The extracorporeal blood circuit features a sterile disposable piston driven pump, and consists of tubing connecting the arterial left femoral vessel via the pump cassette with the special retroperfusion balloon catheter positioned in the coronary vein of the patient. Arterial blood retroperfusate is derived through an 8 French multiple end hole catheter (Retroperfusion Systems Inc.) which is placed percutaneously within the left femoral artery. The pumped retroperfusate flow rate is measured by means of an externally applied electromagnetic flow probe (Transonic Systems Inc.*).

The 50 cm 8 F auto-inflatable balloon catheter was passed through a 9 F sheath inserted via the right internal jugular vein, and was positioned in the coronary sinus under 60° LAO oblique fluoroscopic guidance. Attempts were made always to place the tip of the catheter as deeply as possible, in the coronary sinus preferably in the great cardiac vein. Hand injection of angiographic contrast material confirmed the achieved coronary venous position of the catheter tip (Fig. 2).

When the arterial blood is retrogradely delivered during diastole, it simultaneously inflates the balloon at the tip of the retroperfusion catheter. This brief occlusion of the coronary vein is essential since it minimizes retroperfusate escape via the coronary sinus and maximizes retrograde delivery of arterial blood toward the regionally ischemic myocardium. At end-diastole the balloon is automatically deflated as the retroperfusion pump is stopped in systole, allowing normally phased coronary venous drainage via the coronary sinus into the right atrium. Achievements of proper sequencing has been repeatedly documented in humans by means of fluoroscopic contrast injection.

Protocol (Fig. 3)

Conventional patient preparation for PTCA treatment included oral calcium antagonist and Persantine (started on the day before the procedure), and continuous Nitroglycerine (20 gamma/min) infusion initiated 30 minutes before angioplasty. Following placement of the coronary sinus catheter, Heparin (10 000 I.U.) was injected. The PTCA procedure was performed with conventional balloon catheters, using the right femoral artery. The left femoral artery was also

---

*Transonic Systems Inc.: Ithaca NY 14850, USA.

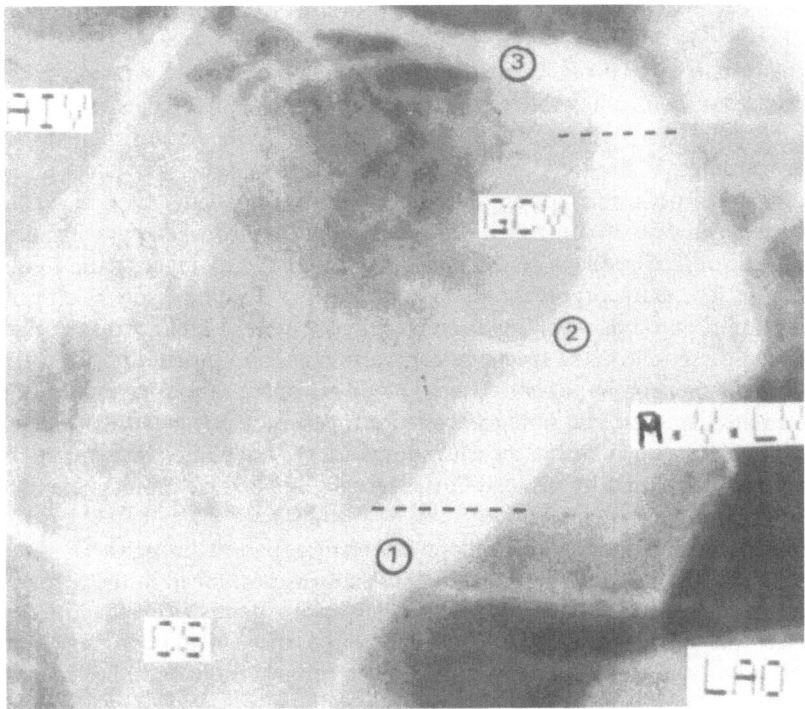

Figure 2.   60° Left anterior oblique cine frame of contrast injection into the coronary sinus.
1 − 2 − 3 = Description of the coronary sinus catheter tip positions. CS = Coronary sinus; GCV = Great cardiac vein; AIV = Anterior interventriculaire vein; M V LV = Marginal vein of the left ventricule.

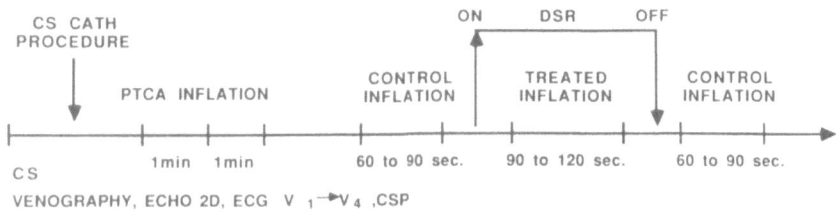

Figure 3.   Study protocol.
CS = Coronary sinus; PTCA = Percutaneous transluminal coronary angioplasty; CSP = Coronary sinus pressure; ECG V1 → V4 = Anterior electrocardiographic recordings; DSR = Diastolic synchronized retroperfusion.

catheterized in order to provide arterial blood for the retroperfusion. After completion of left arterial coronarography, the steerable PTCA balloon catheter was postioned on a guide wire crossing the coronary stenosis. All of the patients first underwent one or two short (< = 60 s) PTCA balloon inflations (without any retroperfusion support) to dilate the stenotic artery and to stabilize the patient's improved coronary function. Five minutes after the last therapeutic PTCA balloon inflation, the retroperfusion study procotol was begun with one initial control (< = 7 atmospheres inflation pressure) PTCA balloon occlusion, lasting 60 to 90 sec, depending upon the patient's tolerance. After balloon deflation, complete recovery from chest pain and ECG changes was achieved wthin 5 min. During this latter recovery period an incremental controlled retroperfusion was initiated and adjusted to provide the highest practicable retroperfusion flow rate, not exceeding a maximum of 150 ml/min. When the retroperfusion flow level reached a plateau, a repeat PTCA inflation with the balloon in the same coronary artery position was performed in the presence of synchronized retroperfusion support. The PTCA balloon inflation was prolonged to two minutes whenever possible depending upon clinical and ECG tolerance. After another recovery period of 5 minutes a second (60 to 90 sec) control PTCA inflation was performed, to assess the reproducibility of ischemia related changes during the comparative untreated control PTCA.

Electrocardiographic recording

Precordial anterior leads V1 to V4 were connected to a Siemens recorder to continuously monitor the anterior wall ECG-changes both during the PTCA balloon inflations and the recovery period. The ECG traces were recorded at 25 mm/sec, and ST elevations (1 mv = 10 mm) were evaluated from each lead with measurements performed 0.08 sec after the J point. The sum of the ECG-ST was computed for every inflation in each patient before coronary artery balloon occlusion and at 30 and 60 sec of the LAD control occlusion, at the maximum PTCA balloon inflation time also, and at 20 sec following initiation of the retroperfusion treatment.

Echocardiography

Each patient was examined before the catheterization procedure to select the best echocardiographic window. 2-D echocardiographic studies were performed immediately before, during, and after untreated control balloon occlusions (controls) and also during the retroperfusion treated PTCA inflation period. Apical four chambers or two chambers views of the left ventricule were recorded and endocardial contours of systolic and diastolic frame images were outlined on transparent paper. From the traced silhouettes, end-diastolic and end-systolic left ventricular areas were computed and the systolic percent change in crossectional area was calculated as an index of global contractile function [% change = (end-diastolic area − end-systolic area) / end-diastolic area]. Wall tracings were studied before the PTCA procedure and at the end of the balloon inflation period during both untreated (control) and retroperfusion treated PTCA balloon occlusion of the LAD coronary artery, with the observer analyzing the echocardiographic frames was blind to treatment or control allocation of the 2D Echo image.

Statistics

All data presented as mean ± standard deviation. Comparisons between the pre-PTCA data, untreated PTCA balloon inflation, and retroperfusion supported PTCA were made by analysis of variance. Statistical significance of ECG changes during equivalent control and treatment periods was also evaluated by analysis of variance.

Results

The coronary angioplasty was successful in all of the 17 patients. No transient coronary artery occlusion, necessitating recrossing of the stenosis was noted, and there was no electrocardiographic or enzyme evidence of persisting myocardial injury as a result of the PTCA procedure.

1. Retroperfusion catheter insertion and coronary vein hemodynamics. In one patient coronary sinus catheterization proved difficult and was abandoned after a 5 min attempt. In the remaining 16 patients (the study population) retroperfusion catheter was positioned within 139 ± 144 sec. Transient atrial fibrillation occured in two of the 16 patients during this catheter manipulation, but these resolved spontaneously without consequences. In four of the patients the coronary sinus tip could not be advanced beyond the proximal portion of the coronary sinus, as shown in Fig. 1 (position 1). In 10 patients the catheter tip was positioned just before the first lateral venous branch (position 2), while in 2 of the 16 patients the retroperfusion catheter tip was located within the great cardiac vein (position 3). Before retroperfusion mean coronary sinus blood pressure in the 16 patients was 4 ± 5 mmHg. As a result of the diastolic coronary venous balloon obstructions and retroperfusate infinous, the mean coronary sinus pressure increased to 16 ± 8 mmHg (diastolic level rose from 4 ± 2.5 to 25 ± 13 mmHg). During the synchronous coronary retroperfusion the mean pumped retroperfusate flow rate was 95 ± 30 ml/min, with a range 50 to 150 ml/min).

2. Clinical and electrocardiographic response in untreated and treated LAD occlusion (Table 1). Forty eight PTCA balloon inflations were analysed for the current study, i.e. 32 untreated controls (before and after treatment) and 16 retroperfusion supported LAD occlusions. Twenty three episodes (72%) of chest pain were encountered during the control PTCA balloon inflations, as compared to 5 of 16 (31%) during retroperfusion support (p < 0.01). Duration of control PTCA balloon inflations was 86 ± 24 sec and this control inflations were significantly shorter than those achieved during retroperfusion supported inflations (101 ± 36 sec; p < 0.01).

Before each of the LAD occlusions, ST segments had returned to normal base line values. At the maximum PTCA balloon inflation time, ST elevations were significantly lower with retroperfusion support (10.4 ± 7.8 mV) as compared to ST changes during the two control inflations immediately before (16.2 ± 7.1 mV) and just after (18.8 ± 10.6 mV; p < 0.01) the retroperfusion supported inflation. There was no significant difference between the above two untreated inflations, confirming the reproducibility of the ECG changes during control occlusion. A typical example of the ST evolution with time is indicated in Fig 4. Comparison between the PTCA balloon inflation induced mean ST elevations, with and without treatment support also shows that retroperfusion delays the development of ST elevations (Fig. 5). During the 32 control LAD occlusions, significant ST elevations were observed at 30 seconds (14.5 ± 7.4 mV; p < 0.05 vs pre-inflation) and found to increase progressively to a peak value 17.5 ± 8.8 mV at the maximum PTCA balloon inflation time. 20 seconds after the balloon deflation (i.e. reperfusion), anterior ST levels were still significantly higher (9.8 ± 6.4 mV) than prior to LAD occlusion (5.5 ± 4 mV; p < 0.01). In contrast, during the retroperfusion supported PTCA balloon inflations the ST changes were significantly lower (p < 0.01) than throughout the untreated control inflations. However, a significant ST elevation was measured at 101 seconds during the retroperfusion treated LAD occlusion (10.4 ± 7.9 mV; p < 0.05 vs occlusion).

3. *Echocardiographic data.* In three patients, sub-optimal echocardiographic views prevented quantitative left ventricular analysis. In one patient (No. 15) transoesophagal echocardiography was performed and M-mode tracings were recorded (Fig. 6). Among striking visual observations, systolic septal wall thickening was generally almost completely lost during untreated LAD balloon occlusion, but remained almost normal with retroperfusion supported LAD occlusions. For the 12 patients studied by 2-D echo (Table 2), the percent left ventricular systolic area changes (area ejection fraction) prior to LAD occlusions averaged 0.32 ± 0.06, decreased to 0.18 ± 0.07 during the first control LAD occlusion, and to 0.17 ± 0.06 during the second untreated LAD occlusion (in both cases, p < 0.001 vs pre-occlusion). There was no significant difference between the two control LAD occlusions. At the peak occlusion time during retroperfusion treated LAD occlusions mean left ventricular systolic area decreased to a significantly lesser extent to 0.25 ± 0.08 (p < 0.05 vs the two untreated control inflations).

Discussion

This study provides clinical documentation of the safety of the new synchronized retroperfusion system, and its effectiveness during PTCA induced LAD occlusions

Table 1. Clinical and electrocardiographic data.

Case No.	Insertion time (sec)	Tip position	Control 1			
			Duration (sec)	CP	ST	
					Base	Inf
1	210	2	45	+	2.5	18
2	90	2	75	+	4.5	22
3	120	1	35	+	4.5	19
4	90	2	60	+	5	16
5	—	—	—	—	—	—
6	120	1	60	0	5	16
7	120	2	90	+	5.5	11.5
8	240	2	120	0	12	15
9	180	2	150	+	2.5	3.5
10	120	1	120	+	9	11.5
11	240	2	60	0	0.5	19
12	180	2	90	+	6	14.5
13	180	2	90	+	0.5	16.5
14	180	1	90	+	2.5	11.5
15	120	2	90	0	3.7	4
16	90	3	90	0	12	31
17	30	3	90	+	10.5	23.5
				11 +		
Mean	139		85		5.4	16.3*
±SD	±144		±29		±3.7	±7

* $p < 0.001$ vs Base.
** $p < 0.001$ vs Control 1 × Control 2.
*** $p < 0.05$ vs Control 1.
**** $p < 0.05$ vs Base.

Insertion time and tip position = Coronary sinus catheter insertion time (sec) and tip position (Fig. 2); Flow = Retroperfusion flow (ml/mn); CP = Typical chest pain; ST Base = Sum of anterior ST elevation beforw LAD occlusion; ST Inf = Sum of anterior ST elevation at maximum inflation time; Control 1 and 2 = Control inflation; Retroperfusion = Inflation supported by retroperfusion.

averaging 90 seconds in duration. Effectiveness was found from delayed appearance and decreased magnitude of electrocardiographic and echocardiographic signs of myocardial ischemia as compared to untreated LAD occlusion. The high success rarte [16/17] of rapid retroperfusion catheterization of the coronary sinus or great cardiac vein, along with the minimal interference with the PTCA procedure, indicates the clinical applicability of the support system. No significant adverse effects of the treatment were noted, confirming previous preclinical studies of the synchronized retroperfusion system [7] and the initial clinical assessment during unstable angina [3] or PTCA [2, 10, 11].

The salutary effects of retroperfusion were evaluated during 90–120 second LAD balloon occlusions, with the treated balloon inflations preceded and also followed by untreated control LAD occlusions. The latter provided evidence of

	Retroperfusion				Control 2			
			ST				ST	
	Duration				Duration			
Flow	(sec)	CP	Base	Inf	(sec)	CP	Base	Inf
120	85	0	2	11	85	+	1.4	19
90	125	0	2.9	9.5	95	+	3	29
120	60	0	3.3	8	60	+	3	25
110	60	+	6	15.5	60	+	5	20
—	—	—	—	—	—	—	—	—
50	60	0	6	15.5	60	0	5	20
90	90	0	6	3	90	+	4	12.5
90	120	0	11	14	120	0	15	17
90	175	0	2.4	2	120	0	2.5	6.5
120	120	+	7	7	120	+	7	9.5
90	60	0	3.5	9.5	60	0	1.5	12.5
50	90	0	3.5	3.5	90	+	3	10.5
90	180	+	1.7	7	90	+	2	20.5
120	90	+	2.5	9	90	+	3	13.5
60	90	0	3.7	4	90	+	3.5	3
50	90	0	15	35	90	0	15	44
70	90	+	9.5	16	90	+	9	30
		5+				11+		
95	101**		5.5	10***	88		5.5	18.9****
±31	±36		±3.7	±8	±20		±4.5	±11

reproducible ECG and echocardiographic changes caused by untreated total occlusion of the LAD coronary artery. Extensive anterior ECG mapping yielded a high electrocardiographic sensitivity, since 13 out of 16 patients (82%) exhibited ECG evidence of myocardial ischemia during LAD occlusion. A similar rate was found by Wohlgelernter [12] when using multiple precordial ECG leads recording during LAD angioplasty in patients without prior history of myocardial infarction. Retroperfusion support delayed the onset of the ECG changes during the LAD occlusions, decreased their magnitude by almost 50%, suggesting significant diminution of the myocardial ischemia. Compared to ECG, changes in left ventricular contraction are considered a more sensitive and precise index of acute myocardial ischemia. Our echocardiographic wall motion study indicates a significantly improved left ventricular contraction and enhances septal wall motion during the retroperfusion treated LAD occlusions. As subjectively evaluated by blinded observation, untreated LAD occlusions (compared to retroperfusion supported), exhibited a significant decrease in systolic left ventricular areas changes generally reflected in absence of contraction of the antero-apical regions. Our quantitative analysis is admittedly relatively simple, and less specific that the more recent method using centerline technique [12]. However a relatively good reproducibility seems to validate our data. These

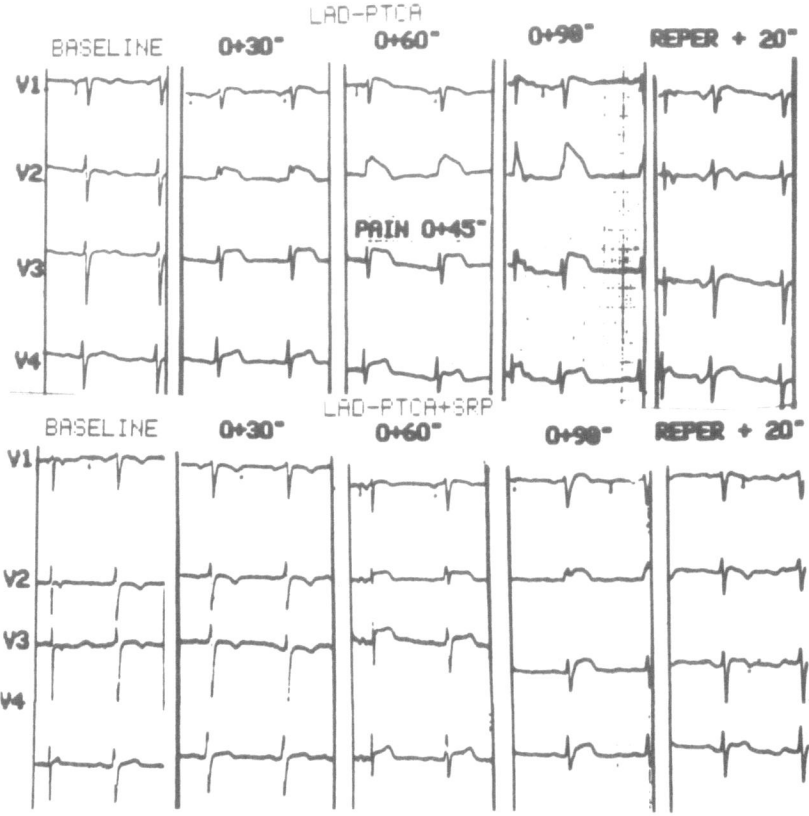

Figure 4. Typical example of electrocardiographic changes during LAD occlusion without (top) and with (bottom) synchronized retroperfusion.
LAD PTCA = Left anterior descending percutaneous transluminal coronary angioplasty; SRP = Synchronized retroperfusion; REPER = Reperfusion; REPER + 20 = Reperfusion + 20; O + 30 = Occlusion + 30 sec.

data are also in agreement those of another group [4] using retroperfusion to protect patients during LAD angioplasty. As reported in a recent abstract, they analyzed the regional left ventricular contractility by the 'centerline method', and found a significant improvement in contraction when LAD balloon occlusion was supported with retroperfusion. Using a different retroperfusion system, K Beatt [13] did not find any beneficial effects on myocardial ischemia when applied during LAD angioplasty. This discrepancy is uncertain (only 3 patients were studied) and could also be ascribed to different characteristics of the early retroperfusion catheters.

The retroperfuson mechanism involved in the observed myocardial tissue preservation and improved function during coronary artery occlusions are not

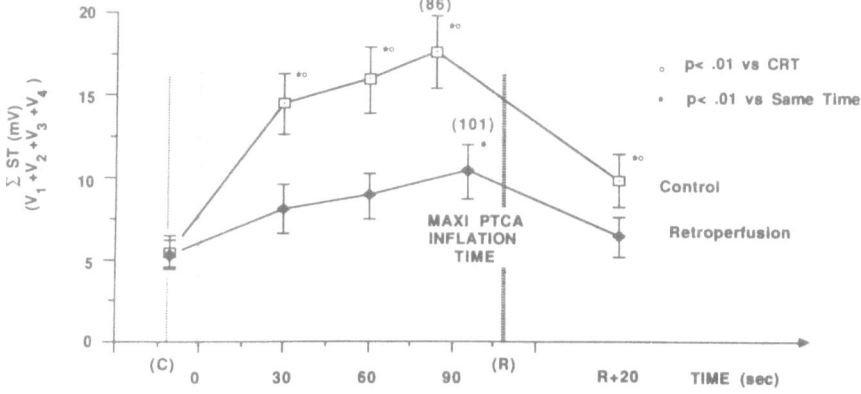

Figure 5. Anterior electrocardiographic ST changes evolution with time during control inflations VS inflations with retroperfusion.
CRT = Control; ST = Sum of anterior V1 to V4 changes (mV).

fully defined. Experimental studies employing acute coronary artery occlusions, indicated that despite some systolic washout of the retroperfused arterial blood, as much as 50% of the retroperfusate may reach the myocardium [14]. If such an arterial blood retrodelivery can be achieved during the short period of PTCA induced myocardial ischemia, a retroperfusion pump flow rate of 90 to 100ml/min should be adequate to maintain contraction, based on experimental indications [15]. Yet another explanation for the observed retroperfusion effectiveness could be a significant enhancement of the toxic metabolite myocardial wash-out from the acutely ischemic myocardium, recently demonstrated by experimental digital angiography [9].

Although this study demonstrates a significant improvement due to retroperfusion support of PTCA balloon occlusion of the LAD, complete protection for the treated 90 seconds LAD occlusion period was not achieved with the system and protocol used. We observed the best results in patients in whom the retroperfusion catheter was inserted far into the coronary sinus, preferably to more selectively retroperfuse the LAD subsewed ischemic region from the great cardiac vein. Unfortunately this selective canulation of the great cardiac vein with the available retroperfusion catheter was not possible in all of the patients. Moreover, during inflation of the balloon placed in the coronary sinus, the balloon catheter tented to move toward the right atrium, in spite of a relative satisfactory initial placement. Problems of this nature could limit the efficacy of retroperfusion and need to be resolved. The limited pumped retroperfusion flow (95 ml/min) could also explain the observed incomplete protection, particularly when the catheter was in the proximal part of coronary sinus. The need for higher developed coronary venous blood pressures and retroperfusion flow was emphasized by the group in Rotterdam. These authors [16] employed only 3 pigs

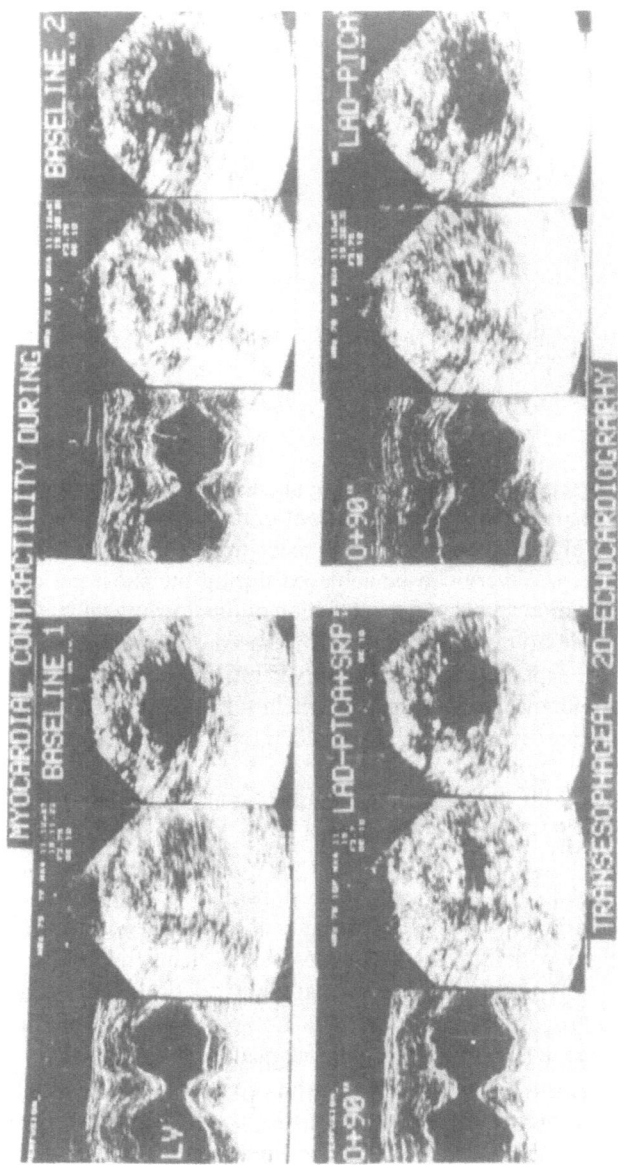

Figure 6. Transoesophageal 2D-echocardiographic during LAD PTCA with and without retroperfusion in patient No. 15.
Left Ventricular (LV) M-Mode Echocardiogram and 2D LV short axis view before occlusion (baseline 1 upper left, baseline 2 upper right) and at 90 sec occlusion with retroperfusion (bottom left) and without retroperfusion (bottom right). The septal motion looks much better with retroperfusion.

Table 2. Echocardiographic left ventricular systolic area changes.

Case No.	Base	Control 1	Retroperfusion	Control 2
2	0.39	0.19	0.35	0.17
3	0.31	0.09	0.20	0.09
4	0.40	0.25	0.22	0.20
6	0.29	0.29	0.36	0.14
7	0.23	0.11	0.11	0.06
8	0.31	0.21	0.36	0.23
9	0.32	0.24	0.31	0.27
12	0.34	0.16	0.29	0.18
13	0.23	0.16	0.20	—
14	0.36	0.16	0.24	0.18
16	0.41	0.26	0.20	0.19
17	0.27	0.14	0.17	0.14

Mean $\pm$ SD 0.31 ± 0.09 0.19 ± 0.07 0.25 ± 0.09 0.18 ± 0.06

$p < 0.001$ $p < 0.05$ $p < 0.01$

$p < 0.05$

$p < 0.001$

Base = Before first control occlusion; Control 1 and 2 = % systolic LV area changes at maximum inflation time during control 1 and control 2 inflations; Retroperfusion = same parameter during inflation treated by retroperfusion.

and demonstrated restoration and maintenance of normal contractility during 10 minute occlusions of the LAD coronary artery, when near systemic systolic and diastolic pressures were achieved in the coronary sinus during synchronized retroperfusion. Based upon the initial clinical data and new experimental indications, a new system with higher retroperfusate tolerated flow rate (up to 250 ml/min) should safely facilitate effective retroperfusion to the ischemic myocardium during coronary vein occlusion.

Conclusion

A new synchronized coronary venous retroperfusion support system was safely applied during LAD PTCA in 16 patients without impending the procedure. Its effectiveness could be demonstrated by a decrease in electrocardiographic and echocardiographic signs of ischemia during retroperfusion support, but substantial variability between patients was noted. To protect the myocardium during prolonged PTCA inflations (> 2 min), improved catheter and pumping systems are currently in experimentation.

Acknowledgements

The authors thank Samuel Meerbaum, M.D. for his advices in reviewing this paper and Mrs Veronique Alix for her assitance in preparing and typing this article.

References

1. Beck CS, Stanton E, Batiuchok W, Leiter E (1978) Revascularization of heart by graft of systemic artery into coronary sinus. *JAMA* 137:435
2. Farcot JC, Berland J, Cribier A, Bourdarias JP, Letac B (1985) Diastolic synchronized retroperfusion in the coronary sinus during percutaneous transluminal angioplasty: Preliminary experience. *Circulation* 72 (Suppl III):470
3. Gore JM, Weiner BH, Benotti JR et al (1986) Preliminary experience with synchronized coronary sinus retroperfusion in humans. *Circulation* 74:381
4. Kar S, Drury JK, Eigler N et al (1988) Amelioration of ischemia during PTCA with diastolic coronary venous retroperfusion (abstract). *J Am Coll Cardiol* 11:64A
5. Meerbaum S, Lang TW, Osher JV et al (1976) Diastolic retroperfusion of acutely ischemic myocardium. *Am J Cardiol* 27:588
6. Farcot JC, Meerbaum S, Lang TW et al (1978) Synchronized retroperfusion of coronary veins for circulatory support of jeopardized ischemic myocardium. *Am J Cardiol* 41:1191
7. Drury JK, Yamazaki S, Fishbein M et al (1985) Synchronized diastolic coronary venous retroperfusion: Results of a pre-clinical safety and efficacy study. *J Am Coll Cardiol* 6:328
8. Yamazaki S, Drury JK, Meerbaum S, Corday E (1985) Synchronized coronary venous retroperfusion: Prompt improvement of left ventricular function in experimental myocardial ischemia. *J Am Coll Cardiol* 5:655
9. Chang BL, Drury JK, Meerbaum S et al (1987) Enhanced myocardial washout and retrograde blood delivery with synchronized retroperfusion during acute myocardial ischemia. *J Am Coll Cardiol* 9:1091
10. Berland J, Farcot JC, Cribier A, Bourdarias JP, Letac B (1986) Clinical evaluation of safety and hemodynamic effects of diastolic coronary venous retroperfusion. In:Mohl W, Faxon D, Wolner E (eds) *Clinics of CSI* pp 281ff Darmstadt: Steinkopff Verlag
11. Weiner BH, Gore JM, Sloan KM, Benotti JR, Gaca JMJ, Okiki ON, Vandersalm TJ, Ball SP, Corrao J, Alpert JS, Dalen JE (1986) Synchronized coronary sinus retroperfusion (SCSR) during LAD angioplasty. *JACC* 7:64A
12. Wohlgelernter D, Cleman M, Highman HA, Fetterman RC, Duncan JS, Zaret BL, Jaffe C (1986) Regional myocardial dysfunction during coronary angioplasty: Evaluation by two-dimensional echocardiography and 12 lead electrocardiography. *JACC* 7:1245
13. Beatt KJ, Serruys PW, De Feyter P., Van Den Brand M, Verdouw PD, Hugenholtz PG (1988) Haemodynamic observations during percutaneous transluminal coronary angioplasty in the presence of synchronized diastolic coronary sinus retroperfusion. *Br Heart J* 59:159
14. Berdeaux A, Farcot JC, Bourdarias JP, Barry M, Bardet J, Giudicelli JF (1981) Effects of diastolic synchronized retroperfusion on regional coronary blood flow in experimental myocardial ischemia. *Am J Cardiol* 47:1033
15. Vatner SF (1980) Correlations between acute reductions in myocardial blood flow and function in conscious dogs. *Cir Res* 47:201
16. Verdouw PD, Beatt K, Berk L, Serruys PW (1988) Does effective diastolic coronary venous retroperfusion depend on arterial-like blood pressure in the coronary sinus? *Am J Cardiol* 61:1148

PART TWO

Non-operative treatment of acute ischemic

23. Coronary angioplasty for unstable angina pectoris

P.J. DE FEYTER, H. SURYAPRANATA and P.W. SERRUYS

Introduction

Coronary atherosclerosis may lead to a variety of syndromes which can affect the same patient at different times. These are stable angina pectoris, unstable angina pectoris, acute myocardial infarction, cardiac failure, arrhythmia and sudden death (not necessarily in that sequence).

Although many studies have been devoted to unstable angina pectoris there is as yet no universally accepted definition and unstable angina is best described as a clinical syndrome between stable angina pectoris and acute myocardial infarction. The syndrome of unstable angina includes many categories of patients, who present with a variable history, who have different laboratory features, in whom varying pathophysiologic mechanisms are operating at different times and who often have an unpredictable outcome [1, 2].

Management of these patients continues to be a problem and a challenge for the physician treating a patient with unstable angina. In the treatment of unstable angina a distinction must be made between the treatment to eliminate acute cardiac ischaemia and maintenance treatment to prevent episodes of ischaemia or to diminish their frequency. It is generally agreed upon that patients with acute ischaemia should be admitted to a coronary care unit. All patients should receive bedrest, sedation and reassurance and precipitating factors such as anaemia, hypertension, tachycardia should be corrected promptly. Since the main causative pathophysiologic mechanisms in a given patient are unknown, treatment is highly pragmatic and consists of a combination of drugs including nitrates, beta blockers and calcium antagonists to increase oxygen supply and to decrease oxygen demand. Usually a step up approach with a combination of these drugs guided by symptoms and haemodynamics of the patients, is advocated to stabilize the acute symptoms [1–3]. Treatment with heparin has been shown beneficial [4] and fibrinolytic treatment may be of value in subgroups of patients with acute ischemia [5–8].

After stabilisation of acute ischemia there appears to be a high propensity of progression to total occlusion of the ischemia related vessel resulting in

P.W. Serruys, R. Simon & K.J. Beatt (eds), Percutaneous Transluminal Coronary Angioplasty. ISBN 0-7923-0346-6.
© *1990 Kluwer Academic Publishers, Dordrecht*

myocardial infarction or cardiac death, which has been shown to be prevented with platelet inhibitors [9, 10].

The treating physician should be aware that many factors may be causative at a particular moment of the disease process and that the very next moment, a different mechanism may prevail or spontaneous improvement can occur. Consequently, to quote PG Hugenholtz: 'there will never be one therapy for every case of unstable angina, nor will there ever be the best therapy for unstable angina; there will only be the optimal therapy for that particular stage of the disease at that particular moment in time for that patient' [11].

However, whatever pathophysiologic mechanism prevails, the common denominator in patients with unstable angina is (sudden) progression of a pre-existing coronary obstruction to a critical obstruction or even to a (intermittent) total occlusion of the ischemia related vessel. Consequently, there is a need for definite revascularization in subgroups of patients. Coronary artery bypass surgery is indicated in patients refractory to intensive drug treatment and in high risk patients after stabilisation of symptoms to (1) prevent new episodes of unstable angina, myocardial infarction or death, or (2) to alleviate symptoms of stable angina who will be often present. Coronary angioplasty has recently gained acceptance as an alternative form of revascularization in patients with unstable angina pectoris. However, it also became evident that angioplasty in these patients is associated with a higher major complication rate compared to angioplasty in stable angina and the precise role of coronary angioplasty in the management of unstable angina is still a matter of debate.

The purpose of this paper is to review recent developments pertaining coronary angioplasty for unstable angina and to establish guidelines for the use of coronary angioplasty in the management of patients with unstable angina pectoris.

Classification of patients with unstable angina pectoris

Unstable angina was classically defined by Paul Wood as follows: 'The onset of acute coronary insufficiency is sudden; a state of normal health or of relatively mild angina of effort, with or without a history of cardiac infarction changing abruptly to one of almost total incapacity. Although the pain is usually provoked by all the familiar triggers (exertion) it may also occur spontaneously, when the patient is sitting quietly in a chair reading the paper, or may wake him repeatedly from sleep. The diagnosis of acute coronary insufficiency denies evidence of coronary infarction.' [12] He believed that coronary insufficiency was a warning sign of impending myocardial infarction. Gazes et al [13] were the first to point out that the natural history of all patients with unstable angina was not uniform. They identified a high-risk subgroup for myocardial infarction and death. High risk patients have frequent, repeated attacks of angina, also in the hospital, accompanied with electrocardiographic ST-T changes and no or little response to treatment.

Due to the fact that unstable angina is a single term used to encompass a number of clinical and physiopathological syndromes we believe that, to evaluate the natural history and the impact of different therapeutic modalities, it is imperative to stratify patients according to clinical subgroups. There appear to be 3 distinct subgroups of patients who have a different prognosis and who require different plans for management:

1. patients with new onset angina of a progressive nature, and those with chronic angina who have a change in their anginal pattern, but no pain at rest or no change on a baseline electrocardiogram. These patients appear to have a more benign course and may only require pharmacologic intervention (including antiplatelet agents) to treat recurrent ischemia or to prevent progression to myocardial infarction and cardiac death.
2. patients with repeated periods of angina at rest or angina at rest with ST-segment or T wave changes on a baseline electrocardiogram. This high risk group appears to have a high incidence of acute myocardial infarction and mortality which requires more agressive interventions.
3. patients with early (within 30 days) postinfarction angina. These patients also appear to have a high incidence of recurrent myocardial infarction and mortality which requires more agressive interventions.

Pathophysiology of unstable angina and the impact of coronary angioplasty

The underlying culprit in coronary artery disease is the atherosclerotic plaque [14–16]. The plaque may or may not cause an important degree of luminal narrowing. Recently it has been recognized that the acute changes which initially occur in the coronary artery endothelium are similar in patients with different acute ischemic syndromes (acute myocardial infarction, unstable angina, sudden death) including endothelial ulceration adjacent to an atherosclerotic plaque, subsequent platelet adhesion and aggregation and eventually thrombosis [14–28]. The initial stimulus that leads to ulceration of the endothelium overlying an atherosclerotic plaque has not been identified. Rheologic, hemodynamic and vasomotor stresses may initiate and propagate plaque damage. Plaque injury exposes circulating blood elements such as platelets to collagen and atherosclerotic debris within the plaque. Interaction at the damaged vessel wall with circulating catecholamines and local release of platelet-derived vasoconstrictor and thrombogenic substances (such as thromboxane A2, leukotrienes, histamine and serotonin) or an imbalance of these relative to vasodilating and antithrombotic substances (such as prostacyclin, endothelial dependant relaxant factor and plasminogen activator) may ultimately lead to a partially or totally occlusive thrombus or to fragmentation of such thrombus with peripheral embolization. Other factors such as the severity of pre-existing stenosis and the extent of collateral flow will also influence the extent of perturbation of coronary blood flow. The (im)balance between these competing forces determines whether the mass of the formed thrombus is partially or totally occlusive, and whether its presence is transient or permanent.

The resulting extent and duration of impaired coronary blood flow will

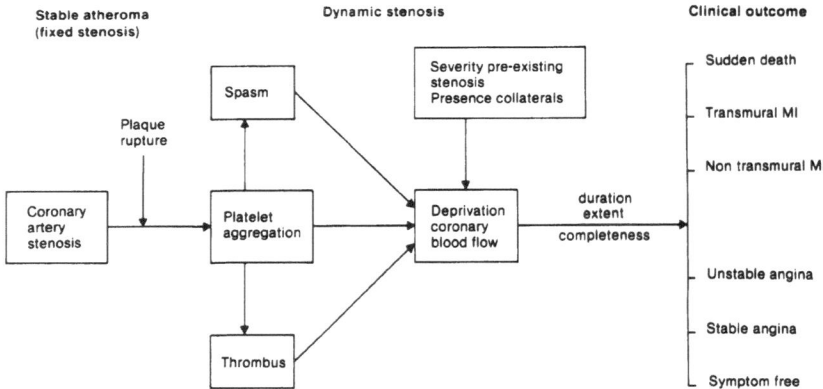

Figure 1. Schematic representation of important pathogenetic factors which lead to a specific clinical outcome.

determine the predominant clinical syndrome: unstable angina, acute myocardial infarction or sudden death (see Fig. 1). In unstable angina the process is limited to endothelial ulceration, platelet aggregation and thrombus formation, which may be intermittent, or more permanent in the presence of an adequate collateral supply. In the majority of the patients with unstable angina the clinical situation stabilizes, the plaque injury heals, but the underlying lesion remains or becomes more severe.

Percutaneous transluminal coronary angioplasty has been shown to be an effective method to enlarge the lumen of stenosed coronary arteries [29] and so it may effectively resolve myocardial ischemia and prevent progression to total occlusion. The mechanism by which the atherosclerotic plaque is reduced involves fracture of the plaque with redistribution within the wall of the coronary artery, and expansion of the external diameter of the artery [30–32]. On the other hand animal studies have shown that endothelial denudation, platelet deposition, mural thrombus and localized vasoconstriction at the site of the arterial injury may all be caused by angioplasty [33–35]. Therefore coronary angioplasty has the potential to intensify the ongoing thrombogenic process in patients with acute ischemic syndromes. Indeed, angioplasty has been shown to induce thrombosis and vasospasm leading to acute closure of the dilated vessel in some patients [36–41]. The picture becomes even more complex when it is realized that restenosis in the first months after angioplasty may result from a complex interaction between platelet accumulation (which is related to the extent of balloon injury), release of platelet derived growth factor, vascular damage and blood flow [35, 42, 43].

It is conceivable that angioplasty causes further injury of the already ulcerated intima in patients with unstable angina, which may lead to an increased platelet accumulation and release of platelet derived growth factor and thus to increased smooth muscle cell proliferation and a higher restenosis rate.

Coronary angioplasty in patients with 'stabilized' unstable angina

Despite a growing experience with coronary angioplasty for the treatment of unstable angina, only a few reports have analyzed the risks and benefits of coronary angioplasty used as an alternative for coronary artery bypass graft surgery in patients who have an initially good response to pharmacological treatment but who are still symptomatic on exertion [44–47]. Although initial pharmacologic treatment may relieve the acute-phase symptoms, patients remain at high risk for progression to myocardial infarction or cardiac death, and the need for CABG surgery is not reduced [48]. The coronary artery obstruction in patients with unstable angina is at risk of becoming a permanent occlusion, leading to myocardial infarction or death [49–51].

Coronary angioplasty, therefore, seems a logical step in an attempt to improve morbidity and mortality. The success and complication rates are listed in Table 1. The initial success rate of coronary angioplasty has been reported between 63% and 90%. These rates are somewhat lower than the 90% success rates achieved in stable angina [52–54]. Procedure-related deaths occurred in 0–4%. The procedure-related myocardial infarction rate was 8–12%. Emergency bypass surgery was deemed necessary in 5–12% of the patients: despite this, the majority had evidence of myocardial infarction [46]. The myocardial infarction rate and emergency bypass surgery rate are definitely higher than for elective angioplasty in patients with stable angina [52–54].

After a successful angioplasty the prognosis is favorable with a low late myocardial infarction rate and low late death rate. Recurrent chest pain was present at 12 months after initially successful coronary angioplasty in 23% [46] and 32% [45] at 14 months.

Currently, data are lacking to compare these results with those obtained with intensive medical treatment or surgery in similar patients groups. Only one observational, nonrandomized study compared the immediate and 18 month results in a comparable group of patients with 1-vessel disease and unstable angina who underwent either CABG surgery or coronary angioplasty [44]. From these data, it appeared that angioplasty compared favorably with bypass surgery. The procedure was associated with similar mortality and morbidity rates, but there was a more marked improvement in symptoms after coronary angioplasty. Eighty-two percent of the patients treated with PTCA and only 63% of the patients treated with CABG surgery were asymptomatic [44].

Coronary angioplasty for refractory unstable angina

Patients with chest pain at rest accompanied by significant ST–T changes in the electrocardiogram and patients with ischemia in spite of treatment with nitrates, beta-blockers, Ca-antagonists and heparin carry an increased risk of mortality and morbidity [11, 55–59] and either bypass surgery or coronary angioplasty is indicated. The advantages of coronary angioplasty over coronary bypass surgery

Table 1. Coronary angioplasty for initially stabilised

Author/Year	No. of patients	Success rate %
Faxon[a] [44] 1983	442	63
Quigley [45] 1986	25	81
de Feyter [46] 1987	71	87
Steffenino [47] 1987	89	90

Definition unstable angina:
Faxon, Quigley: new onset angina, coronary insufficiency, changing pattern of pre-existing angina, angina at rest or variant angina.
de Feyter: chest pain at rest accompanied with ST–T changes.

in these critically ill patients is that the intrinsic risks of major surgery and anesthesia are avoided, it is easy and rapid to implement, and there is a reduction of hospital stay and costs. A major drawback of coronary angioplasty is the early (within 6 months) restenosis rate.

The earlier reported lower success rates of 74 to 76% of coronary angioplasty in patients with unstable angina were achieved with non steerable dilatation catheters [60, 61], whereas the more recent initial success rates of 70–92% were achieved with the more advanced steerable dilatation catheter system [62–65] (Table 2); the latter figure reflects the current state of art. The initial success rate of angioplasty in patients with unstable angina appears to be somewhat lower than the success rate of more than 90% achieved nowadays in patients with stable angina pectoris [52–54]. This is mainly due to the higher procedure related complication rate in patients with unstable angina. The procedure related

Table 2. Coronary angioplasty for refractory unstable

Author/year	No. of patients	Success rate %
Williams[a] [60] 1981	17	76
Meyer[a] [61] 1983	50	74
de Feyter [55] 1985	88	92
Timmis [63] 1987	56	70
Plokker [64] 1988	469	88
Sharma [65] 1988	40	88

[a] PTCA performed with non-steerable dilatation system.

unstable angina pectoris.

Major complication rate			Coronary events after successful angioplasty			Follow-up months mean
death %	MI %	Acute surgery %	Death %	MI %	AP %	
0.9	8	–	1.7	1.5	18	18
4.0	12	12	0.0	0.0	32	14
0.0	10	12	2.0	2.0	23	12
0.0	5	5	0.0	1.5	23	10

Steffenino: worsening in the frequency or severity of chest pain or severe episodes of prolonged pain at rest.
[a] The majority of the patients were initially stabilised.

mortality is reported varying from 0 to 5.4% [Table 2]. A myocardial infarction, which results from a complication during the angioplasty procedure, is reported between 0 and 7% and the need for emergency surgery from 2 to 12.5% (Table 2). The occurrence of major complications is definitely higher in patients with unstable angina than in patients with stable angina [52–54].

The major reason for this high complication rate are related to the underlying pathophysiology leading to clinical instability and an increased risk on abrupt closure due to the formation of an acute occlusive thrombus. After initial successful coronary angioplasty the prognosis is excellent, with a low incidence of late mortality (up to 3.5%) and a low occurrence of late nonfatal myocardial infarction (up to 3.5%). Finally, recurrence of angina after an initial successful coronary angioplasty appears to be comparable to those of patients with stable angina [44, 49, 61, 62, 66].

angina pectoris.

Major complication rate			Coronary events after successful angioplasty			Follow-up months mean
Death %	MI %	Acute surgery %	Death %	MI %	AP %	
0.0	0.0	6.0	0.0	0.0	8	10.5
0.0	4.0	2.0	0.0	0.0	36	6.0
0.0	6.0	7.0	1.0	1.0	20	12.0
5.4	7.1	12.5	3.3	3.3	39	6.0
1.0	4.9	3.0	1.5	0.1	21	19.3
0.0	0.0	12.0	0.0	0.0	34	11.0

Coronary angioplasty for early postinfarction angina

The incidence of early post myocardial infarction angina during the hospitalization period is reported between 18 and 57% [67–75] varying with the patient population. Patients with early postinfarction angina appear to have a poor short and longterm prognosis [67–75]. Postinfarction ischemia may be localized to either the border zone of the infarct ('ischemia in the infarct zone') or to a distant vascular bed ('ischemia at a distance') [71]. The latter patients have been shown to have an extremely worse prognosis. Non-Q wave infarctions are known to be associated with a higher incidence of recurrent infarction [73–75]. The reasons are that patients with a non-Q wave myocardial infarction have more residual jeopardized myocardium within the perfusion zone of the infarct-related vessel than those with a Q wave myocardial infarction and patients with a non-Q wave myocardial infarction and patients with a non-Q wave myocardial infarction have a higher incidence of patent infarct-related vessels, thus providing the stage for a potentially more unstable clinical course [75].

Persistent or recurrent pain early after infarction implies that the cardiac event is not yet complete, and suggests that more aggressive management might improve patients' clinical status and salvage myocardium. The occurrence of

Table 3. Surgical mortality and perioperative myocardial infarction rate in unstable angina and postinfarction unstable angina

Study (author/year)	No. of patients	Perioperative mortality %	Perioperative myocardial infarction %
Unstable angina			
Ahmed [128] 1980	71	4.2	7.0
Brawley [129] 1980	130	7.7	8.0
Rankin [78] 1984	48	4.0	6.1
Rahimtoola [130] 1983	1282	1.8	–
Cohn [131] 1985	222	3.0	1.0
Goldman [132] 1985	299	5.0	16.7
Mc Cormick [133] 1985	3311	3.9	–
Luchi [134] 1987	468	4.1	10.3
Postinfarction unstable angina (< 30 days)			
Nunley [76] 1983	21	0.0	–
Williams [77] 1983	92	2.0	0.0
Molina [82] 1983	38	10.5	–
Rankin [78] 1984	52	4.0	4.0
Baumgartner [84] 1984	34	9.0	15.0
Gertler [80] 1985	44	16.0	–
Singh [79] 1985	108	1.8	4.6
Brower [81] 1985	34	3.0	12.0
Breyer [85] 1985	75	8.0	–
Jones [83] 1987	107	8.5	8.5

severe or refractory postinfarction angina has been a primary indication for urgent revascularization. Recent surgical reports (Table 3) [76–85] have suggested that myocardial revascularisation within the first 30 days after myocardial infarction can be accomplished with an acceptable operative mortality in selected patients, although overall mortality and morbidity rates remain higher than those reported for elective surgery. Accordingly, current strategy for the management of patients with early postinfarction angina is aimed at delaying surgery to such a time when it can be performed with the least inherent risks. This strategy consists of a combined treatment with nitrates, beta-blockers and calcium antagonists, including intra-aortic balloon pump assist. Coronary angioplasty in this situation has been shown to be an attractive alternative to surgical revascularization [86–91] (Table 4). However, the procedural complications are definitely more frequent in this setting than with elective coronary angioplasty [52, 54]. A procedure related mortality is reported up to 2%. A complication resulting in a myocardial infarction occurred in up to 8% and acute surgery was required in up to 12% of the patients. The available data suggest that coronary angioplasty performed early after acute myocardial infarction is an effective procedure in a selected group of patients who have preserved but jeopardized left ventricular function, predominant single vessel disease and an anatomy suitable for coronary angioplasty. However, the procedure is associated with an increased risk of major complications. It remains to be determined whether the same benefits can be achieved in patients with early post infarction angina and multi-vessel disease, or in those who have reduced left ventricular function.

Coronary angioplasty for variant angina

In 1959, Prinzmetal et al [92] described a clinical syndrome characterized by angina at rest with concomitant transient ST-segment elevation on the electro-cardiogram. They suggested that this variant form of angina resulted from temporary occlusion of a large diseased artery due to a normal increase in the tonus of the vascular wall. Gensini [93] documented spontaneously occurring coronary spasm associated with chest pain in a patient with angina pectoris and mild coronary artery disease. The coronary anatomy of patients with variant angina is quite variable, ranging from angiographically normal coronary arteries to severe multivessel disease [94–97]. The majority of patients with variant angina have some degree of organic stenosis, which appears to be the site where spasm occurs in about 90% of the cases [98]. The respective roles of spasm and fixed obstruction in occluding a coronary artery may vary from patient to patient. Significant coronary obstruction or even occlusion can be dynamically produced when superimposed on a fixed atheromatous stenosis. Elimination of the organic stenosis would prevent vasoconstrictive occlusion of the artery and would relieve symptoms in patients with variant angina. Therefore, coronary angioplasty might be considered as an alternative treatment for patients with

Table 4. Coronary angioplasty for early postinfarction

Author/Year	No. of patients	Success rate %
de Feyter [86] 1986	53	89
Holt [87] 1988	70	76
Gotlieb [88] 1987	47	91
Safian[a] [89] 1987	68	87
Hopkins [90] 1988	54	81
Suryapranata[a] [91] 1988	60	85

[a] Coronary angioplasty in post non-Q wave myocardial

variant angina and significant fixed coronary artery stenosis. The initial and late results of coronary angioplasty for variant angina are shown in Table 5. It appears that the initial results are acceptable, with an initial success rate reported between 86 and 95% [99–101]. There was no procedure related death, but a myocardial infarction complicated the procedure in 1 to 9% and acute surgery was necessary in 1 to 10% of the cases. Induction of severe coronary vasospasm by intracoronary manipulation of instruments which might have been expected in patients with variant angina, did not occur as frequently as was anticipated and appears to be of relatively minor concern. Of major concern is the rather high restenosis rate and recurrence of symptoms after initial successful coronary angioplasty which could not be prevented with pharmacologic treatment. In a recent study Bertrand et al [102] demonstrated a high incidence of recurrent angina and angiographically proven restenosis rate of 35% after coronary angioplasty in patients with a dynamic stenosis versus a rate of 22% in those with a fixed coronary stenosis. These results suggest that, not unexpectedly, coronary vasospasm continues after angioplasty, whereas it is also suggested that vasospasm plays a significant role in the recurrence of restenosis. These studies

Table 5. Coronary angioplasty for variant angina pectoris.

Author/Year	No. of patients	Success rate %
Corcos [99] 1985	21	90
Leisch [100] 1986	22	86
Bertrand [101] 1987	102	95

angina pectoris.

Major complication rate			Coronary events after successful angioplasty			Follow-up months mean
Death %	MI %	Acute surgery %	Death %	MI %	AP %	
0	8.0	8.0	0	4	26	9.0
2	5.0	12.0	2	4	21	27.0
2	4.0	2.0	3	3	18	16.3
0	1.5	1.5	0	2	41	17.0
0	0.0	4.0	0	2	25	11.0
0	5.0	7.0	0	5	23	20.0

infarction performed 2.3 months after index infarction.

demonstrate that coronary angioplasty is less satisfactory in patients with variant angina as has also been shown for coronary artery bypass surgery [103].

Coronary angioplasty of only the culprit lesion in patients with unstable angina and multivessel disease

The majority of patients with unstable angina have multivessel disease [48]. Successful multiple dilatations in one angioplasty procedure have been performed with acceptable complication rates in patients with stable angina [104–107]. However, there is less acceptance of and less experience with multivessel dilatation patients with (refractory) unstable angina because multiple dilatations in these clinically unstable patients may increase the risk of major complications. Also there is the risk of performing unnecessary dilatations because of the difficulty in assessing the significance of any additional stenosis in the acute setting. Left ventricular dysfunction occurs in the setting of refractory unstable angina, which is wholly or partially reversible after dilatation of the culprit lesion,

Major complication rate				Coronary events after successful angioplasty			Follow-up months mean
Death %	MI %	Acute surgery %	Spasm	Death %	MI %	AP %	
0	5	10	0	5	16	58	33
0	9	5	14	0	0	47	24
0	1	1	–	0	0	22	6–8

Table 6. Anginal symptoms after PTCA in patients with multivessel disease.

Author/Year	Incomplete revascularization		Complete revascularization		Follow-up months mean
	No. of patients	Angina pectoris %	No. of patients	Angina pectoris %	
Mabin [113] 1985	35	63	31	29	13
Van Dormael [104] 1985	31	35	35	9	6
Ilsley [111] 1986	96	17	78	21	12
de Feyter [110][a] 1986	38	29	98	14	6
Finci [105] 1987	18	56	59	19	24
Thomas [112] 1988	73	37	19	37	12

[a] Patients with unstable Angina.

although this may take a few days to recover after restoration of adequate perfusion [108]. If angina recurs, subsequent dilatation of additional disease can then be performed with less risk. The initial success rate and major complication rate of coronary angioplasty in patients with single vessel disease and dilatation of that particular vessel was comparable to those with multivessel disease and dilatation of only the culprit lesion [109, 110]. However, recurrent or persistent angina pectoris at 6 months follow-up was significantly higher in patients with multivessel disease than in patients with single vessel disease (Table 6) [104, 105, 110–114]. We believe that angioplasty of the culprit lesion in patients with unstable angina and multivessel disease should be regarded as an initial treatment strategy in whom symptoms do not respond adequately to pharmacologic treatment. In most patients, this approach will have a longterm success, but in some further dilations or even bypass surgery will be required, so that this strategy does not provide a definitive longterm treatment in all patients. However, the subsequent interventions can be performed on a more elective basis with less risk.

Thrombolytics in the treatment of unstable angina

The current medical treatment for unstable angina pectoris consists of a combination therapy with nitrates, beta-receptor blockers, calcium channel antagonists and antiplatelet aggregation drugs. The rationale for this approach is based on the recognition of the role of coronary vasospasm, atherosclerosis and platelet aggregation in the pathogenesis of the disease (Fig 1). In addition to these mechanisms, intracoronary thrombosis also plays an important role: consequently, thrombolytic therapy might be indicated for unstable angina. The results of different studies on the use of thrombolytic treatment in patients with unstable angina are presented in Table 7. The results of these studies indicate that thrombolytic treatment can produce additional benefit in, as yet not exactly defined, subsets of patients. The benefit appears to be limited to patients with angiographic evidence of intra-coronary thrombus and it appears to be more

Table 7. Results of thrombolytic treatment in patients with unstable angina.

Study	No. of patients	Treatment	Angiographic evidence of lysis %	Follow-up
Rentrop [115]	5	IC SK	0	
Vetrovec [116]	13	IC SK	77	
Mandelkorn [117]	9	IC SK	44	
Shapiro [118]	18	IC SK	67	
Ambrose [119]	36	IC SK	0	
de Zwaan [8]	38	IC SK(22) rt PA(16)	53	
			Clinical outcome	
Lawrence [5]	20	IV SK (24 hr) + coumadin	5% Sudden death (1 patient)	6 months
	20	coumadin	40% Sudden death (4 pts) infarction (4 pts)	6 months
Gold [6]	24	IV tPA or placebo	40% decrease in recurrent ischemia	7 days
Topol [7]	40	IV tPA or placebo	Improved pacing threshold to ischemia	7 days
Gotoh [120]	21	IC Urokinase	Lysis in 95% Recurrence sympt. 71% Progression to MI: 24%	1 month

effective if the delay between the last attack of chest pain and institution of thrombolytic treatment is short. Thrombolytic treatment appears to be less effective in older thrombus probably due to organization of the thrombus which renders it resistant to thrombolytic therapy. However, even if thrombolytic treatment is effective, there will be a sustained need for definitive coronary revascularization procedures in the majority of patients. The potential benefits of additional treatment with thrombolytic agents have to outweigh the bleeding complications caused by thrombolytic treatment. Future studies will be directed towards defining subgroups of patients with unstable angina who will most likely benefit from thrombolytic therapy, and towards the design of therapeutic schemes associated with a reduced bleeding frequency. Biochemical markers may be useful in clinical practise, not only to detect activation of the clotting system and platelets and an increased risk of bleeding, but also to predict and guide success of thrombolytic treatment.

It is suggested that pretreatment with thrombolytics increases the safety of PTCA for unstable angina, since it may reduce acute closure of the vessel due to acute thrombus formation. Furthermore it has been shown that thrombolytic treatment is of use as a 'bail out' procedure during PTCA in case of abrupt closure due to thrombus formation [121].

Restenosis after coronary angioplasty in patients with unstable angina

The long term outcome after successful coronary angioplasty is still significantly curtailed by the recurrence of stenosis in 12 to 48% of the patients [61, 62, 107,

122–126]. Current data about the restenosis rate after successful coronary angioplasty in patients with unstable angina, compared to the restenosis rate in patients with stable angina, are conflicting. Some reports have indicated that angioplasty for unstable angina is associated with an increased risk of restenosis compared with stable angina [102, 124], whereas others have demonstrated a comparable restenosis rate [45, 61, 62, 123, 107, 127]. However, these conflicting data should be considered with caution, since they might merely reflect the differences between studies in indication and timing of repeat angiography, follow up rate, method of assessment of coronary artery stenosis and patient selection. Furthermore these studies have used visual interpretation of the coronary angiogram, a method which is so seriously hampered by a high intra- an interobserver variability that it is of only limited value for adequate assessment of changes in the severity of coronary lesions. In view of these discrepant results, we have conducted a prospective study at the Thorax Center to compare the incidence of restenosis in stable versus unstable angina pectoris patients [66]. Follow-up angiography was performed in 85% of patients from a consecutive series with a successful coronary angioplasty, irrespective of presence of absence of recurrent ischemic symptoms and the severity of the coronary artery lesions was assessed qualititatively by an automated edge-detection technique. We have shown that the incidence of restenosis in patients with unstable angina pectoris was similar to that of patients with stable angina pectoris.

Proposed management of patients with unstable angina

The relative merits of coronary artery bypass surgery and PTCA in the management of unstable angina are well established. The latest improvements in surgical techniques and myocardial preservation have decreased the operative mortality and morbidity, although those rates are higher than in patients with stable angina (Table 3). Coronary angioplasty has been shown to be an effective method to enlarge the lumen of stenosed coronary arteries. However, careful analysis of the published reports and our own experience indicates that coronary angioplasty in this setting is associated with an increased risk of major complications. The results of coronary angioplasty (Tables 1, 2, 4, 5) cannot be compared with those obtained with surgery (Table 3) since patients who undergo angioplasty are a selection from the whole spectrum of patients with unstable angina. Selected for coronary angioplasty are those with predominantly 1-vessel disease and well preserved left ventricular function. (Table 8) Recent randomized studies aimed at establishing the merits of current pharmacologic treatment, current bypass surgery and coronary angioplasty in the management of patients with unstable angina are lacking. Until further information becomes available we would propose the following practical approach. This approach is based on (a) the history of unstable angina, (b) the time interval between the last attack of chest pain and instituted therapy, (c) the presence of electrocardiographic changes of ST segment and T wave, (d) the response to pharmacologic treatment and (e) the

Table 8. Selection of patients with unstable angina (pain at rest with ST–T wave changes) for coronary angioplasty.

	No. of patients	Vessel involved (No. of patients)				
		0	1	2	3	Left main
Unstable angina[a]						
(total No. of patients)	217	7	75	40	71	24
Coronary angioplasty	93	0	69	18	6	0
Surgery	89	0	4	14	52	19
Pharmacological treatment	35	7	2	8	13	5
Postinfarction unstable Angina[b]						
(total No. of patients)	101	0	37	20	39	5
Coronary angioplasty	53	0	34	14	5	0
Surgery	48	0	3	6	34	5

[a] 217 patients with unstable angina from among 1,283 patients admitted to the CCU from January 1983 to April 1984.
[b] 101 patients with refractory postinfarction unstable angina from among 2,731 patients admitted to the CCU from January 1983 to September 1985.

coronary anatomy and left ventricular function. Patients with unstable angina should initially receive prompt management with stepwise intensification of pharmacologic therapy in an attempt to achieve stability (Table 9). Early angiography and revascularization (coronary angioplasty, or bypass surgery) is indicated if this approach fails and ischemic episodes continue in spite of 'maximum' medical management (Fig. 2). Coronary angioplasty is indicated when a stenosis, technically suitable for dilatation, is found to be responsible for the unstable state. The decision in favour of coronary angioplasty in patients with single vessel disease is easy to make. In the presence of multivessel disease uncertainty remains. Patients with left main stem disease or severe multi-vessel disease should be scheduled for bypass surgery. However, in selected patients with multivessel disease one might prefer dilatation of the ischemia related vessel only, as opposed to total revascularization by multiple dilatation or bypass surgery [109, 110, 114], since this can be performed faster and so reduce hospital

Table 9. Optimal pharmacological treatment for patients with unstable angina.

– Bed rest (CCU) and sedation
– Treatment of precipitating factors (anemia, hypertension, tachycardia)
– Anticoagulant (heparin) or antiplatelet treatment (aspirin)
– Stepwise intensification, with individual tailoring of a pharmacological regimen including adequate administration of:

  • B-Adrenergic blockade to achieve a resting pulse of < 60 bpm
  • Calcium antagonists and nitroglycerin (long acting or IV) to optimize preload (pulmonary capillary wedge pressure < 14 mmHg) and afterload (systolic aortic pressure < 110 mmHg.)

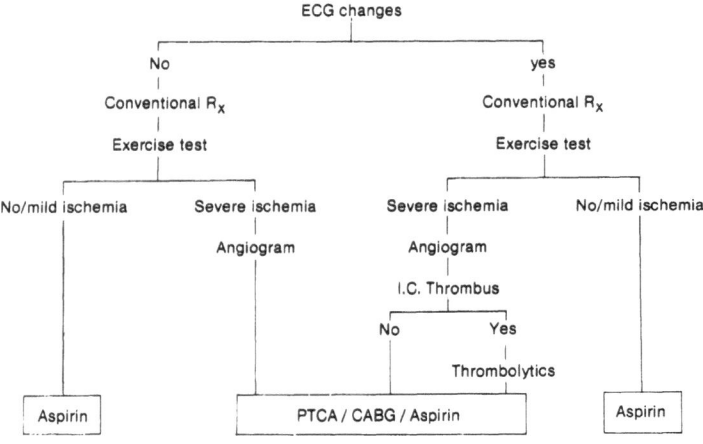

CHEST PAIN AT REST / EARLY POST MI-ANGINA

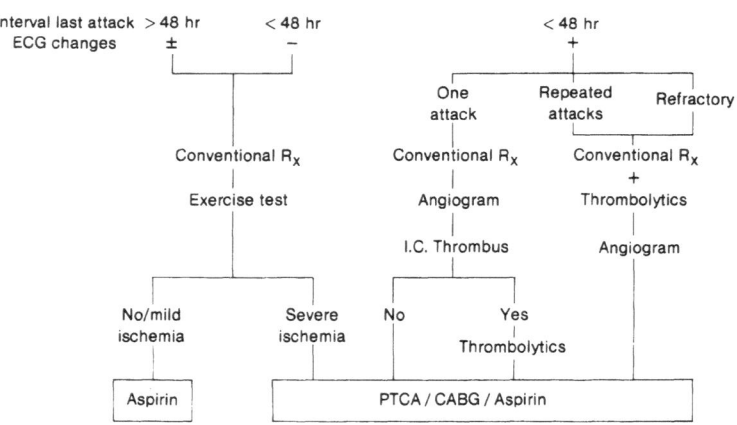

Conventional R_x = nitroglycerin, β-blockers, Ca-antagonists and heparin.

Figure 2. Triage approach to the patient with unstable angina.

stay. The potential of thrombolytic treatment in the management of patients with unstable angina is indicated in Fig. 2 but this needs further study.

References

1. Cairns JA, Fantus IG, Klassen GA (1976) Unstable angina pectoris. *Am Heart J* 92:373–386
2. Scanlon PJ (1982) The intermediate coronary syndrome. *Prog Cardiovasc Dis* 23:351–364
3. Plotnick GD (1979) Approach to the management of unstable angina. *Am Heart J* 98:243–55

4. Telford AM, Wilson C (1981) Trial of heparin versus atenolol in prevention of myocardial infarction in intermediate coronary syndrome. *Lancet* i:1225–1228
5. Lawrence JR, Shepherd JT, Bone I, Rogen AS, Fulton WFM (1980) Fibrinolytic therapy in unstable angina pectoris, a controlled clinical trial. *Thrombos Res* 17:767–777
6. Gold HK, Johns JA, Heinbach RC, Yasuda T, Grossbard E, Zusman R, Collen D (1987) A randomized, blinded, placebo-controlled trial of recombinant tissue-type plasminogen activator in patients with unstable angina pectoris. *Circulation* 75:1192–1199
7. Topol EJ, Nicklas JM, Kander N, Walton JA, Ellis SG, Sanz ML, Gorman L, Pitt B (1988) Need for definitive coronary revascularization despite intravenous tissue plasminogen activator (tPA) for unstable angina: results of a randomized doubleblind, placebo-controlled trial. Submitted
8. de Zwaan C, Bär F, Janssen JHA, de Swart HB, Vermeer F, Wellens HJJ (1988) Effects of thrombolytic therapy in unstable angina: Clinical and angiographic results. *J Am Coll Cardiol* 12:301–9
9. Lewis HD, Davis JW, Archibald DG et al (1983) Protective effects of aspirin against acute myocardial infarction and death in men with unstable angina. *N Engl J Med* 309:396–403
10. Cairns JA, Gent M, Singer J, et al (1985) Aspirin, sulfinpyrazone or both in unstable angina. Results of a Canadian multicenter trial. *N. Engl J Med* 313:1369–1375
11. Hugenholtz PG, Goldman BS (1985) In: *Unstable Angina: Current Concepts and Management*, pp 1–3 Stuttgart – New York: Schattauer
12. Wood P (1961) Acute and subacute coronary insufficiency. *Br Med J* 1:1779–1782
13. Gazes PC, Mobley EM, Farris HM, Duncan RC, Humphries GB (1973) Preinfarction (unstable) angina – a prospective study. Ten year follow-up. *Circulation* 48:331–338
14. Falk E (1983) Plaque rupture with severe pre-existing stenosis precipitating coronary thrombosis: characteristics of coronary atherosclerotic plaques underlying fatal occlusive thrombi. *Br Heart J* 50:127–134
15. Davies MJ, Thomas A (1984) Thrombosis and acute coronary artery lesions in sudden cardiac ischemic death. *N Engl J Med* 310:1137–1140
16. Levin DC, Fallon JT (1982) Significance of angiographic morphology of localized coronary stenoses. Histopathologic correlations. *Circulation* 66:316–320
17. Laffel GL, Braunwald E (1984) Thrombolytic therapy: A new strategy for the treatment of acute myocardial infarction. *N. Engl J Med* 311:710–717 and 770–776
18. Rentrop P (1985) Thrombolytic therapy in patients with acute myocardial infarction. *Circulation* 71:627–631
19. De Wood MA, Spores J, Notske R, Mouser RT, Burroughs R, Golden MS, Lang HT (1980) Prevalence of total coronary occlusion during the early hours of transmural myocardial infarction. *N Engl J Med* 303:897–902
20. Gorlin R, Fuster V, Ambrose JA (1986) Anatomic-physiologic link between acute coronary syndromes. *Circulation* 74:6–9
21. Sherman CT, Litvack F, Grundfest W et al (1986) Coronary angioscopy in patients with unstable angina pectoris. *N Engl Med* 315:913–919
22. Fitzgerald DG, Roy L, Catelle F, Fitzgerald GA (1986) Platelet activation in unstable coronary disease. *N Engl J Med* 315:983–993
23. Fuster V, Chesebro JH (1986) Mechanisms of unstable angina. *N Engl J Med* 315:1023–1025
24. Maseri A, L'Abbate, Baroldi G. et al. (1978) Coronary vasospasm as a possible cause of myocardial infarction: a conclusion derived from the study of 'preinfarction' angina. *N Engl J Med* 229:1271–1277
25. Davies MJ, Thomas AC (1985) Plaque fissuring – the cause of acute myocardial infarction, sudden ischemic death and crescendo angina. *Br Heart J* 53:363–373
26. Falk E (1985) Unstable angina with fatal outcome: dynamic coronary thrombosis leading to infarction or sudden death. *Circulation* 71:699–708
27. Davies MJ, Thomas AC, Knapman PA, Hangartner JR (1986) Intramyocardial platelet aggregation in patients with unstable angina suffering sudden ischemic cardiac death. *Circulation* 73:418–428
28. Epstein SE, Talbot TL (1981) Dynamic coronary tone in precipitation, exacerbation and relief of angina pectoris. *Am J Cardiol* 48:797–803

29. Gruentzig AR, Senning A, Siegenthaler WE (1979) Nonoperative dilatation of coronary artery stenoses – percutaneous transluminal coronary angioplasty. *N Engl J Med* 301:61–68
30. Castaneda-Zuniga WR, Formanek A, Tadavarthy M, Vlodaver Z, Edwards JE, Zollikofer C, Amplatz K (1980) The mechanism of balloon angioplasty. *Radiology* 135:565–571
31. Block PC, Myler RK, Stertzer S, Fallon JT (1981) Morphology after transluminal angioplasty in human beings. *J Engl J Med* 305:382–385
32. Ryan TJ (1983) The mechanism of transluminal angioplasty: evidence for formation of aneurysms in experimental atherosclerosis. *Circulation* 68:1136–1140
33. Pasternak RC, Baughman KL, Fallon JT, Block PC (1980) Scanning electron microscopy after coronary transluminal angioplasty of normal coronary arteries. *Am J Cardiol* 45:591–598
34. Lam JYT, Chesebro JH, Steele PM, Badimon L, Fuster V (1987) Is vasospasm related to platelet deposition? Relationship in a porcine preparation of arterial injury in vivo. *Circulation* 73:243–248
35. Wilentz JR, Sanborn TA, Haudenschild CC, Valeri CR, Ryan T, Faxon DP (1987) Platelet accumulation in experimenal angioplasty: time course and relation to vascular injury. *Circulation* 75:636–642
36. Hollman J, Gruentzig AR, Douglas JS, King SB, Ischinger T, Meier B (1983) Acute occlusion after percutaneous transluminal coronary angioplasty: A new approach. *Circulation* 68:725–732
37. MacDonald RG, Feldman RL, Conti CR, Pepine CJ: Thrombo-embolic complications of coronary angioplasty. *Am J Cardiol* 54:916–917
38. Mabin TA, Holmes DR, Smith HC, Vlietstra RE, Bove AA, Reeder GG, Chesebro J, Bresnahan JF, Orszulak TA (1985) Intracoronary thrombus: Role in coronary occlusion complicating percutaneous transluminal coronary angioplasty. *J Am Coll Cardol* 5:198–202
39. Cowley MJ, Dorros G, Kelsey SF, van Raden M, Detre K (1984) Acute coronary events associated with percutaneous transluminal coronary angioplasty. *Am J Cardiol* 53:12C–6C
40. Ischinger T, Gruentzig AR, Meier B, Galan K (1986) Coronary dissection and total coronary occlusion associated with percutaneous transluminal coronary angioplasty: Significance of initial angiographic morphology of coronary stenosis. *Circulation* 74:1371–1379
41. Sugrue D, Holmes DR, Smith HC, Reeder GS, Lare GE, Vlietstra RE, Bresnahkan JF (1986) Coronary artery thrombus as a risk factor for acute vessel occlusion during percutaneous transluminal coronary angioplasty: improving results. *Br Heart J* 56:62–66
42. Austin GE, Ratliffe NB, Hollman J, Tabei S, Phillips DF (1985) Intimal proliferation of smooth muscle cells as an explanation for recurrent coronary artery stenosis after percutaneous transluminal coronary angioplasty. *J Am Coll Cardiol* 6:369–375
43. Ross R, Glomset JA, Kariya B, Harker LA (1972) A platelet dependent factor that stimulates the proliferation of arterial smooth muscle cells in vitro. *Ann NY Acad Sci* 201:22–29
44. Faxon DP, Detre KM, McGabe CH et al (1983) Role of percutaneous trasluminal coronary angioplasty in the treatment of unstable angina. Report from the National Heart, Lung and Blood Institute Percutaneous Transluminal Coronary Angioplasty and Coronary Artery Surgery Study Registries. *Am J Cardiol* 53 (12):131C–35C
45. Quigley PJ, Erwin J, Maurer BJ, Walsh MJ, Gearty GF (1986) Percutaneous transluminal coronary angoplasty in unstable angina. Comparison with stable angina. *Br Heart J* 55:227–230
46. de Feyter PJ, Serruys PW, Suryapranata H, Beatt K, van den Brand M (1987) PTCA early after the diagnosis of unstable angina. *Am Heart J* 114:48–54
47. Steffenino G, Meier B, Finci L, Rutishauer W (1987) Follow-up results of treatment of unstable angina by coronary angioplasty. *Br Heart J* 57:416–419
48. Rahimtoola SH (1984) Coronary bypass surgery for unstable angina. *Circulation* 69:842–848
49. Neill WA, Wharton TP, Fluri-Lundeen J, Cohen JS (1980) Acute coronary insufficiency: Coronary occlusion after intermittent ischemic attacks. *N Engl J Med* 302:1157–1162
50. Moise A, Theroux P, Taeymans Y, Descoings B, Lesperance J, Waters DD, Pelletier GB, Bourassa MG (1983) Unstable angina and progression of coronary atherosclerosis. *N Engl J Med* 309:685–689
51. Rafflenbeul W, Smith LR, Rogers WJ, Mantle JA, Rackley CE, Russel RO (1979) Quantitative coronary arteriography. Coronary anatomy of patients with unstable angina pectoris re-

examined 1 year after optimal medical therapy. *Am J Cardiol* 43:699–708
52. Anderson HV, Roubin GS, Leimgruber PP, Douglas JS, King SB, Gruentzig AR (1985) Primary angiographic success rates of percutaneous transluminal coronary angioplasty. *Am J. Cardiol* 56:712–717
53. Block PC (1985) Percutaneous transluminal coronary artery disease. *Circulation* 7 (Suppl V): V-161–165
54. de Feyter PJ, van den Brand M, Serruys PW, et al (1988) Increase of initial success rate and safety of single vessel PTCA in 1371 patients: A seven year experience. *J Intervent Cardiol* 1:3–11
55. Harris PH, Harrell FE, Lee KL, Behar VS, Rosati RA (1979) Survival in medically treated coronary artery disease. *Circulation* 60:1259–1269
56. Duncan B, Fulton M, Morrison SL, Lutz W, Donald KW, Kerr F, Kirby BJ, Julian DG, Oliver MF (1976) Prognosis of new and worsening angina pectoris. *Br Med J* 1:981–985
57. Roberts KB, Califf RM, Harrell FE, Lee KL, Pryor DB, Rosati RA (1983) The prognosis for patients with new onset angina who have undergone cardiac catheterization. *Circulation* 68:970–978
58. Olson HG, Lyons KP, Aronow WS, Stinson RJ, Kuperus J, Waters HJ (1981) The high-risk angina patients. *Circulation* 64:674–684
59. Lubsen J, Tijssen JGP, Kerkkamp HJJ (Hint Research Group) (1986) Early treatmet of unstable angina in the coronary care unit: A randomised double blind, placebo controlled comparison of recurrent ischemia in patients treated with nifedipine of metoprolol or both. *Br Heart J* 56:400–413
60. Williams DO, Riley RS, Singh AK, Gewirtz H, Most AS (1981) Evaluation of the role of coronary angioplasty in patients with unstable angina pectoris. *Am Heart J* 102:1–9
61. Meyer J, Schmitz HJ, Kiesslich T et al (1983) Percutaneous transluminal coronary angioplasty in patients with stable and unstable angina pectoris: Analysis of early and late results. *Am Heart J* 106:973–980
62. de Feyter PJ, Serruys PW, Brand van den M, Balakumaran K, Mochtar B, Soward AL, Arnold AER, Hugenholtz PG (1985) Emergency cornary angioplasty in refractory unstable angina. *N Engl J Med* 313:342–347
63. Timmis AD, Griffin B, Crick JCP, Sowton E (1987) Early percutaneous transluminal coronary angioplasty in the management of unstable angina. *Int J Cardiol* 14:25–31
64. Plokker HWT, Ernst SMPG, Bal ET, van den Berg ECJM, Mast GEG, Feltz TA, Ascoop CAPL (1988) Percutaneous transluminal coronary angioplasty in patients with unstable angina pectoris refractory to medical therapy. *Cath Cardiovasc Diagn* 14:15–18
65. Sharma B, Wyeth RP, Kolath GS, Gimenez HJ, Franciosa JA (1988) Percutaneous transluminal coronary angioplasty of one vessel for refractory unstable angina pectoris: Efficacy in single and multivessel disease. *Br Heart J* 59:280–286
66. Luyten HE, Beatt KJ, de Feyter PJ, van den Brand M, Reiber JC, Serruys PW (1988) Angioplasty for stable versus unstable angina pectoris: Are unstable patients more likely to get restenosis. *Int J Cardiac Imaging* (in press)
67. Stenson RE, Flamm MD, Zaret BL, McGowan RL (1975) Transient ST segment elevation with postmyocardial infarction angina: Prognostic significance. *Am Heart J* 89:449–454
68. Marmor A, Sobel BE, Roberts R (1981) Factors presaging early recurrent myocardial infaction ('Extension'). *Am J Cardol* 48:603–610
69. Fioretti P, Brower RW, Balakumaran K (1986) Early post-infarction angina. Incidence and prognostic relevance. *Eur Heart J* 7 (Suppl C): 73–77
70. Fraker TD, Wagner GS, Rosati RA (1979) Extension of myocardial infarction: Incidence and prognosis. *Circulation* 60:1126–1129
71. Schuster EH, Bulkley BH (1981) Early postinfarction angina: Ischemia at a distance and ischemia in the infarct zone. *N Engl J Med* 305:110–115
72. Bosch X, Theroux P, Waters D, Pelletier GB, Roy D (1987) Early postinfarction ischemia: clinical, angiographic, and prognostic significance. *Circulation* 75:988–995
73. Madigan NP, Rutherford BD, Frye RL (1976) The clinical course, early prognosis and coronary anatomy of subendocardial infarction. *Am J Med* 60:635–641

74. Hutter AM, De Sanctis RW, Flynn T, Yeatman LA (1981) Nontransmural myocardial infarction: A comparison of hospital and late clinical course of patients with that of matched patients with transmural anterior and transmural inferior myocardial infarction. *Am J Cardiol* 48:595–602

75. Gibson RS, Beller Ga, Gheorghiade M, Nygaard TW, Watson DD, Huey BL, Sayre SL, Kaiser DL (1986) The prevalence and clinical significance of residual myocardial ischemia 2 weeks after uncomplicated non Q wave infarction: A prospective natural history study. *Circulation* 73:1186–1198

76. Nunley DL, Grunkemeier GL, Teply JF, Abbruzzese PA, Savis JS, Khonsari S, Starr A (1983) Coronary bypass operation following acute complicated myocardial infarction. *J Thorac Cardiovasc Surg* 85:485–491

77. Williams DB, Ivey TD, Bailey WW, Irey SJ, Rideout JT, Stewart D (1983) Postinfarction angina: Results of early revascularization. *J Am Coll Cardiol* 2:859–864

78. Rankin JS, Newton JR, Califf RM, Jones RH, Wechsler AS, Oldham HN, Wolfe WG, Lowe JE (1984) Clinical characteristics and current management of medically refractory unstable angina. *Ann Surg* 200:475–464

79. Singh AK, Rivera R, Cooper GN, Karlson KE (1985) Early myocardial revascularization for post infarction angina: Results and longterm follow-up. *J Am Coll Cardiol* 6:1121–1125

80. Gertler JP, Elefteriades JA, Kopf GS, Hashim SW, Hammond GL, Geha AS (1985) Predictors of outcome in early revascularization after acute myocardial infarction. *Am J Surg* 149:441–444

81. Brower RA, Fioretti P, Simoons ML, Haalebos M, Rulf ENR, Hugenholtz PG (1985) Surgical versus non surgical management of patients soon after acute myocardial infarction. *Br Heart J* 54:460–465

82. Molina JE, Dorsey JS, Emanuel DA, Reyes J (1983) Coronary bypass operation for early postinfarction angina. *Surg Gynaecol and Obstr* 157:455–460

83. Jones RN, Pifarre R, Sullivan HJ, Montoga A, Bakhos M, Grieco JG, Foy BK, Wyatt J (1987) Early myocardial revascularization for postinfarction angina. *Ann Thorac Surg* 44:159–162

84. Baumgartner WA, Borkon AM, Zibulewsky J, Watkins L, Gardner TJ. Bulkley BH, Achuff SC, Baughman KL, Traill TA, Gott VL, Reitz BA (1984) Operative intervention for postinfarction angina. *Ann Thorac Surg* 38:265–267

85. Breyer RH, Engelman RM, Rousou JA, Lemeshow S (1985) Postinfarction angina: an expanding subset of patients undergoing bypass surgery. *J Thorac Cardiovasc Surg* 90:532–540

86. de Feyter PJ, Serruys PW, Soward A, Brand van den M, Bos E, Hugenholtz PG (1986) Coronary angioplasty for early postinfarction unstable angina. *Circulation* 54:460–465

87. Holt GW, Gersh BJ, Holmes DR, Vlietstra RE, Bresnahan JF, Reeder GS, Smith HC (1988) Results of percutaneous transluminal coronary angioplasty for angina pectoris early after acute myocardial infarction. *J Am Coll Cardiol* 61:1238–1242

88. Gottlieb SO, Brim KP, Walfod GD et al (1987) Initial and late results of coronary angioplasty for early postinfarction unstable angina. *Cath Cardiovasc Diagn* 13:93–99

89. Safian RD, Snyder D, Synder BA, McKay RG, Corell BH, Aroesty M, Pasternak RC, Bradley AB, Monrad S, Baim DS (1987) Usefulness of PTCA for unstable angina pectoris after non Q-wave acute myocardial infarction. *Am J Cardiol* 59:263–266

90. Hopkins J, Savage M, Zaluwski A, Dervan JP, Goldberg S (1988) Recurrent ischemia in the zone of prior myocardial infarction: Results of coronary angioplasty of the infarct related artery. *Am Heart J* 115:14–19

91. Suryapranata H, Beatt K, de Feyter PJ, Verroste J, van den Brand M, Zijlstra F, Serruys PW (1988) Percutaneous transluminal coronary angioplasty for angina pectoris after a non-q-wave acute myocardial infarction. *Am J Cardiol* 61:240–243

92. Prinzmetal M, Kennamer R, Merliss R, Wada T, Bor N (1959) Angina pectoris. A variant form of angina pectoris. *Am J Med* 27:375–388

93. Gensini GG, DiGiorgi S, Murad NS (1962) Arterio graphic demonstration of coronary spasm and its release after the use of a vasodilator in a case of angina pectoris. *Angiology* 13:550–553

94. Cheng TO, Bashour T, Kelser GA, Weiss L, Bacos L (1973) Variant angina of Prinzmetal with normal coronary arteriogram. *Circulation* 47:476–485

95. Severi S, Davies G, Maseri A, Marzillo P, L'Abbate A (1980) Longterm prognosis of 'variant' angina with medical treatment. *Am J Cardiol* 46:226–232
96. Shubrooks SJ, Bete JM, Hutter AM. et al (1975) Variant angina pectoris clinical and anatomic spectrum and results of coronary bypass surgery. *Am J Cardiol* 36:142–147
97. Johnson AD, Stroud HA, Viewig WVR, Ross (1978) Variant angina pectoris, clinical presentations, coronary angiography patterns and the results of medical and surgical management in 42 consecutive patients. *Chest* 73:786–794
98. Mac Alpin RN (1980) Relation of coronary arterial spasm to site of organic stenosis. *Am J Cardiol* 46:146–153
99. Corcos T, David PR, Bourassa MG, Guiteras P, Robert J, Mata LA, Waters DA (1985) Percutaneous transluminal coronary angioplasty for the treatment of variant angina. *J. Am Coll Cardiol* 5:1046–1054
100. Leisch FB, Schutzenberger W, Kerschner K, Herbinger W (1986) Influence of a variant angina on the results of percutaneous transluminal coronary angioplasty. *Br Heart J* 56:341–345
101. Bertrand ME, Lablanche JM, Fourrier JL, Traisnel G (1987) Percutaneous transluminal coronary angioplasty in patients with spasm superimposed on atherosclerotic narrowing. *Br Heart J* 58:469–472
102. Bertrand ME, Lablanche JM, Thieuleux FA, Fourrier JL, Traisnel G, Asseman P (1986) Comparative results of percutaneous transluminal coronary angioplasty in patients with dynamic versus fixed coronary stenosis. *J Am Coll Cardiol* 8:504–508
103. Gaasch W, Lufschavoski R, Leachman RD, Alexander JK (1974) Surgical management of Prinzmetal's variant angina. *Chest* 66:614–617
104. van Dormael MG, Chaitman BR, Ischinger T, Aker UT, Harper M, Hernandez J, Deligonul U, Kennedy HL (1985) Immediate and short-term benefit of multi lesion coronary angioplasty: influence of degree of revascularization. *J Am Coll Cardiol* 6:983–991
105. Finci L, Meier B, de Bruyne B, Steffenino G, Divernois J, Rutishauser W (1987) Angiograhic follow-up after multivessel percutaneous transluminal coronary angioplasty. *Am J Cardiol* 60:467–470
106. Dorros G, Lewin RF, Janke L (1987) Multiple Lesion transluminal coronary angioplasty in single and multivessel coronary artery disease. *J Am Coll Cardiol* 10:1007–1013
107. Myler RK, Topol EJ, Shaw RE, Stertzer SH, Clark DA (1987) Multiple vessel coronary angioplasty: Classification, results and patterns of restenosis in 494 consecutive patients. *Cath Cardiovasc Diagn* 13:1–15
108. de Feyter PJ, Suryapranata H, Serruys PW, Beatt K, van den Brand M, Hugenholtz PG (1987) Effects of successful Percutaneous Transluminal Coronary Angioplasty on global and regional left ventricular function in unstable angina pectoris. *Am J Cardiol* 60:993–997
109. de Feyter PJ, Suryapranata H, Serruys PW, Beatt K, van Domburg R, van den Brand M, Tijssen JJ, Azar AJ, Hugenholtz PG (1988) Coronary angioplasty for unstable angina: Immediate and late results in 200 consecutive patients with identification of risk factors for unfavorable early and late outcome. *J Am Coll Cardiol* 12:324–333
110. de Feyter PJ, Serruys PW, Arnold A, et al (1986) Coronary angioplasty of the unstable angina related vessel in patients with multivessel disease. *Eur Heart J* 7:460–467
111. Ilsley CAJ, Ablett MB (1986) Percutaneous transluminal coronary angioplasty in multi lesion disease: Complete versus incomplete revascularization. *Texas Heart Institute J* 13:371–376
112. Thomas ES, Most AS, Williams DO (1988) Coronary angioplasty for patients with multivessel coronary artery disease: Follow-up clinical status. *Am Heart J* 115:8–13
113. Mabin TA, Holmes DR, Smith HC et al (1985) Follow-up clinical results in patients undergoing percutaneous transluminal coronary angioplasty. *Circulation* 71:754–760
114. Wohlgelernter D, Cleman M, Highman HA, Zaret BL (1986) Percutaneous transluminal coronary angioplasty of the 'culprit reason' for management of unstable angina pectoris in patients with multivessel coronary artery disease. *Am J Cardiol* 58:460–464
115. Rentrop P, Blanke H, Karsch KR, Kaiser H, Kostering H, Leitz K (1981) Selective intracoronary thrombolysis in acute myocardial infarction and unstable angina pectoris. *Circulation* 63:307–317

116. Vetrovec GW, Leinbach RC, Gold HK, Cowley MJ (1982) Intracoronary thrombolysis in syndromes of unstable ischemia: Angiographic and clinical results. *Am Heart J* 104:946–952
117. Mandelkorn JB, Wolf NM, Singh S, Shechter JA, Kersh RI, Rodgers DM, Workman MB, Bantivoglio LG, La Porte SM, Meister SG (1983) Intracoronary Thrombus in nontransmural myocardial infarction and in unstable angina pectoris. *Am J Cardiol* 52: 1–6
118. Shapiro EP, Brinker JA, Gottlieb SO, Gusman PA, Bulkley BH (1985) Intracoronary thrombolysis 3 to 13 days after acute myocardial infarction for postinfarction angina pectoris. *Am J Cardiol* 55:1453–1458
119. Ambrose JA, Hjemdahl-Monsen C, Borrico S et al (1987) Quantitative and qualitative effects of i.c. streptokinase in unstable angina and non-q wave infarction. *J Am Coll Cardiol* 9:1156–1165
120. Gotoh K, Minamino T, Katoh O et al (1988) The role of i.c. thrombus in unstable angina: angiographic assessment and thrombolytic therapy during ongoing anginal attacks. *Circulation* 77:526–534
121. Suryapranata H, de Feyter PJ, Serruys PW (1988) Coronary angioplasty in patients with unstable angina pectoris: Is there a need for thrombolysis? *J Am Coll Cardiol* (in press)
122. Kaltenbach M, Kober G, Scherer D, Vallbracht C (1985) Recurrence rate after successful coronary angioplasty. *Eur Heart J* 6:276–281
123. Holmes Jr DR, Vlietstra RE, Smith HC, Vetrovec GW, Kent KM, Cowley MJ, Faxon DP, Gruntzig AR, Kelsey SF, Detre KM, Van Raden MJ, Mock MB (1984) Restenosis after percutaneous transluminal coronary angioplasty (PTCA). A report from the PTCA Registry of the National Heart, Lung and Blood Institute. *Am J Cardiol* 53:77C–81C
124. Leimgrüber PR, Roulin GS, Hollman J, Meier B, Douglas JS, King III SB, Gruntzig AR (1986) Restenosis after successful coronary angioplasty in patients with single-vessel disease. *Circulation* 73:710–717
125. Levine S, Ewels CJ, Rosing DR, Kent KM (1985) Coronary angioplasty: Clinical and angiographic follow-up. *Am J Cardiol* 55:673–676
126. Serruys PW, Luijten HE, Beatt KJ, Geukens R, Feyter PJ de, Brand M van den, Reiber JHC, Katen HJ ten, Es GA van, Hugenholtz PG (1988) Incidence of restenosis after successful coronary angioplasty: A time-related phenomenon. *Circulation* 77:311–371
127. Ernst J, Feltz TA, Bal ET, Bogeryn L, Berg EJM, Ascoop CAPL, Plokker HWM (1987) Longterm angiographic follow-up, cardiac events and survival in patients undergoing percutaneous transluminal coronary angioplasty *Br Heart J* 57:220–225
128. Ahmed M, Thompson R, Seabra-Gomes R,Rickards A, Yacoub M (1980) Unstable angina: A clinico arteriographic correlation and longterm results of early myocardial revascularization. *J Thorac Cardiovasc Surg* 79:609
129. Brawley RK, Merrill W, Gott VL, Donahoo JS, Watkins L, Gardner TJ (1980) Unstable angina pectoris: Factors influencing operative risk. *Ann Surg* 19:745
130. Rahimtoola SH, Nunley D, Grunkemeier G, Tepley J, Lambert L, Starr A (1983) Ten year survival after coronary bypass surgery for unstable angina. *Engl J Med* 308:676–681
131. Cohn LH, O'Neill A, Collins JJ (1985) Surgical treatment of unstable angina up to 1984. In: Hugenholtz PG, Goldman BS (eds), *Unstable Angina: Current Concepts and Management*, pp. 279–286. New York – Stuttgart: Schattauer 279–286
132. Goldman HE, Weisel RD, Christakis G, Katz A, Scully HE, Mickleborough LM, Baird RJ (1985) Predictors of outcome after coronary artery bypass graft surgery for stable and unstable angina pectoris. In: Hugenholtz PG, Goldman BS (eds), *Unstable Angina-Current Concepts and Management*, pp. 319–329. New York – Stuttgart: Schattauer
133. Mc Cormick JR, Schick EC, Mc Gabe CH, Kronmal RA, Ryan TJ (1985) Determinants of operative mortality and longterm survival in patients with unstable angina. *J Thorac Cardiovasc Surg* 89:683–699
134. Luchi RJ, Scott SM, Deupree RH et al (1987) Comparison of medical and surgical treatment for unstable angina. *NEJM* 316:977–984

24. Coronary angioplasty in patients with non-Q wave myocardial infarction

HARRY SURYAPRANATA, PIM J. DE FEYTER and
PATRIC W. SERRUYS

Introduction

The clinical course of patients with non-Q wave myocardial infarction (MI) has
been the subject of interest. Natural history studies have suggested that non-Q
wave MI is associated with less necrosis, better left ventricular function and
a lower in-hospital mortality compared with Q-wave MI. Despite this more
favourable initial prognosis, long-term survival for patients with non-Q wave MI
appears to be similar to or even less than that in patients with Q-wave MI [1–26].
The relatively high mortality rate of patients with non-Q wave MI seems to be
related to unstable angina or subsequent recurrent MI in the same area [1, 4, 6–8,
16, 19, 23–26] and may be preventable if recurrent MI can be averted with
revascularization. These findings have understandably led some to recommend
more agressive evaluation and treatment strategies for survivors of non-Q wave
MI, particularly since the benefit of prophylactic pharmacologic treatment is
unproven in this subset of patients [27–30].

The present paper reviews the natural history, pathogenesis, and the short and
long-term results of coronary angioplasty in patients with non-Q wave MI.

Natural history

The reported incidence of non-Q wave MI varies between 4–41% of all acute MI
(Table 1) and seems to be increasing [18] probably as a result of therapeutic
interventions employed before or during the acute symptomatic phase of MI that
may minimize the extent of acute myocardial damage. Although non-Q wave MI
and Q wave MI as classified by electrocardiographic results cannot always be
anatomically differentiated [7, 37], it seems likely that they differ clinically,
physiologically and prognostically as discussed by Spodick [38]. In particular,
non-Q wave MI is generally associated with smaller amounts of myocardial
necrosis, better left ventricular function and a lower incidence of in-hospital
mortality when compared with Q wave MI (Table 2). But despite this initially

P.W. Serruys, R. Simon & K.J. Beatt (eds), Percutaneous Transluminal Coronary Angioplasty. ISBN 0-7923-0346-6.
© *1990 Kluwer Academic Publishers, Dordrecht*

Table 1.   Incidence of non-Q wave myocardial infarction (NQMI).

	N	NQMI	%
Abbot 1973 [31]	230	78	35
Madias 1974 [5]	104	43	41
Rigo 1975 [12]	159	48	31
Genovese 1976 [32]	500	22	4
Cannom 1976 [11]	188	40	21
Rothkopf 1979 [33]	43	10	23
Fabricius 1979 [20]	276	98	36
Thanavaro 1980 [15]	745	124	17
Mahony 1980 [23]	635	141	22
Marmor 1981 [1]	200	58	29
BHAT Trial 1982 [27]	3837	806	21
Krone 1983 [24]	593	94	16
Coll 1983 [34]	458	28	6
Maisel 1985 [8]	1253	227	22
Connolly 1985 [13]	1221	353	29
Theroux 1986 [35]	448	157	35
Boden 1986 [36]	538	194	36
Gibson 1986 [16]	241	87	36
Huey 1987 [9]	150	35	23
Goldberg 1987 [18]	2451	882	36

Table 2.   Short-term mortality.

	Q-Wave MI patients (% mortality)	Non-Q wave MI patients (% mortality)
Norris [39]	437 (31)*	205 (12)
Schor [40]	1970 (23)*	142 (8)
Szklo [10]	953 (30)*	283 (18)
Connolly [13]	482 (24)*	422 (13)
Boxall [41]	259 (11)*	70 (1)
Thanavaro [15]	621 (11)*	125 (3)
Hutter [7]	129 (20)*	67 (9)
Bagley [42]	223 (8)*	61 (0)
Marmor [6]	215 (23)	125 (10)
Goldberg [18]	1577 (25.2)	882 (12)

Only studies with > 50 patients with non-Q-wave MI.
* p < 0.05 compared with patients with non-Q-wave MI.

favourable prognosis, evidence has accumulated that long-term mortality in these patients is similar to or even greater than that in patients with Q wave MI (Tables 3 and 4).

Despite marked improvement in pharmacologic therapy, non-Q wave MI is frequently associated with subsequent unstable angina, recurrent MI, and death. In a prospective study designed to determine the prognosis of 50 consecutive patients with non-Q wave MI, Madigan et al [17] found that unstable angina occurred in 46% of patients before discharge and that recurrent MI occurred in

Table 3. Long-term mortality.

	Follow-up months	Q-Wave MI patients (% mortality)	Non-Q wave MI patients % mortality)
Norris [39]	72	308 (48)	206 (46)
Szklo [10]	36	953 (27)	283 (28)
Fabricius-Bjerre [20]	60	127 (41)	98 (48)
Boxall [41]	32	259 (22)	70 (16)
Mahony [23]	30	342 (34)	152 (45)
Pohjola [43]	60	418 (34)	213 (20)
Hutter [7]	29	129 (42)	67 (52)
Marmor [6]	9	215 (30)	125 (27)
Krone [24]	56	499 (20)	94 (16)
Maisel [8]	12	959 (18)	277 (16)
Gibson [16]	27	154 (8)	87 (9)
Theroux [35]	12	291 (6)	157 (6)
Goldberg [18]	12	1201 (12)	792 (15)

Only studies with > 50 patients with non-Q-wave MI.

Table 4. Non-Q wave myocardial infarction (NQMI): incidence of reinfarction (RE-MI) and mortality.

	NQMI	RE-MI %	Mortality %			
			Early	1 year	2 years	5 years
Abbott 1973 [31]	78	—	23	—	—	—
Madias 1974 [5]	43	—	9	—	—	—
Rigo 1975 [12]	48	—	13	—	19	—
Madigan 1976 [17]	50	—	2	—	—	—
Cannom 1976 [11]	40	—	8	—	33	—
Kossowsky 1976 [22]	35	35	11	—	—	—
Szklo 1978 [10]	283	—	18	—	28	—
Fabricius 1979 [20]	98	—	—	—	—	49
Rothkopf 1979 [33]	10	20	—	—	—	—
Poehllman 1980 [21]	50	13	8	—	—	—
Thanavaro 1980 [15]	124	—	3	—	—	—
Hutter 1981 [7]	67	57	9	—	—	52
Marmor 1981 [1]	58	43	12	—	—	—
Hollander 1984 [25]	38	18	—	—	21	—
Maisel 1985 [8]	277	8	8	12	—	—
Connolly 1985 [13]	353	—	6	—	—	—
Zema 1985 [44]	28	—	4	—	—	—
Gibson 1986 [16]	87	18	—	9	—	—
Gibson 1986 [45]	576	7	4	—	—	—
Goldberg 1987 [18]	882	—	12	15	21	41

21% of the patients. The reported incidence of recurrent MI remains high at 6 to 86% and is associated with a poor prognosis [1, 7, 8, 10–12, 16, 22, 25, 46–48]. Maisel et al [8] reported a high mortality, both early and late, for patients with subsequent extension following a non-Q wave MI. In-hospital mortality rate in this subset of patients was 43%, while in those with Q wave MI was 15%. The one year cumulative survival rates for patients with Q vs non-Q wave MI without extension were similar: 82 and 84%. For those with extension, however, one year survival rates were 66 and 35%, respectively. This finding was supported by others [1, 6, 25, 47, 49].

Pathogenesis

The pathophysiologic basis of the apparent greater clinical instability after non-Q wave MI and the reason for loss of the initial prognostic advantage are not completely understood. The long-term prognosis of patients with non-Q wave MI may be related to the degree of potentially jeopardized myocardium. Patients with non-Q MI, appear to have more residual myocardial mass at risk as determined by exercise scintigraphy [9, 16] for subsequent ischemia or necrosis. The prevalence and extent of quantitatively determined 201-thallium redistribution within the infarct zone on exercise scintigraphy was greater in patients with non-Q wave MI than those with Q wave MI (60% vs 36%) [16]. Furthermore, a recent study [50] of regional myocardial metabolism and blood flow assessed by positron emission tomography demonstrated metabolic integrity (residual viable tissue) in 91% of infarcted regions without Q waves, whereas only 36% of the infarcted regions with Q waves showed metabolic activity. This jeopardized myocardium may be tenuously preserved by the collateral circulation, thereby favouring the development of angina, recurrent MI, and malignant ventricular arrhythmias. This hypothesis has been supported by several studies that found greater rates of angina, recurrent MI and sudden death among hospital survivors of non-Q wave MI than among those with Q wave MI [7, 11, 19].

The pathogenesis of non-Q wave MI may involve spontaneous coronary reperfusion characterized by a shorter time to peak CK level and lower peak CK values, as well as a higher prevalence of patent infarct related vessel, which may result in better left ventricular function and regional perfusion when compared to the Q wave MI [9]. Figures approach the findings in our recent thrombolytic trial [51, 52]. In this controlled randomized trial of intracoronary streptokinase, it was found that recanalization of an initially occluded infarct-related vessel was associated with a significant improvement in resting regional myocardial function of the infarct zone, implying reperfusion-related limitation in infarct size. However, the incidence of recurrent MI in the same area as the initial injury was found higher after successful thrombolytic therapy compared with control group. Of note, data from another intracoronary streptokinase study [53] also indicated more extensive exercise-induced peri-infarction ischemia in patients with open versus closed infarct-related vessel at 5 to 6 weeks after onset of MI. These findings suggest similarities between thrombolysis-treated infarcts and the naturally evolving non-Q wave MI. As such, it seems likely that as fibrinolytic therapy becomes more widely used, the pool of patients with incomplete infarctions who are at increased risk of recurrent MI will increase. The beneficial results of coronary angioplasty in acute MI [54–57], suggest that reperfusion may need to be supplemented by additional intervention following successful thrombolysis.

There is also evidence that suggests that non-Q wave MI and unstable angina share a common pathogenesis. Several studies have emphasized the important pathophysiologic link between unstable angina and non-Q wave MI [14, 58–63]. In unstable angina, the pathophysiologic process is limited to endothelial ulceration, platelet aggregation and thrombus formation, which may be intermittent, or more permanent in the presence of an adequate collateral supply. MI is related to the same process but with the formation of a totally occlusive thrombus. When the balance between intracoronary thrombus and antithrombotic natural and pharmacologic factors lean toward continued thrombus formation, persistent total coronary occlusion leading to acute MI may occur. If the coronary artery remains occluded for a long period (more than 15 min), then myocardial necrosis will occur. If very early cloty lysis occurs with or without embolization to the distal coronary bed, or if an adequate collateral supply is present, infarction will be limited (non-Q wave MI), whereas it will be extended (Q-wave MI) when no or late clot lysis occurs. The beneficial results of coronary angioplasty in patients with unstable angina have recently been reported [64].

Angiographic findings

Schulze [2] examined angiographic findings in 31 patients with Q and 17 with non-Q wave MI. There was no difference between groups with respect to the prevalence of single-, double-, or triple- vessel disease. This finding is consistent with a recently published study in 154 patients with Q wave and 87 with non-Q wave MI [65]. In contrast to Q wave MI, total coronary occlusion of the infarct-related vessel is infrequently observed in the early hours of a non-Q wave MI, but it increases moderately in frequency over the next several days [14]. Several angiographic studies [9, 14, 16, 17, 66] have demonstrated that patients with non-Q wave MI had a lower incidence of a totally occluded infarct related vessel, ranging from 32 to 48%, when compared to those with Q wave MI. The incidence of collateral circulation to the area supplied by occluded vessel in this subset of patients was higher, ranging from 85 to 93%, when compared to those with Q wave MI. The essential finding of these studies is that some degree of perfusion, either antegrade or by means of collateral vessels, is present soon after non-Q wave MI, although it is insufficient to prevent the initial necrosis. Thus, it appears that the anatomical distribution of coronary artery disease in those with non-Q wave MI resembles that of patients with Q wave MI, but that viable amounts of myocardium may be protected from further necrosis by the presence of a subtotal occlusion or collateral circulation. These findings have been supported by post mortem studies [67, 68].

Furthermore, a specific angiographic morphology frequently present in patients with unstable angina, as described by Ambrose et al, is also found in patients with non-Q wave MI [62]. This eccentric convex intraluminal obstruction with a narrow neck resulting from one or more irregular overhanging edges was found in 65% of ischemia-related coronary arteries in patients with non-Q wave MI [62]. This similarity in coronary morphology suggests once again a similar pathogenesis as previously suggested. Therefore, the management of patients with non-Q wave MI should be similar to patients with unstable angina.

Therapeutic implications

Presently, there is little proven specific pharmacologic therapy for patients with non-Q wave MI. Randomized trials in postinfarction patients using long-term beta-adrenergic blockade have yielded confliction results when data are analyzed according to the presence or absence of electrocardiographic Q waves. The Beta-blocker Heart Attack Trial [27] demonstrated reduced mortality with propranolol compared with placebo in 2858 patients with Q wave MI, but showed no effect in 873 patients with non-Q wave MI. By comparison, the Norwegian Timolol Trial [30] found prolonged survival in timolol-treated patients regardless of infarct type; however, the incidence of reinfarction was reduced only in patients with Q wave MI. Although several animal studies have shown that calcium-channel blockers can protect ischemic myocardium at risk for MI [69–71], only a few clinical trials of patients with non-Q wave MI have been reported. The results of a recently published study indicated that treatment with diltiazem for up to 14 days has a protective effect against reinfarction and severe angina [45].

The problems of definitive therapy and the timing of therapy are more difficult. The high incidence of recurrent MI and unstable angina in patients with non-Q wave MI support the concept of myocardial salvage through recanalization, for one might postulate that these patients were left with an "incomplete MI" and an area of the myocardium "at risk", and have understandably led some to recommend more aggressive evaluation and treatment strategies for survivors of non-Q wave MI. Several investigators suggest that coronary bypass surgery or coronary angioplasty is feasible and safe for patients with angina after non-Q wave MI [72–76].

The first reports [77–84] of patients undergoing surgical revascularization early after myocardial infarction noted an increased operative mortality compared with that in other patients undergoing revascularization months or years after MI. Patients treated surgically within the first 7 days after MI experienced twice the mortality of those treated surgically after 8 to 30 days and more than threefold the mortality of those treated surgically more than 30 days after MI [82]. However, continuing improvement in surgical techniques, development of effective methods of intraoperative myocardial protection and improvement in postoperative care, associated with the consequent lower mortality and better long-term results [85–88], have restored enthusiasm among some surgeons for revascularization in patients with angina early after MI. Several investigators [74–76] have demonstrated that surgical intervention is feasible and safe early in the course of non-Q wave MI with the incidence of perioperative MI between 1 to 10.7%, incidence of in-hospital death between 1.9 to 3.6%, late death in 1% and angina-free survival between 68 to 96% during follow-up period of 15 to 29 months. In fact, Aintablian [75] found no difference in early graft closure rate, improvement in wall motion, development of new Q wave, or angina-free survival when compared to the group of patients undergoing bypass surgery for stable or unstable angina. Williams [76] have shown that revasvularization can be accomplished with acceptable mortality even within 30 days of acute MI.

In the ten years since the beginning of coronary angioplasty [89], this technique has expanded from a curiosity to a major therapeutic alternative for patients needing revascularization. Recently, the initial restricted indications have been widened to include dilatation of complex lesions, multivessel lesions and vein graft. The results of two recently published data [72, 73] suggest that coronary angioplasty is an effective initial treatment strategy in the management of patients with non-Q wave MI. Safian et al [72] reported the short- and long-term results of coronary angioplasty in 68 consecutive patients with angina, an average of 2.3 months, after non-Q wave MI (41 anterior and 27 inferior). Coronary angioplasty was successful in 87% of the patients. Long-term follow-up (average 17 ± 10 months) was obtained in patients in whom coronary angioplasty was successful. Recurrent angina developed in 41% (24/58), but was relieved by repeat coronary angioplasty in 14, by late coronary artery bypass surgery in 4 and by pharmacologic therapy in 6. There was one non-fatal MI, due to progressive disease in a non-dilated vessel, and one non-cardiac death. At last follow-up, 79% of the patients with initially successful angioplasty were asymptomatic.

Between January 1982 and January 1987, 116 patients underwent coronary angioplasty in our institution, for angina either at rest or during submaximal exercise despite optimal pharmacologic therapy, a median of 31 (range 2–362) days after a non-Q wave MI. They represented 8% of our total coronary angioplasty population during the study period. Non-Q wave MI was defined as prolonged chest pain compatible with acute MI, associated with electrocardiographic ST-segment and T-wave abnormalities without progression to pathologic Q-waves, but with abnormal elevation of the creatinine kinase level (at least twice of the normal value) before any intervention. Post-infarction angina was considered unstable if it occurred at rest lasting for at least 15 min, associated with electrocardiographic manifestations of myocardial ischemia without evidence of further myocardial necrosis. Patients were selected for coronary angioplasty if the ischemia-related lesion was suitable for dilatation. The selection was based only on the symptoms and the coronary anatomy and was not influenced by left ventricular function. Angioplasty was considered successful when a reduction of the severity of the obstruction to less than 50% luminal diameter narrowing was achieved with abolition of acute ischemic symptoms without progression to MI, emergency surgery, or death. Clinical and angiographic data are summarized in Table 5.

Table 5. Clinical characteristics.

N	116
Male/Female	89/27
Age (median, yr)	57 (range 31–74)
Previous CABG	4
Previous PTCA	9
Anterior/Inferior non-Q MI	74/42
Peak CK enzyme level (median, U/1)	357 (range 206–972)
Stable angina pectoris	62
Unstable angina pectoris	54
Median time from MI to PTCA (days)	31 (range 2–362)
Single/double/triple vessel disease	75/33/8
Total occlusion	22
Single vessel dilatation	101
Multivessel dilatation	15
Initial global ejection fraction (%)	58 ± 8 (range 32–71)

Abbreviations: CABG = coronary artery bypass graft; PTCA = percutaneous transluminal coronary angioplasty; MI = myocardial infarction; CK = creatinine phosphokinase.

Table 6. Angiographic data.

PTCA vessel	N	Primary success
LAD	79	71 (90%)
RCA	31	27 (87%)
LCX	20	16 (80%)
Bypass graft	2	1 (50%)
Total	132	115 (87%)

Abbreviations: LAD = left anterior descending coronary artery; RCA = right coronary artery; LCX = left circumflex.

From the 116 patients who underwent coronary angioplasty for angina after a non-Q wave MI, 132 lesions were dilated (Table 6). Success was achieved in dilating the obstructed vessel in 99 patients (115 lesions). Fig. 1 shows the clinical outcome of all patients. Electrocardiographic exercise testing was obtained in 71% (70 of 99) of the patients, 8 (range 1 to 49) months, after initially successful angioplasty (Fig 2). The average maximum workload achieved, predicted for age, sex, and height, was 98% (range 54 to 131%).

Clinical follow-up was obtained in all patients, at a mean interval of 20 (3–59) months, and summarized in Table 7. If coronary artery bypass surgery, recurrent MI, death or recurrent angina requiring pharmacologic therapy are considered events, 74% of the patients were event-free at 20 months after successful angioplasty, while if any cardiac recurrence, including repeat coronary angioplasty, are considered events, only 63% of patients were event-free during follow-up (Fig 3).

In addition, sequential left ventricular angiograms, before and 6 (range 2–8) months after coronary angioplasty, of adequate quality sufficient to allow

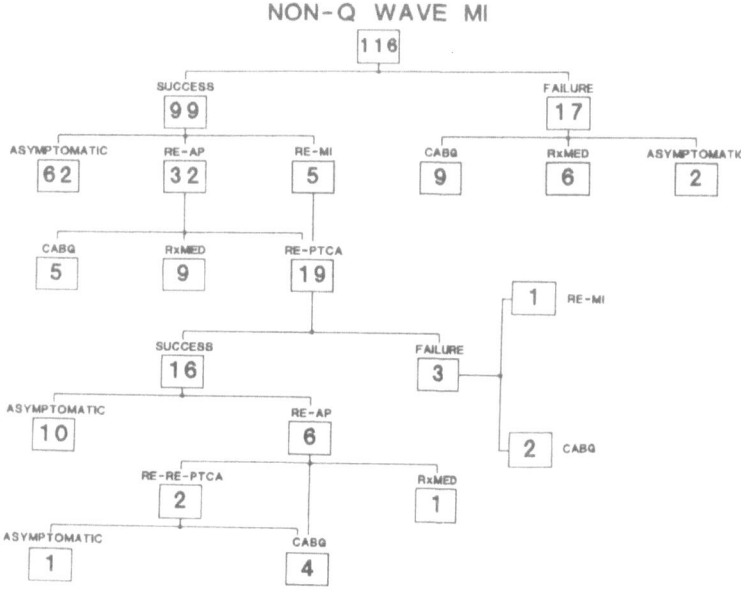

Figure 1. Short- and long-term (mean of 20 months) follow-up in 116 patients undergoing coronary angioplasty (PTCA) for severe angina (AP) after a non-Q wave myocardial infarction (MI). CABG = coronary artery bypass grafting; Rx Med = controlled by pharmacologic treatment.

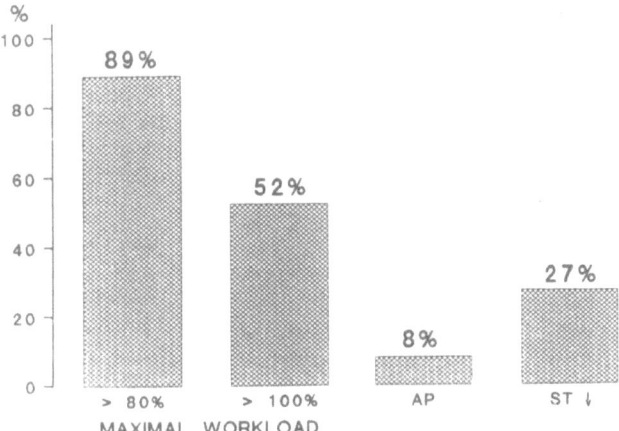

Figure 2. Results of electrocardiographic exercise testing (n = 70), 8 (range 1–49) months after initially successful angioplasty. A maximum workload of >80% and >100% predicted for age, sex and height was achieved in 89% and 52% of the patients, respectively. The majority of the patients (92%) were symptom-free during the test; ST-segment depression was documented in 27%.

Table 7. Mean clinical follow-up of 20 (range 3–59) months.

	Initial success n = 99	Failure n = 17
Death	0	1
Emergency CABG	0	7
MI related to PTCA	0	5
Late recurrent MI	6	0
Repeat PTCA	13	0
Repeat PTCA + CABG	6	0
Late CABG	5	2
Pharmacologic therapy	9	6
Event-free	62	2

Abbreviations: See Table 5.

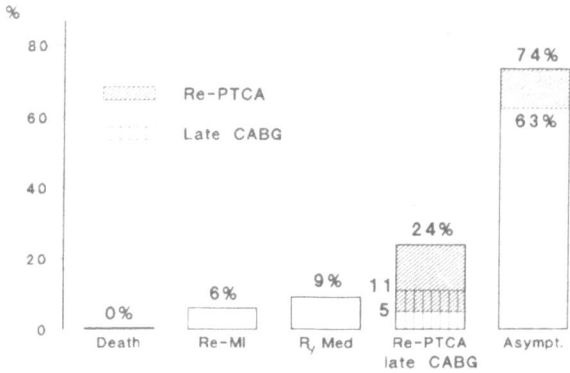

Figure 3. If coronary artery bypass surgery (CABG), recurrent myocardial infarction (re-MI), death or recurrent angina requiring pharmacologic therapy (R/Med) are considered events, 74% of the patients were event-free (Asympt.) at 20 months after initially successful angioplasty, while if any cardiac recurrence, including repeat coronary angioplasty (Re-PTCA) is considered an event, only 63% of patients were event-free.

quantitative analysis of global and regional left ventricular function [90] were obtained in a subset of patients undergoing successful coronary angioplasty [91]. Table 8 shows the sequential changes in the global and regional left ventricular function before coronary angioplasty and at follow-up angiography [91]. The global ejection fraction increased significantly from $60 \pm 9\%$ to $67 \pm 6\%$ (p = 0.0003), and this was due to significant decrease in end-systolic volume from 29 ± 12 to $24 \pm 6 \, ml/m^2$. This significant increase in the global ejection fraction was primarily due to a significant improvement in the regional contribution to ejection fraction of the infarct zone, as shown in Table 8.

Table 8. Global and regional left ventricular function (n = 36).

	Before PTCA	At 6 months follow-up	p-value
Global LV function			
EDV ml/m²	73 ± 17	71 ± 15	ns
ESV ml/m²	29 ± 12	24 ± 6	0.006
SV ml/m²	44 ± 12	47 ± 11	0.08
EF %	60 ± 9	67 ± 6	0.0003
Regional LV function			
Infarcted area (%)	12.6 ± 4.8	20.1 ± 7.7	10^{-8}
Non-infarcted area (%)	46.4 ± 11.9	44.5 ± 11.9	0.007

Abbreviations: PTCA = percutaneous transluminal coronary angioplasty, EDV = end-diastolic volume; ESV = end-systolic volume; SV = stroke volume; EF = global ejection fraction.

Conclusion

The results indicate not only that coronary angioplasty can be performed safely and effectively in patients with angina early after a non-Q wave MI, but also that the incidence of late recurrent MI and cardiac death are lower than expected. However, recurrent angina occurred in 32% of our patients after initially successful angioplasty, figures similar to that reported for stable angina [92]. All were satisfactorily treated by repeat coronary angioplasty, coronary bypass surgery or pharmacologic therapy. Furthermore, detailed analysis of serial global and regional left ventricular function demonstrated the additional benefit of correcting the residual obstructive lesion. This finding confirmed once again the hypothesis that these patients were left with an incomplete MI and an area of the myocardium at risk as determined by exercise thallium scintigraphy [16] and by positron emission tomography [50].

The benefits of coronary angioplasty after a non-Q wave MI are limited, when the artery is occluded at the time of attempted angioplasty, even when recanalization is initially successful [73]. In keeping this in mind, together with the fact that recurrent MI occurred early after a non-Q wave MI [25], suggest that coronary angioplasty should be performed early after a non-Q wave MI.

Although the majority of patients undergoing angioplasty following non-Q wave MI had a single-vessel disease with relatively small to moderate enzymatic infarct size and might be expected to have a favorable outcome. These patients constitute a high-risk subgroup because of the presence of ongoing angina, either at rest or during submaximal exercise, despite optimal pharmocologic therapy. The incidence of angina recurring after acute MI varies from 18 to 57% [1, 7, 16, 17, 45, 46, 49]. Such early post MI angina carries a poor short-and long-term prognosis [1, 7, 10–12, 16, 46, 47]. Persistent or recurrent angina after MI implies that the cardiac event is not yet complete and suggests that more aggressive invasive management might improve clinical status and might salvage myocardium. Our policy over the last few years has been to offer coronary angioplasty to selected patients with angina, who early after acute MI are either refractory to pharmacologic therapy or who experience angina induced by mild exertion despite initial response to maximal pharmacologic therapy. A randomized study between early angioplasty and continued medical management is perhaps the only way to provide clear insight into the relative merits of early angioplasty. Nevertheless, selected patients in whom pharmacologic therapy has failed can undergo coronary angioplasty early after a non-Q wave MI.

References

1. Marmor A, Sobel BE, Roberts R (1981) Factors presaging early recurrent myocardial infarction ('extension'). *Am J Cardiol* 48:603–610
2. Schulze RA, Pitt B, Griffith LSC, Ducci HH, Achuff SC, Baird MG, Humphries J (1978) Coronary angiography and left ventriculography in survival of transmural and non transmural myocardial infarction. *Am J Med* 64:108–113
3. Geltman EM, Ehsani AA, Campbell MK, Schechtman K, Roberts R, Sobel BE (1979) The influence of location and extent of myocardial infarction on long term ventricular dysrhytmia and mortality. *Circulation* 60:805–814
4. Friedberg CK (1972) Introduction to symposium on myocardial infarction. *Circulation* 45:179–188
5. Madias JE, Chahine RA, Gorlin R, Blacklow DJ (1974) A comparison of transmural and nontransmural acute myocardial infarction. *Circulation* 49:498–507
6. Marmor A, Geltman EM, Schechtman K, Sobel BE, Roberts R (1982) Recurrent myocardial infarction: Clinical predictors and prognostic implications. *Circulation* 66:415–421
7. Hutter AM, De Sanctis RW, Flynn T, Yeatman LA (1981) Nontransmural myocardial infarction: A comparison of hospital and late clinical course of patients with that of matched patients with transmural anterior and transmural inferior myocardial infarction. *Am J Cardiol* 48:595–602
8. Maisel AS, Ahnve S, Gilpin E, Henning H, Goldberger AL, Collins D, Le Winter M, Ross J Jr (1985) Prognosis after extension of myocardial infarct: the role of Q-wave or non-Q wave infarction. *Circulation* 71:211–217
9. Huey BL, Gheorghiade M, Crampton RS, Beller GA, Kaiser DL, Watson DD, Nygaard TW, Craddock GB, Sayre SL, Gibson RS (1987) Acute non-Q wave myocardial infarction associated with early ST segment elevation: Evidence for spontaneous coronary reperfusion and implications for thrombolytic trials. *J AM Coll Cardiol* 9:18–25
10. Szklo M, Goldberg R, Kennedy HL, Tonascia JA (1978) Survival of patients with nontransmural myocardial infarction: A population-based study. *Am J Cardiol* 42:648–652
11. Cannom DS, Levy W, Cohen LS (1976) The short- and long-term prognosis of patients with transmural and nontransmural myocardial infarction. *Am J Med* 61:452–458
12. Rigo P, Murrary M, Taylor DR, Weisfeldt ML, Strauss HW, Pitt B (1975) Hemodynamic and prognostic findings in patients with transmural and nontransmural infarction. *Circulation* 51:1064–1070
13. Connolly DC, Elveback LR (1985) Coronary heart disease in residents of Rochester, Minnesota VI: Hospital and post hospital course of patients with transmural and subendocardial myocardial infarction. *Mayo Clin Proc* 60:375–381
14. De Wood MA, Stifter WF, Simpson CS, Spores J, Eugster GS, Judge TP, Hinnen ML (1986) Coronary arteriorgraphic findings soon after non-Q wave myocardial infarction. *N Engl J Med* 315:417–423

15. Thanavaro S, Krone RJ, Kleiger RE, Province MA, Miller JP, Demello VR, Oliver GC (1980) In-hospital prognosis of patients with first nontransmural and transmural infarctions. *Circulation* 61:29–33

16. Gibson RS, Beller GA, Gheorghiade M, Nygaard TW, Watson DD, Huey BL, Sayre SL, Kaiser DL (1986) The prevalence and clinical significance of residual myocardial ischemia 2 weeks after uncomplicated non-Q wave infarction: A prospective natural history study. *Circulation* 73:1186–1198

17. Madigan NP, Rutherford BD, Frye RL (1976) The clinical course, early prognosis and coronary anatomy of subendocardial infarction. *Am J Med* 60:634–641

18. Goldberg RJ, Gore JM, Alpert JS, Dalen JE (1987) Non-Q wave myocardial infarction: Recent changes in occurrence and prognosis. A community-wide perspective. *Am Heart J* 113:273–279

19. Lekakis J, Katsoyanni K, Trichopoulos D, Tsitouris G (1984) Q-versus non-Q wave myocardial infarction: Clinical characteristics and 6-month prognosis. *Clin Cardiol* 7:283–288

20. Fabricius-Bjerre N, Munkvad M, Knudsen JB (1979) Subendocardial and transmural myocardial infarction: a five year survival study. *Am J Med* 66:986–990

21. Poehlman JH, Silverman ME (1980) Clinical characteristics, electrocardiographic and enzyme correlations, and long-term prognosis of patients with chest pain associated with ST depression and/or T wave inversion. *Am Heart J* 99:173–180

22. Kossowsky WA, Mohr BD, Rafii S, Lyon AF (1976) Superimposition of transmural infarction following acute subendocardial infarction: How frequent? *Chest* 69:758–761

23. Mahony C, Hindman MC, Aronin N, Wagner GS (1980) Prognostic differences in subgroups of patients with electrocardiographic evidence of subendocardial or transmural myocardial infarction. *Am J Med* 69:183–186

24. Krone RJ, Friedman E, Thanavaro S, Miller JP, Kleiger RE, Oliver GC (1983) Long-term prognosis after first Q-wave (transmural) or non-Q-wave (nontransmural) myocardial infarction: analysis of 593 patients. *Am J Cardiol* 52:234–239

25. Hollander G, Ozick H, Greengart A, Shani J, Lichstein E (1984) High mortality early reinfarction with first nontransmural myocardial infarction. *Am Heart J* 108:1412–1416

26. Löfmark R (1979) Clinical features in patients with recurrent myocardial infarction. *Acta Med Scand* 206:367–370

27. Beta-Blocker Heart Attack Research Group (1982) A randomized trial of propranolol in patients with acute myocardial infarction: Mortality results. *JAMA* 247:1707–1714.

28. Norwegian Multicenter Study Group (1981) Timolol-induced reduction in mortality and reinfarction in patients surviving acute myocardial infarction. *N Engl J Med* 304:801–807

29. Miami Trial Research Group (1985) Metoprolol in acute myocardial infarction: mortality. *Am J Cardiol* 56:15G

30. Overskeid K, Abrahamsen AM, Frisvold OJ, von der Lippe G, Lund-Johansen P, Pedersen S (1981) Timolol after myocardial infarction. *N Engl J Med* 305:407–408

31. Abbot JA, Scheinman MM (1973) Nondiagnostic electrocardiogram in patients with acute myocardial infarction. *Am J Med* 55:608–613

32. Genovese MG, Salaki JS, Kennedy RJ, Grace WJ (1976) Subendocardial infarction: what happens later. *Am Heart J* 72:542–543

33. Rothkopf M, Boerner J, Stone MJ, Smitherman TC, Buja LM, Parkey RW, Willerson JT (1979) Detection of myocardial infarct extension by CK-B radioimmunoassay. *Circulation* 59:268–274

34. Coll S, Castaner A, Sanz G, Roig E, Magrina J, Navarro-Lopez F, Betriu A (1983) Prevalence and prognosis after a first nontransmural myocardial infarction. *Am J Cardiol* 51:1584–1588

35. Theroux P, Kouz S, Bosch X, Waters DD, Roy D, Pelletier GB, Dyrda I (1986) Clinical and angiographic features of non-Q-wave and Q-wave myocardial infarction (abstr). *Circulation* 74 (II):303

36. Boden WE, Kleiger RE, Capone RJ et al. (1986) Sequential ECG, enzymatic and demographic features in a large prospective randomized trial of 538 non-Q wave myocardial infarction patients (abstr). *Clin Res* 34:284A

37. Savage RM, Wagner GS, Ideker RE, Podolsky SA, Hackel DB (1977) Correlation of postmortem anatomic findings with electrocardiographic changes in patients with myocardial infarction:

retrospective study of patients with typical anterior and posterior infarcts. *Circulation* 55:279–285

38. Spodick DH (1983) Q-wave infarction versus ST infarction: Non-specificity of electrocardiographic criteria for differentiating transmural and nontransmural lesions. *Am J Cardiol* 51:913–915

39. Norris RM, Caughey DE, Deeming LW, Mercer CJ, Scott PJ (1970) Coronary prognostic index for predicting survival after recovery from acute myocardial infarction. *Lancet* 2:485

40. Schor S, Shani M, Modan B (1975) Factors affecting immediate mortality of patients with acute myocardial infarction: a nationwide study. *Chest* 68:217

41. Boxall J, Saltups A (1980) A comparison of nontransmural and transmural myocardial infarction. *Aust NZ J Med* 10:176

42. Bagley N, Hung D, Pennington C, Sloman JG (1982) Subendocardial myocardial infarction. *Aust NZ J Med* 12:166

43. Pohjola A, Siltanen P, Romo M (1980) Five-year survival of 728 patients after myocardial infarction. A community study. *Br Heart J* 43:176

44. Zema MJ (1985) Q-wave, ST segment, and T-wave myocardial infarction. *Am J Med* 78:391–398

45. Gibson RS, Borden WE, Théroux P, Strauss HD, Pratt CM, Gheorghiade M, Capone RJ, Crawford MH, Schlant RC, Kleiger RE, Young PH, Schechtman K, Perryman MB, Roberts R, and the Diltiazem Reinfarction Study Group (1986) Diltiazem and reinfarction in patients with non-Q-wave myocardial infarction: results of a double-blind, randomized multicenter trial. *N Engl J Med* 315:423–429

46. Stenson RE, Flamm MD, Zaret BL, McGowan RG (1975) Transient ST-segment elevation with postmyocardial infarction angina: Prognostic significance. *Am Heart J* 89:449–454

47. Fraker TD, Wagner GS, Rosati RA (1979) Extension of myocardial infarction: incidence and prognosis. *Circulation* 60:1126–1129

48. Reid PR, Taylor DR, Kelly DT (1974) Myocardial infarct extension detection by precordial ST-segment mapping. *N Engl J Med* 290:123–128

49. Buda AJ, MacDonald IL, Dubbin JD, Orr SA, Strauss HD (1983) Myocardial infarct extension: prevalence, clinical significance, and problems in diagnosis. *Am Heart J* 105:744–749

50. Hashimoto T, Kambara H, Fudo T, Hayashi M, Tamaki S, Tokunaga S, Tamaki N, Yonekura Y, Konishi J, Kawai C (1988) Non-Q wave versus Q wave myocardial infarction: regional myocardial metabolism and blood flow assessed by positron emisson tomography. *J Am Coll Cardiol* 12:88–93

51. Simoons ML, Serruys PW, van den Brand M, Res J, Verheugt FWA, Krauss XH, Remme WJ, Bär F, De Zwaan C, van der Laarse A, Vermeer F, Lubsen J (1986) Early thrombolysis in acute myocardial infarction: limitation of infarct size and improved survival. *J Am Coll Cardiol* 7:717–728.

52. Serruys PW, Simoons ML, Suryapranata H, Vermeer F, Wijns W, van den Brand M, Bär F, Krauss XH, Remme WJ, Res J, Verheugt FWA, van Domburg R, Lubsen J, Hugenholtz PG (1986) Preservation of global and regional left ventricular function after early thrombolysis in acute myocardial infarction. *J Am Coll Cardiol* 7:729–742

53. Melin JA, DeCoster PM, Renkin J, Detry J-MR, Beckers C, Col J (1985) Effects of intracoronary thrombolytic therapy on exercise-induced ischemia after acute myocardial infarction. *Am J Cardiol* 56:705

54. Meyer J, Merx W, Schmitz H, Erbel R, Kiesslich T, Dörr R, Lambertz H, Bethge C, Krebs W, Bardos P, Minale C, Messmer BJ, Effert S (1982) Percutaneous transluminal coronary angioplasty immediately after intracoronary streptolysis of transmural infarction. *Circulation* 66:905–913

55. Erbel R, Pop T, Henrichs KJ, Olshausen K von, Schuster CJ, Rupprecht HJ, Stekernagel C, Meyer J (1986) Percutaneous transluminal coronary angioplasty after thrombolytic therapy: A prospective controlled randomized trial. *J Am Coll Cardiol* 8:485–495

56. O'Neill W, Timmis GC, Bourdillon PD, Lai P, Ganghadsran V, Walton J, Ramos R, Laufer N, Gordon S, Schork A, Pitt B (1986) A prospective randomized clinical trial of intracoronary versus coronary angioplasty for acute myocardial infarction. *N Engl J Med* 314:812–818

57. Suryapranata H, Serruys PW, de Feyter PJ, van den Brand M, Beatt K, van Domburg R, Kint

PP, Hugenholtz PG (1988) Coronary angioplasty immediately after thrombolysis in 115 consecutive patients with acute myocardial infarction. *Am Heart J* 115:519–529

58. Davies MJ, Thomas DC (1985) Plaque fissuring: The cause of acute myocardial infarction, sudden ischemic death and crescendo angina. *Br Heart J* 53:363–371
59. Falk E (1985) Unstable angina with fatal outcome: Dynamic coronary thrombosis leading to infarction or sudden death. *Circulation* 71:699–708
60. Ambrose JA, Winters SL, Arora RR, Heft JL, Goldstein J, Rentrop KP, Gorlin R, Fuster V (1985) Coronary angiographic morphology in myocardial infarction: A link between the pathogenesis of unstable angina and myocardial infarction. *J Am Coll Cardiol* 6:1233–1238
61. Gorlin R, Fuster V, Ambrose JA (1986) Anatomic-physiologic link between acute coronary syndromes. *Circulation.* 74:6–9
62. Ambrose JA, Hjemdahl-Monsen CE, Borrico S, Gorlin R, Fuster V (1988) Angiographic demonstration of a common link between unstable angina pectoris and non-Q wave acute myocardial infarction. *Am J Cardiol* 61:244–247
63. Mandelkorn JB, Wolff NM, Singh S, Schechter JA, Kersh RI, Rodgers DM, Workman MB, Bentivoglio LG, La Porte SM, Meister SG (1983) Intracoronary thrombus in nontransmural myocardial infarction and in unstable angina pectoris. *Am J Cardiol* 52:1–6
64. de Feyter PJ, Serruys PW, van den Brand M, Balakumaran K, Mochtar B, Soward AL, Arnold AER, Hugenholtz PG (1985) Emergency coronary angioplasty in refractory unstable angina. *E Engl J Med* 313:342–347
65. Gibson RS (1987) Clinical, functional, and angiographic distinctions between Q wave and non-Q wave myocardial infarction: Evidence of spontaneous reperfusion and implications for intervention trials. *Circulation* 75(V):128–138
66. Nicholson MR, Roubin GS, Bernstein L, Harris PJ, Kelly DT (1983) Prognosis after initial non-Q wave myocardial infarction related to coronary arterial anatomy. *Am J Cardiol* 52:462–465
67. Davies MJ, Woolf N, Robertson WB (1976) Pathology of acute myocardial infarction with particular reference to occlusive coronary thrombi. *Br Heart J* 38:659–664
68. Freifeld AG, Schuster EH, Bulkley BH (1983) Nontransmural versus transmural myocardial infarction. A morphologic study. *Am J Med* 75:423–432
69. Yellon DM, Hearse DJ, Maxwell MP, Chambers DE, Downey JM (1981) Sustained limitations of myocardial necrosis 24 hours after coronary artery occlusion: verapamil infusion in dogs with small myocardial infarcts. *Am J Cardiol* 51:1409
70. Klein HH, Schubothe M, Nebendahl K, Kreuzer H (1984) The effects of two different diltiazem treatments on infarct size in ischemic, reperfused porcine hearts. *Circulation* 69:1000
71. Melin JA, Becker LC, Hutchins GM (1984) Protective effects of early and late treatments with nifedipine during myocardial infarction in the conscious dog. *Circulation* 69:131
72. Safian RD, Snyder LD, Synder BA, McKay RG, Lorell BH, Aroesty JM, Pasternak RC, Bradley AB, Monrad ES, Baim DS (1987) Usefulness of percutaneous transluminal coronary angioplasty for unstable angina pectoris after non-Q wave acute myocardial infarction. *Am J Cardiol* 59:263–266
73. Suryapranata H, Beatt K, de Feyter PJ, Verrostte J, van den Brand M, Zijlstra F, Serruys PW (1988) Percutaneous transluminal coronary angioplasty for angina pectoris after a non-Q acute infarction. *Am J Cardiol* 61:240–243
74. Madigan NP, Rutherford BD, Barnhorst DA, Danielson GK (1977) Early saphenous vein grafting after subendocardial infarction: Immediate surgical results and late prognosis. *Circulation* 56 (suppl II):1–3
75. Aintablian A, Hamby RI, Weiss D, Hoffman I, Voleti CO, Wisoff BG (1978) Results of aortocoronary bypass surgery grafting in patients with subendocardial infarction: Late follow-up. *Am J Cardiol* 42:183–186
76. Williams DB, Ivey TD, Bailey WW, Irey SJ, Rideout JT, Stewart D (1983) Postinfarction angina: Results of early revascularization, *J Am Coll Cardiol* 2:859–864
77. Johnson WD, Flemma RJ, Lepley D Jr (1970) Direct coronary surgery utilizing multiple-vein bypass grafts. *Ann Thorac Surg* 9:436–444
78. Cohn LH, Fogarty TJ, Daily PO (1972) Emergency coronary artery bypass. *Surgery* 10:821–829

79. Favaloro RG, Effler DB, Cheanvechai C (1971) Acute coronary insufficiency (impending myocardial infarction and myocardial infarction): surgical treatment by the saphenous vein graft technique. *Am J. Cardiol* 28:598–613

80. Piffarre R, Spinazzola A, Nemickas R, Scanlon PJ, Tobin JR (1971) Emergency aorto-coronary bypass for acute myocardial infarction. *Arch Surg* 103:525–528

81. Sustaita H, Chatterjee K, Matloff JM (1972) Emergency bypass surgery in impending and complicated acute myocardial infarction. *Arch Surg* 105:30–35

82. Dawson JT, Hall RJ, Hallman GL, Cooley DA (1974) Mortality in patients undergoing coronary artery bypass surgery after myocardial infarction. *Am J Cardiol* 33:483–486

83 Hill JD, Kerth WJ, Kelly JJ, et al. (1971) Emergency aortocoronary bypass for impending or extending myocardial infarction. *Circulation* 43, 44 (suppl:I):105–110

84. Reul GJ, Morris GC, Howell JF, Crawford ES, Sterlter WJ (1973) Emergency coronary artery bypass grafts in the treatment of myocardial infarction. *Circulation* 47, 48 (suppl III):127–131

85. Levine FH, Gold HK, Leinbach RC, Daggett WM, Austen WG, Buckley MJ (1979) Safe early revascularization for continuing ischemia after acute myocardial infarction. *Circulation* 60 (suppl I):5

86. Jones EL, Waites TF, Craver JM, Bradford JM, Douglas JS, King SB, Bone DK, Dorney ER, Clements SD, Thompkins T, Hatcher CR (1981) Coronary bypass for relief of persistent pain following acute myocardial infarction. *Ann Thorac Surg* 32:33

87. Nunley DL, Grunkemeier GL, Teply JF, Abbruzzese PA, Savis JS, Khonsari S, Starr A (1983) Coronary bypass operation following acute complicated myocardial infarction. *J Thorac Cardiovasc Surg* 85:485

88. Singh AK, Rivera R, Cooper GN, Karlson KE (1985) Early myocardial revascularization for post-infarction angina: Results and longterm follow-up. *J Am Coll Cardiol* 6:1121–1125

89. Gruntzig AR, Senning A, Siegenthaler WE (1979) Non-operative dilatation of coronary artery stenosis: Percutaneous transluminal coronary angioplasty. *N Engl J Med* 301:61–67

90. Slager CJ, Hooghoudt TEH, Serruys PW, Schuurbiers JCH, Reiber JHC, Meester GT, Verdouw PD, Hugenholtz PG (1986) Quantitative assessment of regional left ventricular motion using endocardial landmarks. *J Am Coll Cardiol* 7:317–326

91. Suryapranata H, Serruys PW, Beatt K, de Feyter PJ, van den Brand M, Roelandt J (1989) Recovery of regional myocardial dysfunction following successful coronary angioplasty early after a non-Q wave myocardial infarction. *Am Heart J* (in press)

92. Meier B, King SB, Gruentzig AR (1984) Repeat coronary angioplasty. *J Am Coll Cardiol* 4:463–466

25. Thrombolytic therapy and PTCA in acute myocardial thrombosis

M.L. SIMOONS, P.J. DE FEYTER and H. SURYAPRANATA

The role of reperfusion by thrombolytic therapy in patients with evolving myocardial infarction has been established by a large number of trials [1–7]. Myocardial infarction is caused in most patients by thrombotic occlusion of a major coronary vessel. Timely lysis of this thrombus results in salvage of myocardial tissue, preservation of regional myocardial function and thus in improved early- and long-term survival. However, in many patients a severe stenosis remains after thrombolytic therapy which may result in recurrent ischemia, reinfarction, and loss of the initial gain of thrombolysis. PTCA immediately after thrombolysis can reduce this residual stenosis and further improve coronary blood flow [8, 9]. Furthermore PTCA can be used to perforate persistent occlusions and reperfuse the myocardium when thrombolysis fails. Thus immediate PTCA would be expected to result in a higher rate of coronary patency then thrombolytic therapy. After PTCA the improved coronary blood flow might further limit infarct size and preserve left ventricular function. Furthermore the rate of recurrent ischemia and reinfarction would be reduced and survival improved. In clinical practice however, these expectations were not fulfilled. In this review the effects of early PTCA in patients with coronary thrombosis on the above mentioned factors are analysed.

Coronary patency after thrombolysis and PTCA

Intracoronary- or intravenous infusion of a thrombolytic drug causes gradual resolution of intracoronary thrombus [10]. The number of patients with a patent infarct related vessel in a given study will depend not only on the drug used, its doses and the mode of administration, but also on the timing of angiography. Unfortunately, non-invasive signs to estimate coronary patency are unreliable, and angiography remains mandatory to establish patency after administration of a thrombolytic drug [11]. In Table 1, the results of early angiography during or after various interventions in patients with evolving myocardial infarction are presented [12–26]. The highest patency figures have been reported after

P.W. Serruys, R. Simon & K.J. Beatt (eds), Percutaneous Transluminal Coronary Angioplasty. ISBN 0-7923-0346-6.
© *1990 Kluwer Academic Publishers, Dordrecht*

Table 1. Patency of the infarct related vessel.

		Patency %	References
No thrombolysis		20	[12, 13]
Streptokinase	iv	40–60	[13, 14, 15]
Streptokinase	ic	70–90	[1, 13, 16, 17]
Double chain rt-PA	iv	65–75	[14, 15, 18]
Single chain rt-PA	iv	70–90	[19, 20, 21, 22]
APSAC	iv	64	[23]
Direct PTCA		83–95	[24, 25, 26]

Patency of the infarct related coronary artery at angiography 60 to 90 minutes after initiation of thrombolytic therapy, or after direct PTCA without thrombolysis.

intracoronary streptokinase and after intravenous administration of (predominantly) single chain rt-PA. When PTCA is applied instead of thrombolytic therapy to reperfuse evolving myocardial infarction, the 'success rate' is approximately 85% [24–26] which is similar to or slightly better than intracoronary streptokinase and intravenous rt-PA. Since precious time is lost by preparation of the catheterisation laboratory and introduction of the catheters, a combination therapy was developed including intravenous administration of a thrombolytic drug to achieve early reperfusion in part of the patients followed by PTCA [8, 16, 17, 19, 20, 21] in order to perforate persisting occlusions and to reduce residual stenosis. PTCA is then performed at a time when the drug is still acting, and in the presence of residual thrombus at the infarct related segment. Experience with PTCA in patients with unstable angina has shown that complication rate is higher, and that sudden reocclusion occurs more frequently when a thrombus is present [27]. Thus the clinical benefit of combined thrombolytic therapy ànd PTCA should be assessed carefully.

A few randomised trials have compared thrombolytic therapy with streptokinase or rt-PA and the same therapy combined with immediate PTCA. Early- and late patency figures from these trials are presented in Table 2. In three trials [19, 28, 29] patients were selected with patent vessels, in whom PTCA seemed feasible according to the operator. In these trials PTCA did reduce the residual diameter stenosis in most patients. However, in a few cases the artery occluded during the procedure [19, 28]. Three other groups of investigators attempted PTCA in all patients, unless angiography revealed no significant stenosis of the infarct related segment [17, 21, 25]. In most patients occlusions which were present prior to PTCA could be perforated and the residual lesion could be dilated. In a few however, the occlusion persisted or reocclusion occurred. Again, the residual stenosis was less severe after PTCA although the number of patients with a patent vessel was not greater after PTCA then after continuation of thrombolytic therapy without PTCA. At pre-discharge angiography in 4 studies the number of patients with a patent vessel was not enhanced by immediate PTCA [17, 21, 28, 29].

Table 2.

Thrombolytic regimen	Number of patients		Early patency %		Late patency %		References
	T	PTCA	T	PTCA	T	PTCA	
SK-ic	79	83	90	86	77	78	Erbel [17]
SK-ic	36	36	100	94	86	82	Vermeer [28]
SK-ic	27	29	85	83	—	—	O'Neill [25]
rt-PA iv	13	15	100	100	100[a]	80	Topol [29]
rt-PA iv	98	99	100	91	—	—	Topol [19]
rt-PA iv	184	183	—	90	90	84	Simoons [21]

Angiographic results of thrombolytic therapy (T) with intracoronary streptokinase (SK-ic), in part of the patients preceeded by intravenous streptokinase [17, 28] or with intravenous rt-PA. In one study SK-ic was combined with mechanical perforation of the thrombus [17]. In one other study intracoronary Streptokinase therapy was compared with immediate PTCA without thrombolysis [25].
[a] including 3 patients with PTCA before discharge because of recurrent ischemia due to reocclusion.

In Fig. 1 the percentage diameter stenosis and the TIMI perfusion score are presented as observed in the trial by the European Cooperative Study Group comparing thrombolytic therapy with rt-PA and an invasive approach of rt-PA, angiography and PTCA [21]. This figure illustrates that immediate PTCA indeed opened vessels which were still occluded at angiography, and that the number of patients without a severe stenosis predischarge was greater after PTCA then after rt-PA alone. However, the distribution of the perfusion scores before discharge was similar in both groups. Furthermore it is apparent that reocclusion occurred in part of the patients after PTCA, in spite of concommitant therapy with heparin and acetyl salicylic acid.

Infarct size and left ventricular function after thrombolysis and PTCA

Infarct size was estimated from myocardial HBDH-enzym release in the studies by the Interuniversity Cardiology Institute of the Netherlands [28] and by the European Cooperative Study Group [21]. Neither observed any difference between infarct size after thrombolysis compared with thrombolysis with immediate PTCA. Furthermore peak CK values were similar in the two patient groups reported by Erbel et al [17]. Infarct size after thrombolytic therapy is 15% (iv Streptokinase), 20% (iv rt-PA) or even 30% (ic Streptokinase) smaller then after conventional therapy [2, 7, 30]. However, no further limitation of infarct size was observed when immediate PTCA was performed during thrombolytic therapy.

Global left ventricular function was studied before hospital discharge, between 7 days and 3 weeks after admission by different investigators. Left ventricular

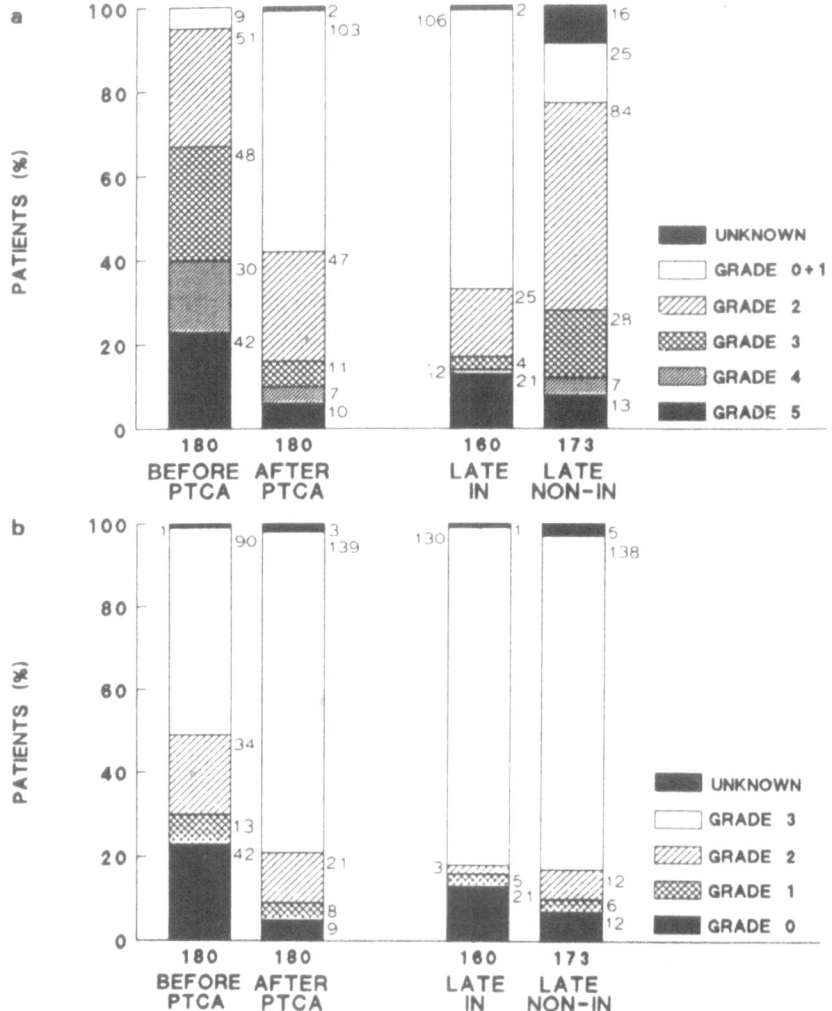

Figure 1. Grades of stenosis (a) and perfusion (b) of infarct related vessel before and after PTCA and after 10–22 days in patients allocated to invasive (IN) and non-invasive (non-IN) therapy.
Unknown = patients in whom the infarct-related segment (a) or artery (b) could not be identified in the angiogram. The number of patients with angiography is given under each bar: numbers next to the bars represent the number of patients in that particular subgroup (Reproduced from the Lancet [21]).

ejection fraction by contrast angiography or by radionuclide angiography was not greater after immediate PTCA compared with thrombolytic therapy without PTCA. Although the change in ejection fraction [24, 28, 29] as well as regional wall motion [17, 29, 31] appeared to be somewhat better after PTCA.

Clinical course and survival after thrombolysis and PTCA

The initial clinical course after immediate PTCA was not more favourable then after thrombolytic therapy [21]. Bleeding at the puncture site occurred more frequently after PTCA then in patients who did not undergo angiography, and more blood transfusions were given in the former group [21]. Early reocclusion was relatively frequent in spite of PTCA [17, 19, 24]. However, reinfarction after 24 hr seemed less frequent after PTCA [21, 28]. Also (re) PTCA or bypass surgery were performed less frequent after immediate PTCA (Table 3). On the other hand, mortality was not reduced by immediate PTCA. In some studies, mortality appeared even higher after PTCA then after thrombolytic therapy, although these differences were statistically not significant [19, 21].

Immediate PTCA: a reappraisal

In contrast to the expectations when the studies were initiated, immediate PTCA appeared not to be of advantage during thrombolytic therapy. The number of patent vessels was not enhanced (Table 2), infarct size was not reduced further and only small benefits, if any, were observed in left ventricular function, while mortality was not reduced (Table 3). The need for late PTCA was reduced in several studies. However, it is inefficient to attempt immediate PTCA in all (or most) patients with myocardial infarction in order to reduce the need for late interventions which can usually be done electively, and which are required in part of the patients only. Thus the single remaining benefit of immediate PTCA is the lower incidence of reinfarction in some studies ([21, 28] Table 3).

The reason for the lack of benefit of immediate PTCA is the high rate of early thrombotic reocclusion. This occurs particularly when rt-PA has been administered as thrombolytic agent [19, 21], while early reocclusion after PTCA seems

Table 3.

Late PTCA/CABG		Reocclusion/ re-infarction		Mortality		Follow up	References
T	PTCA	T	PTCA	T	PTCA		
		14[a]	12[a]	13	10	22 d	Erbel [17]
14	7	11	5	4	2	3 jr	Vermeer [28]
15	7	4[a]	2[a]	1	2	10 d	O'Neill [25]
		2	0	0	1	10 d	Topol [29]
29	13	13[a]	11[a]	1	4	10 d	Topol [19]
33	20	18	12	6	15	3 m	Simoons [21]

Clinical follow up of the studies presented in Table 2. The numbers of patients who underwent PTCA or bypass surgery (CABG) are presented as well as the numbers of patients with reocclusion and/or reinfarction and those who died within the specified follow up periods.
[a] reocclusion of the infarct related vessel.

less frequent when streptokinase [17, 31] or after rt-PA with urokinase [32] are used. It should be realised that in most patients the thrombotic occlusion is caused by rupture of a pre-existing atherosclerotic plaque. The exposed plaque remains present during and after the intervention, and endothelial damage by PTCA may further activate platelet aggregation. This can be prevented in part by acetyl salicylic acid [21], while Streptokinase and Urokinase may prevent rethrombolysis in part of the patients by breakdown of clotting factors. Nevertheless in many patients the thrombotic tendency prevails, and negates the potential benefits of immediate PTCA. Unfortunately this applies in particular to patients with persistent occlusion in spite of thrombolytic therapy [33]. It is possible that rethrombosis after thrombolytic therapy and PTCA can be prevented by newer drugs, such as antiplatelet antibodies [34] or thromboxane receptor blockers [35]. The clinical value of such approaches remains to be established.

Systematic delayed PTCA

In order to reduce the late sequellae of myocardial infarction, it has been proposed to perform coronary angiography a few days after admission, to select patients for further revascularisation procedures. The TIMI-II studies were designed to assess the value of elective delayed PTCA of the infarct related vessel [36]. Such approach cannot contribute to limitation of the infarct size, but it might facilitate recovery of left ventricular function and prevent recurrent ischemia and reinfarction. In the pilot study 6 weeks non fatal reinfarction rate was only 9% (23 out of 253 patients) after delayed, 18 to 48 hr, PTCA; compared with 16% (5 out of 31) without PTCA and 21% (7 out of 33) after immediate PTCA. The highest mortality occurred after immediate PTCA (3 out of 33 patients = 9%), while 6 weeks mortality in patients allocated to delayed PTCA was 5% (13 out of 253). The TIMI-IIA protocol, comparing immediate PTCA and delayed PTCA in 389 patients showed no difference between these to strategies, neither in left ventricular function, nor in mortality (7.2% vs 5.7%), or reinfarction (6.7% vs 4.1%). On the other hand transfusions and bypass surgery were required more frequently after immediate PTCA [37]. The comparison between 'conservative' therapy with rt-PA in 1636 patients and rt-PA followed by systematic PTCA after 18 to 48 hours in 1626 patients was reported at the 1988 American Heart Association Sessions. In the 'conservative' group PTCA and/or bypass surgery for recurrent ischemia were performed in 16% respectively 10% within 6 weeks after infarction. In the PTCA group these figures were 61% and 12%. In spite of allocation to delayed PTCA no intervention was done in 39% of the patients, because of absence of a significant stenosis (13%), total occlusion of the infarct related vessel (12%) or unsuitable anatomy (13%). In this study again no benefit of systematic PTCA appeared. In both patient groups global left ventricular ejection fraction was the same, while mortality (4.7 vs 5.2%) and non-fatal reinfarction (5.4% vs 5.9%) were even somewhat lower after 'conservative' management [38].

From these data it is apparent that neither immediate PTCA, nor systematic angiography followed by PTCA in suitable patients, have any benefits over non invasive ('conservative') therapy with an effective thrombolytic drug such as rt-PA.

The treatment strategy in acute myocardial infarction

Treatment of patients with acute myocardial infarction has improved greatly in recent years. In addition to detection and treatment of life threatening arrhythmias and timely correction of an impaired hemodynamic state (beta blockers, iv nitrates), in mortality can be reduced, and long term outcome can be improved by thrombolytic therapy. Furthermore administration of acetyl salicylic acid reduces reinfarction and mortality both after thrombolytic therapy and without [5]. Combination of such measures with thrombolytic therapy and with prompt angiography followed by PTCA or bypass surgery in patients with recurrent ischemia results in low mortality and low reinfarction rates [7, 21]. The complications of such initially non-invasive approach are so infrequent that it becomes unlikely that these can be improved by an initially invasive approach including angiography and PTCA, even if the early thrombotic complications of PTCA could be prevented. The invasive approach to myocardial infarction has greatly improved our knowledge and understanding of the pathophysiology, but it is doubtful whether such invasive approach will ever be cost-effective in clinical practice.

A practical and cost-effective strategy for treatment of myocardial infarction contains four 'decision points' (Table 4). Immediately upon hospital admission, or if possible immediately upon arrival of the ambulance service at the patients home, the diagnosis 'myocardial infarction' should be established. Thrombolytic therapy is indicated in patients with electrocardiographic evidence of evolving infarction, and in patients with a clinical diagnosis of infarction in whom the ECG cannot be interpreted such as those with left bundle branch block. At the Thoraxcenter thrombolytic therapy is initiated in all patients admitted within 3 hr after the onset of symptoms with at least 0.2 mV ST segment elevation in leads V_1 to V_4 or with 0.1 mV ST segment elevation in two other leads, and in patients with 0.3 mV ST segment elevation in $V_1 - V_4$ and/or 0.2 mV ST segment elevation in other leads admitted within 6 hr after the onset of symptoms (= coronary occlusion).

If no contraindications are present, therapy with rt-PA, Heparin and Aspirin is given at the Thoraxcenter. In other clinics APSAC or Streptokinase may be used as initial therapy, although these are probably less effective than rt-PA (Table 1). In patients who meet the criteria for thrombolytic therapy, but who also have contraindications (Table 4) immediate PTCA can be performed without thrombolytic therapy.

The patient is re-assessed between 12 and 48 hr after admission. In those patients with a small rise in serum enzymes and no Q wave development, in spite of extensive ST segment elevation upon admission (large area at risk), early

Table 4.   Clinical decisions regarding reperfusion therapy in acute myocardial infarction

I.   *Verify indications*

Onset of symptoms suggesting myocardial infarction less than 6 hr before admission with ECG signs of a large infarction:

ST segment elevation >0.3 mV in 2 leads V_1-V_4

or ST segment elevation >0.2 mV in 2 other leads

or ST segment elevation >0.1 mV in II, III or AVF

with ST segment depression >0.3 mV in 2 leads V_1-V_4 indicating posterior wall ischemia

Onset of symptoms suggesting myocardial infarction less than 3 hr before admission with ECG signs of a moderate infarction:

ST segment elevation >0.2 mV in 2 leads V_1-V_4

or ST segment elevation >0.1 mV in 2 other leads.

Clinical signs of myocardial infarction starting less than 6 hr before admission, with uninterpret--abel ECG (e.g. left bundle branch block)

Verify contraindications

Respirator required

Transmural myocardial infarction less than 14 days ago (Q waves)

Recent trauma (head!)

Recent puncture in a non compressible vessel (subclavian vein)

Intramuscular injection

Pregnancy or current menstruation

Known bleeding disorder

Major surgery less than 3 months ago

Cerebro vascular accident less than 3 months ago

Gastrointestinal bleeding less than 3 months ago

Genito-urinary bleeding less than 3 months ago

Known major hepatic disease (alcoholism)

Persistent hypertension at admission despite treatment (systolic >200 mmHg)

II.   *Choice of thrombolytic therapy*

rt-PA   10 mg bolus injection

50 mg in first hour

40 mg in subsequent 2 hr

or

APSAC   30 mg in 5 min i.v.

or

Streptokinase 1.500.000 U in 30 to 60 min i.v.

In patients with an indication for thrombolytic therapy and contra-indications present immediate PTCA without thrombolysis is recommended.

III.   *Assessment after 12–48 hours*

In patients with extensive myocardial ischemia upon admission and no or small rise in serum enzymes (small infarction or unstable angina with large area at risk) perform angiography followed by PTCA or bypass surgery as indicated.

IV.   *Assessment before discharge*

In patients with recurrent chest-pain and/or electrocardiographic signs of myocardial ischemia and

in patients with myocardial ischemia during pre-discharge exercise stress test perform angiography followed by PTCA or bypass surgery as indicated.

angiography is performed, followed by PTCA or surgery as indicated. Other patients are maintained on Aspirin and Heparin or oral anticoagulants during in-hospital rehabilitation.

Patients with recurrent angina are referred for angiography followed by PTCA or surgery as appropriate. Other patients undergo a pre discharge exercise test. Again, patients with exercise induced ischemia are referred for angiography and PTCA or surgery.

After hospital discharge all patients are treated with beta blockers, unless contraindicated, and with Aspirin. In those patients with a large akinetic or dyskinetic segment as judged by echocardiography, oral anticoagulants are prescribed in stead of Aspirin in order to prevent intraventricular thrombus formation.

When this strategy is followed between 25 and 50% of patients with myocardial infarction are referred for angiography, PTCA or surgery.

References

1. Kennedy JW, Ritchie JL, Davis KB, Fritz JK (1983) Western Washington randomized trial of intracoronary streptokinase in acute myocardial infarction. *N Engl J Med* 309:1477–1482
2. Simoons ML, Serruys PW, Brand M vd et al (1985) Improved survival after early thrombolysis in acute myocardial infarction. *Lancet* ii:578–582
3. Gruppo Italiano per lo studio della streptochinasi nell'infarto miocardico (GISSI) (1986) Effectiveness of intravenous thrombolytic treatment in acute myocardial infarction. *Lancet* i:397–401
4. AIMS Trial Study Group (1988) Effect of intravenous APSAC on mortality after acute myocardial infarction: Preliminary report of a placebo-controlled clinical trial. *Lancet* i: 545–549.
5. ISIS-2 (Second International Study of Infarct Survival) Collaborative Group (1988) Randomized trial of intravenous streptokinase, oral aspirin, both, or neither among 17 187 cases of suspected acute myocardial infarction: ISIS-2. *Lancet* ii:349–360
6. Wilcox RG, Lippe G vd, Olsson CG, Jensen G, Skene AM, Hampton JR (1988) Trial of tissue plasminogen activator for mortality reduction in acute myocardial infarction. Anglo-Scandinavian Study of Early Thrombolysis (ASSET). *Lancet* 525–530
7. Werf F van de, Arnold AER and the European Cooperative Study Group for Recombinant Tissue-type Plasminogen Activator (rTPA) (1988) Effect of intravenous tissue plasminogen activator on infarct size, left ventricular function and survival in patients with acute myocardial infarction. *Br Med J* 297:1374–1379
8. Meyer J, Merx W, Schmitz H, et al. (1982) Percutaneous transluminal coronary angioplasty immediately after intracoronary streptolysis of transmural myocardial infarction. *Circulation* 66:905–916
9. Serruys PW, Wijns W, Brand M vd et al (1983) Is transluminal coronary angioplasty mandatory after successful thrombolysis? *Br Heart J* 50:257–265
10. Mueler HS, Rao AK, Forman SA et al (1987) Thrombolysis in myocardial infarction (TIMI): comparative studies of coronary reperfusion and systemic fibrinogenolysis with two forms of recombinant tissue-type plasminogen activator. *J Am Coll Cardiol* 10:479–490
11. Califf RM, O'Neil W, Stack RS et al (1988) Failure of simple clinical measurements to predict perfusion status after intravenous thrombolysis. *Ann Int Med* 108:658–662
12. De Wood MA, Spores J, Notske R et al (1980) Prevalence of total coronary occlusion during the early hours of transmural myocardial infarction. *N Engl J Med* 303:897–902

13. Rentrop KP (1985) Thrombolytic therapy in patients with acute myocardial infarction. *Circulation* 71:627–631
14. Verstraete M, Bernard R, Bory M, et al. (1985) Randomized trial of intravenous recombinant tissue-type plasminogen activator versus intravenous streptokinase in acute myocardial infarction. *Lancet* i: 842–47
15. Cheseboro JH, Knatterud G, Roberts R, et al (1987) Thrombolysis in myocardial infarction (TIMI) trial, phase I: A comparison between intravenous tissue plasminogen activator and intravenous streptokinase. *Circulation* 76:146
16. Serruys PW, Simoons ML, Suryapranata H, et al (1986) Preservation of global and regional left ventricular function after early thrombolysis in acute myocardial infarction. *J Am Coll Cardiol* 112:672–681
17. Erbel R, Pop T, Henrichs KJ et al (1986) Percutaneous transluminal coronary angioplasty after thrombolytic therapy: a prospective controlled randomized trial. *J Am Coll Cardiol* 8:485–495
18. Topol EJ, Morris DC, Smalling RW, et al (1987) A multicenter, randomized, placebo-controlled trial of a new form of intravenous recombinant tissue-type plasminogen activator (Activase) in acute myocardial infarction. *J Am Coll Cardiol* 9:1205–1213
19. Topol EJ, Califf RM, George BS, et al and the TAMI Study Group (1987) A randomized trial of immediate versus delayed elective angioplasty after intravenous tissue plasminogen activator in acute myocardial infarction. *N Engl J Med* 317:581–588
20. Williams DO, Borer J, Braunwald E, et al (1986) Intravenous recombinant tissue-type plasminogen activator in patients with acute myocardial infarction: a report from the NHLBI thrombolysis in myocardial infarction trial. *Circulation* 73:338–346
21. Simoons ML, Arnold AER, Betriu A, et al (1988) Thrombolysis with tissue plasminogen activator in acute myocardial infarction: No additional benefit from immediate percutaneous coronary angioplasty. *Lancet* i:197–203
22. McNeill AJ, Shannon JS, Cunningham SR, et al (1988) A randomised dose ranging study of recombinant tissue plasminogen activator in acute myocardial infarction. *Br Med J* 296: 1768–1771
23. Bonnier HJRM, Visser RF, Klomps HC, et al (1988) Comparison of intravenous anisoylated plasminogen streptokinase activator complex (APSAC) and intracoronary streptokinase in acute myocardial infarction. *Am J Cardiol* (in press)
24. O'Neill W, Timmis GC, Bourdillon PD, et al (1986) A prospective randomized clinical trial of intracoronary streptokinase versus coronary angioplasty for acute myocardial infarction. *N Engl J Med* 314: 812–818
25. Rothbaum DA, Linnemeier TJ, Landin RJ, et al (1987) Emergency percutaneous transluminal coronary angioplasty in acute myocardial infarction: a 3 year experience. *J Am Coll Cardiol* 10:264–272
26. Rutherford BD, Harzler GO, McConahay DR, Johnson WL (1986) Direct balloon angioplasty in acute myocardial infarction without prior use of streptokinase (abstract). *J Am Coll Cardiol* 7:149A
27. Ellis SG, Roubin GS, King SB, et al (1988) Angiographic and clinical predictors of acute closure after native vessel coronary angioplasty. *Circulation* 77:372–379
28. Vermeer F, Simoons ML, Feyter PJ de, et al (1988) Immediate PTCA after successful thrombolysis with intracoronary streptokinase, three years follow up. *Eur Heart J* 9:346–353
29. Topol EJ, O'Neill WW, Langburd AB, et al (1987) A randomized, placebo-controlled trial of intravenous recombinant tissue-type plasminogen activator and emergency coronary angioplasty in patients with acute myocardial infarction. *Circulation* 75:420–428
30. The ISAM Study Group (1986) A prospective trial of intravenous streptokinase in acute myocardial infarction mortality, morbidity, and infarct size at 21 days. *N Engl J Med* 314:1465–1470
31. Suryapranata H, Serruys PW, Vermeer F, et al (1987) Value of immediate coronary angioplasty following intracoronary thrombolysis in acute myocardial infarction. *Cath Cardiovasc Diagn* 13:223–232
32. Topol EJ, Califf RM, George BS, et al (1988) Coronary arterial thrombolysis with combined

infusion of recombinant tissue-type plasminogen activator and urokinase in patients with acute myocardial infarction. *Circulation* 77:1100–1107

33. Califf RM, Topol EJ, George BS, et al (1988) Characteristics and outcome of patients in whom reperfusion with intravenous tissue-type plasminogen activator fails: Results of the Thrombolysis and Angioplasty in Myocardial Infarction (TAMI) I trial. *Circulation* 77:1090–1099
34. Gold HK, Coller BS, Yasuda T, et al (1988) Rapid and sustained coronary artery recanalization with combined bolus injection of recombinant tissue-type plasminogen activator and monoclonal antiplatelet GPIIb/IIIa antibody in a canine preparation. *Circulation* 77:670–677
35. Golino P, Ashton JH, Glas-Greenwalt P, et al (1988) Mediation of reocclusion by thromboxane A_2 and serotonin after thrombolysis with tissue-type plasminogen activator in a canine preparation of coronary thrombosis. *Circulation* 77:678–684
36. Passamani E, Hodges M, Herman M, et al (1987) The thrombolysis in myocardial infarction (TIMI) phase II pilot study: Tissue plasminogen activator followed by percutaneous transluminal coronary angioplasty. *J AM Coll Cardiol* 10:51B–64B
37. TIMI-IIA (1988) Immediate vs delayed catheterization and angioplasty following thrombolytic therapy for acute myocardial infarction. *JAMA* 260:2849–2858
38. TIMI Study Group (1989) Comparison of invasive and conservative strategies after treatment with intravenous tissue plasminogen activator in acute myocardial infarction. *N. Engl J Med* 320:618–627

26. The United States thrombolysis and angioplasty trials for acute myocardial infarction

JOSEPH M. SUTTON and ERIC J. TOPOL

Introduction

There has been intense interest and clinical trial work in the United States to determine the optimal integrated strategy of intravenous thrombolysis and coronary angioplasty for acute myocardial infarction (AMI). Randomized, controlled trials have been performed by the Thrombolysis and Angioplasty in Myocardial Infarction (TAMI) study group, the Thrombolysis in Myocardial Infarction (TIMI) study group, and the Johns Hopkins University investigators. A series of trials have been performed which prospectively evaluate therapy with intravenous tissue plasminogen activator (t-PA) in combination with coronary angioplasty or as a sole intervention. Further, the precise timing of angioplasty has been considered, ranging from the immediate phase of infarction, to 18–48 hr, 72 hr, and 7 days. In this review the United States trials will be presented in detail. Using this as a foundation, the results will be compared with other similar studies and a consensus of findings will be developed.

Pilot study

In a small, randomized study of 50 patients receiving either intravenous rt-PA or placebo within a mean of 3.8 hours after the onset of AMI symptoms, 28 patients among the 84% of those achieving successful thrombolysis were determined to have a residual stenosis of at least 50% and were randomized to immediate PTCA (15 patients) or no PTCA (13 patients) [3]. In this subset of patients, subsequent ischemic events tended to occur less frequently among patients who underwent PTCA, and there was a notable reduction in documented reinfarction between the two groups, with 13% (2/15) patients undergoing immediate PTCA versus 54% (7/13) of patients treated with rt-PA alone, suffering reinfarction. There was no difference detected in global left ventricular function between these two groups, and followup angiography 7 days following therapy, demonstrated no difference in patency rate of the infarct vessel among patients treated with

P.W. Serruys, R. Simon & K.J. Beatt (eds), Percutaneous Transluminal Coronary Angioplasty. ISBN 0-7923-0346-6.
© *1990 Kluwer Academic Publishers, Dordrecht*

rt-PA who underwent immediate PTCA, compared with those patients who received rt-PA alone. When regional wall motion was assessed in the area of the infarction, a significant improvement was noted in the patients randomized to immediate PTCA. Further, the regional infarct zone wall motion was improved in patients not experiencing recanalization despite rt-PA therapy who were treated with rescue PTCA and among patients treated with placebo, who underwent PTCA as a primary reperfusion procedure.

The improvement in regional infarct zone wall motion in the PTCA group may have resulted from increased blood flow through infarct arteries with reduced residual stenoses, suggesting that there may be improved myocardial performance when treatment of the residual anatomic lesion accompanies successful thrombolysis, or when PTCA results in primary recanalization of a persistently closed vessel despite pharmacologic therapy.

Again, the timing of therapy or the patient profile that would optimize the risk to benefit ratio for acute intervention in AMI remained largely undefined.

Thrombolysis and angioplasty in myocardial infarction (TAMI)

Results of the Thrombolysis and Angioplasty in Myocardial Infarction (TAMI) trial are summarized in tables 1 and 2 [4–6]. The study was designed to determine whether immediate or deferred PTCA was preferable subsequent to successful thrombolytic therapy. A total of 386 patients were enrolled and treated at a mean of 2.9 hr from symptom onset with 150 mg of intravenous rt-PA over 6 to 8 hr. The results of initial thrombolytic therapy were assessed by coronary angiography within 90 min, and patients were then assigned to various subgroups within the study according to the initial coronary anatomy and clinical response to rt-PA (TAMI patient groups A–C). (Fig. 1) The overall reperfusion rate achieved with intravenous rt-PA thereapy was similar to results reported by the TIMI-I study, with 75% of patients found to have TIMI grade 2 or 3 flow at initial catheterization [1, 6].

Thrombolysis resistant group

TAMI group-A included all 96 patients in whom thrombolytic therapy was unsuccessful [4]. Clinical judgment regarding suitability of the infarct lesion for immediate PTCA was applied to each case. Among the 96 patients in this group, 86 (90%) were subjected to rescue PTCA, with a resulting residual stenosis below 50% achieved in 73% of these patients.

Overall mortality among patients in the TAMI-A group was 10.4%, with the highest rate of death occurring in the group of 9 patients in whom attempted PTCA was completely unsuccessful (44%). Mortality was substantially altered in patients with partially successful PTCA (residual stenosis >50%) at 14%, compared with a 6% mortality rate among patients with successful PTCA and

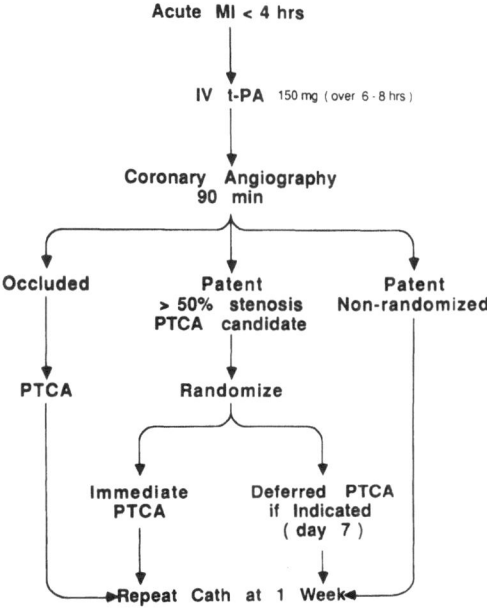

Figure 1. The Thrombolysis and Angioplasty in Myocardial Infarction (TAMI) Phase-I protocol. Cath = cardiac catheterization; IV t-PA = intravenous tissue-type plasminogen activator (150 mg over 6 to 8 hr); MI = myocardial infarction; PTCA = percutaneous transluminal coronary angioplasty. The patients with occluded vessels comprise group A, group B consists of those patients randomized for PTCA, while group C patients were excluded from randomization (Reproduced with permission from Topol et al [4–6]).

lesser (< 50%) residual stenosis of the infarct vessel. There were no deaths among the patients from this group who did not undergo PTCA. This disproportionate mortality rate is due, in part, to the triage process, with more critical patients undergoing attempted PTCA in the presence of persistent life-threatening coronary artery occlusion. Additionally, patients with occluded infarct arteries, presenting with cardiogenic shock, were not excluded from this therapeutic approach if they had coronary artery lesions approachable by PTCA. Only 2 of the 10 patients from TAMI group-A not subjected to PTCA were excluded for critical anatomy that was unapproachable by the procedure, while 6 of these 10 patients were felt to have small, uncomplicated completed infarcts due to occlusion of a small branch artery, and 2 patients experienced thrombolysis just beyond the initial 90 minute assessment point. Thus, 80% of patients in the subset not undergoing PTCA were believed to have no myocardium at risk of further infarction, while patients with life-threatening cardiogenic shock were emergently treated if they were found to have coronary anatomy suitable for angioplasty.

The early, in-hospital reocclusion rate among patients in whom rescue

PTCA was considered successful was inordinately high (29%), despite the use of standard anticoagulant and antiplatelet agents. There was no improvement in pre-discharge left ventricular ejection fraction, compared with the initial baseline study. Although successful reduction in luminal stenosis by PTCA was followed by a high incidence of complications, including restenosis, the incidence of emergency or urgent coronary artery bypass surgery (CABG) tended to be lower among patients in whom PTCA after thrombolytic therapy failure was attempted (4% vs 10%).

Better thrombolytic agents or pharmacologic regimens, or the identification and modification of factors predisposing to poor thrombolytic efficacy in this group of patients is needed to impart a better prognosis among patients in whom a t-PA regimen fails to achieve early thrombolysis.

Randomized patients

Patients entering the TAMI study, who experienced successful thrombolysis and had residual lesions suitable for PTCA, were randomized to immediate PTCA (99 patients) at the time of the initial catheterization, or to deferred PTCA at 7 days (98 patients) [5, 6]. Successful minimalization of residual lesions was achieved with similar frequency in both groups (90% for immediate PTCA, versus 94% for deferred PTCA). Likewise, the rate of reocclusion following successful PTCA was nearly the same in both groups (11% reocclusion for immediate PTCA, vs 13% after deferred PTCA). Among patients in the deferred PTCA group, an additional 15% of patients were found to have minimal disease when reevaluated at 7 days, presumably because of continued thrombolysis beyond 90 min into thrombolytic therapy. This represents an important subset of patients who would have otherwise undergone emergency coronary angioplasty on the basis of a tight residual stenosis. While baseline left ventricular ejection fractions tended to be lower in the immediate PTCA group (52.0% vs 55.0%), there was no significant difference in the degree of improvement of left ventricular function recovery (mean increase of 1.1% vs 1.3%). (Fig. 2).

There was an 18% incidence of recurrent ischemic events in the deferred PTCA group, prompting emergency PTCA or CABG prior to the planned day 7 procedure. This higher incidence of recurrent ischemia following interruption of AMI by thrombolytic therapy, necessitates close observation and prompt availability of emergency revascularization capability. Of note, the overall requirement for CABG was similar in both groups, 14.7% among immediate PTCA patients, versus 15.5% in the deferred PTCA group, with a slightly higher rate of emergency surgery occurring in the immediate PTCA group. Of note and concern, there was a higher mortality rate for the immediate versus the deferred PTCA strategy (4% versus 1%, respectively), but this difference did not achieve statistical significance.

Thus, immediate PTCA was associated with a higher mortality rate and a higher emergency CABG frequency. Although delayed PTCA resulted in

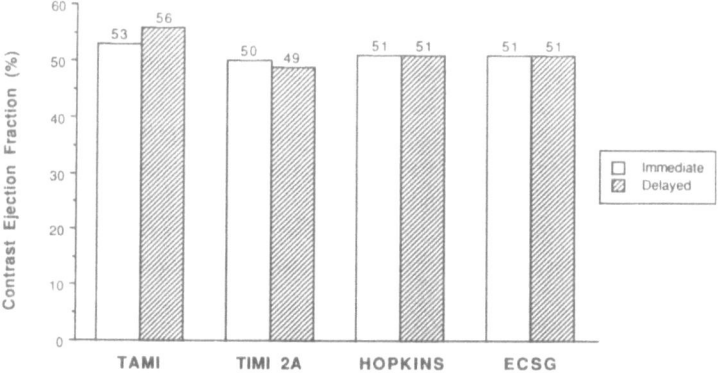

Figure 2. Pre-discharge ejection fraction. No differences in left ventricular function were observed at the time of hospital discharge between patients undergoing early versus delayed coronary angioplasty as late as 3 days after thrombolytic therapy.
TAMI = Thrombolysis and Angioplasty in Myocardial Infarction study; TIMI 2A = Thrombolysis In Myocardial Infarction study; HOPKINS = The Johns Hopkins University study; ECSG = European Co-operative Study Group. (Adapted from Topol et al [4–6], TIMI study group [2], Guerci et al [7], Simoons et al [8]).

a higher incidence of early recurrent ischemic events, these untoward events were not reflected in either a higher mortality rate or any compromise of left ventricular ejection fraction. In fact, the pre-discharge left ventriculograms in the deferred PTCA group were obtained prior to any revascularization procedure in 82% of these patients.

The study demonstrated the lack of need for emergency angioplasty among patients in whom thrombolytic therapy is successful. While the deferred approach to subsequent revascularization appears to be associated with a favorable clinical outcome, early angiography may still have a role in identifying the approximate 25% of patients who do not experience recanalization with thrombolytic agents, who might benefit from immediate PTCA or those patients in high risk anatomic subsets such as left main or equivalent stenoses, who may be triaged to CABG.

Patients unsuitable for randomization

Clinical judgement following successful thrombolysis, defined 90 patients as unsuitable for PTCA. This group (TAMI group-C) included patients with infarct anatomy best suited for CABG surgery because of left main or left main equivalent coronary artery disease (22%), diffuse multivessel lesions (39%), or coronary anatomy resulting in cardiogenic shock despite successful recanalization of the infarct vessel (4%). In 25% of patients in this group, a minimal residual stenosis (< 50% luminal occlusion) was present after thrombolysis, and uncertainty regarding the infarct vessel due to ambiguous electrocardiogram findings accounted for the exclusion of 3% of patients in this group. The remaining 7% were excluded from randomization for miscellaneous reasons.

Mortality in this subset of patients was higher (11.0%) than in any of the other groups. This mortality rate was chiefly influenced by the inclusion of patients with very high risk underlying anatomy including left main disease, left main equivalent, or diffuse multilesional, multivessel coronary artery disease, as well as patients in whom myocardial necrosis by the time of successful recanalization was extensive enough to cause cardiogenic shock. These patients collectively comprised 65% of patients not randomized.

In the absence of other revascularization options, patients in the TAMI-C group underwent CABG surgery about three times as frequently other patients, with 47% (38/81 with significant residual coronary artery disease) undergoing the surgery prior to hospital discharge, compared with 12% of patients in the TAMI-A group, 15% in the TAMI-B, immediate PTCA group, and 16% in the TAMI-B, deferred PTCA group. Emergency CABG was performed in 12 patients from this group, with no intraoperative deaths. Overall mortality among these 12 patients, and 12 additional patients undergoing emergency CABG because of unsuccessful PTCA attempts was 12.5% (3/24), despite an incidence of preoperative cardiogenic shock in 33% (8/24) of these patients.

While thrombolysis was successful in patients triaged to this group, the role of PTCA in the setting of multivessel disease is not well defined. During the acute phase of AMI, only the infarct vessel would be approached, however in patients with multivessel disease and positive functional test results before hospital discharge, the non-infarct vessels may need to be considered for revascularization. As experience with PTCA has accumulated and confidence in selecting approach able lesions increases, the procedure has been used increasingly in patients with multiple lesions, more diseased vessels, and poorer left ventricular function [9]. The ongoing United States Bypass Angioplasty Revascularization Investigation (BARI), and other multicenter randomized PTCA versus CABG trials, may define patients with this clinical outcome to thrombolytic therapy who could safely undergo PTCA of the infarct and non-infarct vessels several days to weeks after successful thrombolytic therapy.

In the TAMI-C group of 24 patients found to have minimal residual lesions after successful thrombolysis, 1 patient from this category accounted for one of the five late deaths following hospital discharge. Although there is angiographically no significant fixed stenosis of the infarct vessel, there was sufficient underlying pathology to cause the initial presentation of AMI. It is likely that this minimal disease syndrome results from coronary artery vasospasm and in situ thrombosis; another possible etiology is rupture of a minimal plaque. We have found this syndrome to be more common among females, younger patients, and those without a prodrome of angina. They have been empirically managed with aspirin and calcium channel blockade.

TIMI phase II

Phase II of the TIMI trial was designed to determine the role of early PTCA as an adjunct to rt-PA therapy [2]. Two treatment strategies were devised to complement thrombolytic therapy. In the TIMI-IIa subtrial, patients were randomized to immediate PTCA within 2 hr of initiating t-PA infusion or to early deferred angiography and angioplasty, if appropriate, at 18 to 48 hr.

A pilot study for TIMI-II was undertaken to determine the feasibility of the complex protocol design. Prior to initiating the randomized trial, a total of 317 patients presenting within a mean of 2.7 hr from the onset of AMI received 150 mg or intravenous t-PA over 6 hours. Patients were then treated in a nonrandom fashion with no followup angiography, or PTCA at either 2 hr or 18 to 48 hr beyond initiation of rt-PA infusion (Tables 1 and 2). The patients were not randomized to the various treatment approaches, but rather entered the protocols dependent upon the assignment of the particular center to which they presented.

Mortality was the only evaluated end point for the 31 patients treated entirely by noninvasive thrombolytic therapy. There were no deaths reported with this approach, however clinical reocclusion, ischemia and reinfarction tended to be higher for this group (16.0%). Neither the extent of residual disease, nor the efficacy of thrombolytic therapy were known because of the noninvasive approach. A total of 33 patients underwent immediate PTCA within 2 hr (mean 1 hr) of thrombolytic therapy. This approach was associated with a slightly higher mortality rate (9.1%), but a lower rate of reocclusion (8%). Mortality in the largest arm of the study was 6.3% among the 253 patients undergoing PTCA at 18 to 48 hr beyond initiation of rt-PA. This mortality rate is affected by the larger number of patients in this group, and is difficult to compare with results among the markedly smaller number of patients treated with the alternative strategies. The delayed approach with angioplasty success rates similar to those achieved with the more immediate procedure, however there was an insignificant trend towards a higher reocclusion rate. Successful thrombolysis occurred in over 82 and 89% of patients undergoing immediate and delayed PTCA respectively. Because of 5 cases of intracranial hemorrhage associated with the 150 mg dose, a change in dose to 100 mg was initiated near the end of the study.

The preliminary results of the randomized implementation of the TIMI phase-IIA proved to be similar. In the group randomized to immediate PTCA, 195 patients received intravenous rt-PA a mean of 2.8 hr following the onset of symptoms, and underwent PTCA, if suitable anatomy was present, within 2 hr of thrombolytic treatment. Successful thrombolysis was achieved in 75% of patients, and PTCA proved successful at reducing the residual coronary lesion in over 90% of the 137 patients with suitable coronary anatomy who actually underwent the procedure. Of the 194 patients randomly assigned to have PTCA performed at 18 to 48 hr, 82% had successful reperfusion of the infarct vessel, and 102 of these patients eventually underwent the delayed procedure with successful

Table 1. rt-PA clinical trials.

	TAMI				TIMI II pilot		
	A	B₁	B₂	C	2 hr	18–48 hr	NI
No. of patients	96	99	98	90	33	253	31
Time to therapy (hr)	└──────── 2.9 ────────┘				└──────── 2.7 ────────┘		
Reperfusion rate (%)	└──────── 75 ────────┘				82	87	NA
Mortality (%)	10.4	4.0	1.0	11.0	9.1	6.3	0.0
Bleeding complications							
Minor (%)	└──────── 7.5 ────────┘				└──────── 9.0 ────────┘		
Major (%)	└──────── 0.5 ────────┘				└──────── 1.5 ────────┘		
Reocclusion (%)							
Post tPA	—	—	13.0	—	—	—	16.0
Post PTCA	29	11.0	—	—	8.0	14.0	—
Time to initial angiogram	└──────── 60—90 min ────────┘				2 hr	32 hr	NA

Abbreviations:
TAMI = Thrombolysis and Angioplasty in Myocardial Infarction Trial.
I   = tPA reperfusion failure group.
IIa   = tPA, successful reperfusion, early PTCA.
IIb   = tPA, successful reperfusion, delayed PTCA.
III   = tPA successful, excluded from PTCA randomization.
TIMI = Thrombolysis in Myocardial Infarction Study.
NI   = noninvasive.
JHH = Johns Hopkins Hospital Study.
ECSG = European Cooperative Study Group.
NA   = Not assessed.

results similar to the 2 hr PTCA group (96%). There was no difference in either mortality or left ventricular performance between the two groups.

The differing thrombolytic rates reflect the occurrence of additional, late thrombolysis during the 30 hr time delay to catheterization in the PTCA-deferred group. There were more hemorrhagic complications associated with PTCA performed 2 hr into the 6 hr rt-PA infusion, and the overall mortality was 8%. Immediate PTCA afforded successful reperfusion in 91% of cases in which thrombolytic intervention was unsuccessful at the time of the initial catheterization. While these patients benefit from hastened myocardial reperfusion, there remains no reliable clinical means of identifying patients in whom thrombolysis does not occur expeditiously.

The study indicated that immediate PTCA following administration of rt-PA is not required in the presence of successful chemical thrombolysis. The clinical outcome appeared unaltered by deferring the procedure up to 48 hours in these patients, with no demonstrable difference in pre-discharge left ventricular

TIMI I		TIMI IIa		JHH		ECSG
tPA	SK	2 hr	18–48 hr	tPA	Placebo	
99	115	195	194	72	66	367
└── ≤7 ──┘		2.8	2.9	3.2	3.1	2.6
66	36	72	82	66	24	89
5.0	8.0	8.0		5.6	7.6	5.2
6.0	10			9.8	7.6	
6.0	0			0.0	0.0	
11	14			5.6	10.6	
—	—			NA	NA	
90 min		1.8 hr mean	32.6 hr	└── 1–6 hr ──┘ 2.5 mean		42 min

performance. The benefit of early angiography to allow identification and early mechanical revascularization of patients in whom there is a delay or absence of thrombolysis was illustrated, especially given the high efficacy of PTCA reported for this group of patients (91%). As in the TAMI study, there were no overall differences in left ventricular ejection fractions between patients undergoing immediate PTCA and those randomized to the deferred strategy. Further, the deferred approach did not allow timely identification of those patients with unsuccessful chemical thrombolysis was not demonstrated.

The ongoing TIMI-IIb subtrial is designed to compare early PTCA at 18 to 48 hr with conservative thrombolytic therapy alone. Therapy with t-PA is followed by randomization to immediate or deferred beta blocker therapy in eligible patients. All groups are then randomized to undergo either no PTCA or early PTCA 18 to 48 hr subsequent to initiating t-PA therapy (Fig. 3). The larger group of patients treated with a conservative, non-invasive strategy, will allow a meaningful comparison of this approach with the outcome of patients undergoing PTCA after thrombolytic therapy. This trial is addressing the fundamental question of the absolute need for coronary angioplasty following thrombolytic therapy. The conservative 'wait-and-see' approach is compared to an empiric, prophylactic strategy of cardiac catheterization at 48 to 72 hr.

The Johns Hopkins trial

To determine the general benefit of early deferred compared with elective PTCA, following intravenous rt-PA therapy, 72 patients treated with 80 to 100 mg of the

Table 2.   Angioplasty following tPA therapy.

	TAMI				TIMI II pilot		
	A	B₁	B₂	C	2 hr	18–48 hr	NI
No. of patients	96	99	98	90	33	253	31
tPA							
Time to therapy (hr)		⎣———— 2.9 ————⎦				⎣———— 2.7 ————⎦	
Dose (mg)		⎣———— 150 ————⎦				⎣———— 150 ————⎦	
Reperfusion success rate (%)		⎣———— 75 ————⎦			82	89	NA
PTCA							
Time		60–90 min	7–10 days	—	2 hr	18–48 hr	NA
Early							
n =	86	99	—	—	23	128	NA
LVEF							
Early	51.5	52.0	—	—			
Late	51.0	53.2	—	—			
Reocclusion	29%	11%	—	—	8%	14%	NA
-Mortality (%)	10.4	4.0	—	—	9.1	6.3	0.0
None or Delayed							
n =	—	—	98	—			
LVEF							
Early	—	—	55.0	—		⎣———— NR ————⎦	
Late	—	—	56.4	—		⎣———— NR ————⎦	
Reocclusion	—	—	13%	—	—	—	
Mortality (%)	—	—	1.0	11.0			16.0

NI = noninvasive.
NR = not reported.
*   = the last 2/3 of patients entered in TIMI IIa received 100 mg.
       the first 1/3 of patients entered in TIMI IIa received 150 mg.
**   = 42 randomized, 4 excluded.
LVEF = Left Ventricular Ejection Fraction.

drug over three hours within a mean of 3.2 hr from the onset of AMI were evaluated by coronary angiography a mean of 2.5 hr into therapy [7]. A placebo-treated control group of 66 patients with similar clinical characteristics, were enrolled following a mean of 3.1 hr from initial symptoms. The 85 patients from both groups found to have coronary anatomy suitable for angioplasty, were randomized to undergo the procedure either on the third day following medical therapy (42 patients), or to await further intervention until the conclusion of the ten day study (43 patients). Improvement of left ventricular ejection fraction by the tenth day of the trial was used as indicators of successful therapy and infarct size reduction.

Patent infarct vessels were found in 66% of patients treated with rt-PA, while only 24% of patients in the placebo group had open infarct arteries at the time of

TIMI IIa		JHH		ECSG
2 hr	18–48 hr	tPA	Placebo	
195	194	72	66	367
2.8	2.9	3.2	3.1	<5
└— 100, 150* —┘		100	—	150
75	82	66	24	89
2 hr	18–48 hr	└— 48–72 hrs —┘		18–48 hr
137	102	└— 38** —┘		183
		└— 51.3 —┘		—
50	49	└—51.2—┘		51
└—NR—┘		NR	NR	12.5%
└—8.0—┘		NR	NR	7.0
		└— 96 —┘		184
		└— 49.2 —┘		—
		└— 50.5 —┘		51
		7.3		11.0%
		5.6	7.6	3.0

the early angiogram. Although a closed infarct artery was not a considered a contraindication for exclusion from randomization to early angioplasty, no patient underwent the procedure immediately for direct recanalization. Overall mortality was lower among patients treated with rt-PA (5.6%), than in the placebo group (7.6%), and the incidence of congestive heart failure was more than twice as common in the placebo group – 33% vs 14% respectively.

Left ventricular function, measured by gated blood pool imaging, assessed at days one and ten, demonstrated a dichotomy of left ventricular ejection fraction trends. Patients treated with rt-PA, experienced an average increase in resting left ventricular function of 3.6%, while the ejection fraction diminished by a mean of 4.7% during the course of the study among those patients randomized to placebo. Although there was no difference in resting left ventricular performance between the early angioplasty group and the elective treatment group (mean improvement of 1.9% in the elective group, and 1.1% in the angioplasty group), there was improved augmentation of ejection fraction with maximal exercise in the patients treated with early PTCA (8.1% augmentation, vs 1.2%, $p < 0.02$, Fig. 4).

There was no stratification of clinical outcome with respect to thrombolytic

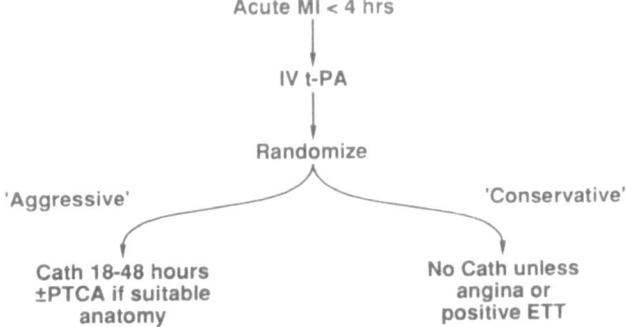

Figure 3. The Thrombolysis In Myocardial Infarction (TIMI) Phase-2B study design. Early angioplasty, compared with conservative management after thrombolytic therapy.
MI = myocardial infarction; IV t-PA = intravenous tissue-type plasminogen activator; Cath = cardiac catheterization; PTCA = percutaneous transluminal cororary angioplasty; ETT = graded exercise tolerance test.

treatment success; thus it was not noted whether the subgroup of patients with unsuccessful thrombolysis benefited from the earlier approach to PTCA. Early deferred PTCA was associated with a reduction in recurrent ischemic events from 19 to 5%, and only two patients awaiting the end of the trial before further consideration for PTCA, had to undergo the procedure emergently. Additionally,

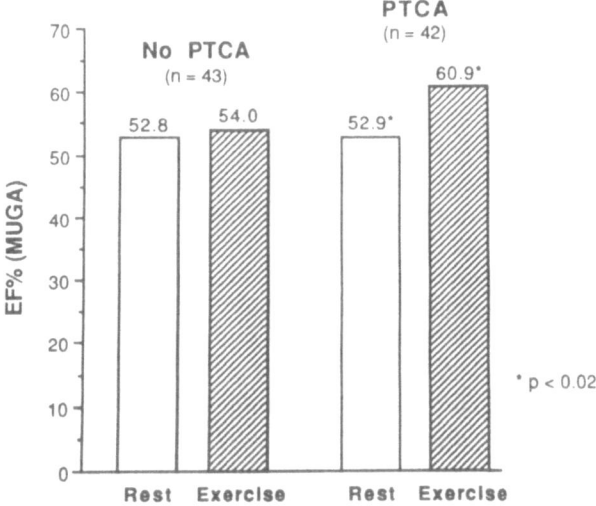

Figure 4. Rest and exercise left ventricular function for patients randomized to either early angioplasty or no angioplasty after thrombolytic therapy in the Johns Hopkins study.
MUGA = gated blood pool scintigraphy (Adapted from Gueric et al [7]).

deferring PTCA by 3 days, resulted in further reduction of residual stenosis in 2 patients, who no longer needed to be subjected to the procedure according to the protocol design.

The study concluded that early treatment with intravenous rt-PA could be safely followed in many patients with residual stenoses by deferred PTCA. Although the study also reported that early angiographic evaluation of thrombolytic results was unnecessary, the outcome of this late triage approach in patients with persistently closed infarct arteries despite early medical therapy was not evaluated [10]. This strategy of immediate thrombolytic intervention and angiography with or without coronary angioplasty at 3 days is widely transferable. The question remains, however, of the definite need for angioplasty for asymptomatic patients who have high grade residual stenoses, and whether coronary angiography should even be performed.

TAMI phase-II

No additional benefit could be demonstrated in terms of acute infarct vessel patency with combination thrombolytic therapy using t-PA with urokinase in TAMI phase-II [12]. The maximal patency rate achieved, despite combination therapy at high doses was found to be 75%. No synergism could be demonstrated; there appears to be a limit to the extent of early recanalization achievable with thrombolytic agents alone, with about 25% of patients proving resistant to current pharmacologic intervention (Fig. 5).

Among patients with unsuccessful thrombolysis, this combination treatment

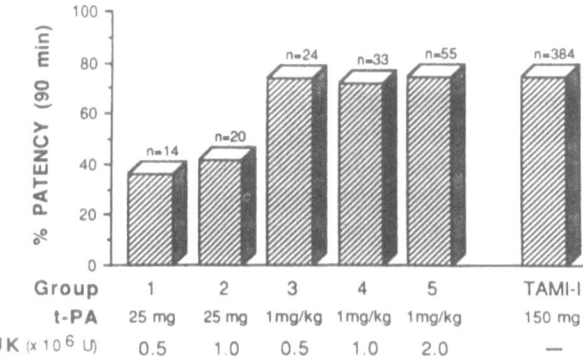

Figure 5. Infarct vessel patency at 90 minutes for the five dose combinations of urokinase and t-PA in the Thrombolysis and Angioplasty in Myocardial Infarction (TAMI) Phase 2 study. No synergism was observed with combination therapy. A plateau recanalization response beyond which additional thrombolysis could not be achieved.

t-PA = tissue-type plasminogen activator; UK = urokinase (Reproduced with permission from Topol et al [12]).

was associated with a significantly higher late patency rate in those who underwent "rescue" angioplasty, with 96% (22/23) of patients treated with both agents compared with 69% (56/81) of those receiving t-PA alone (TAMI-I patients) having persistantly patent vessels at repeat angiography (p=0.017) (Table 2).

This combined t-PA and urokinase approach resulted in a eghtfold elevation in fibrin degradation products which may impart important antiplatelet effects, as well as systemic fibrinogen depletion which may have some role in diminishing plasma viscocity. There was no significant increase in bleeding complications associated with combined thrombolytic therapy, however there was a trend towards lower in-hospital mortality (0/27 vs 10.4% (10/96) of patients treated with t-PA alone, p=0.075).

In summary, immediate coronary angioplasty following thrombolytic therapy may be associated with a more favorable outcome when non-fibrin specific or a combination of thrombolytic agents are used [12, 15].

The role of angioplasty in myocardial infarction

Cumulative experience with elective PTCA has resulted in improved patency rates, with increased successful lesion reduction (by at least 20%) achieved in 78.3% of cases, compared with the previously observed success rate of 61.0%, and mortality associated with the procedure remains low at 1%. A high technical PTCA success rate has also been noted in patients with acute myocardial infarction [9].

Direct angioplasty

Since its conception, angioplasty has played a controversial role in the treatment of coronary artery lesions associated with acute myocardial infarction. Direct PTCA of a closed infarct vessel observed angiographically early in the course of AMI is associated with a high success rate of over 90%. If the procedure is performed in the absence of thrombolytic therapy, the bleeding complication rate is low. Direct PTCA of an infarct lesion is impractical, as the acute event is almost uniformly diagnosed outside the catheterization laboratory and requires rapid access to and mobilization of an angioplasty team, as well as available emergency surgical backup.

The practical aspects of a direct PTCA approach compared with intra-coronary streptokinase were illustrated by the study of O'Neill et al [13]. The mean time to recanalization was similar in the two groups, yet the mean time from presentation of the patient to achieved reperfusion among both groups was 1.2 h. Reperfusion can be achieved more rapidly by the intravenous infusion of rt-PA within 60 min in about 70 to 80% of patients [1, 3, 5, 6]. This reduction in time to successful recanalization is significant for reducing infarct size.

Direct PTCA has merit as an alternative strategy to achieve reperfusion in a few important subsets. First, patients with a contraindication to thrombolysis may benefit from mechanical recanalization. Such patients are frequently encountered, including those with refractory hypertension, recent bleeding or trauma, or previous stroke. Second, patients in whom direct PTCA can be performed very rapidly may benefit from more timely reperfusion as compared with intravenous thrombolysis. Third, patients with an unclear diagnosis, such as an atypical history or patients with underling left bundle branch block may benefit from immediate angiography and a direct angioplasty approach, thus sparing the patient from unnecessary thrombolytic therapy if acute coronary artery occlusion is not present.

Immediate angioplasty

Immediate PTCA following successful thrombolytic therapy has not yielded a favorable mortality rate or augmentation of left ventricular function as compared with a delayed procedure (Table 2).

The European cooperative study randomized 183 patients to undergo immediate PTCA or delayed angiography prior to assessing of thrombolytic results. The mortality differences in this trial achieved statistical significance, with a 3% mortality rate for patients allocated to non-invasive therapy versus 7% among patients undergoing early angiography at 6 to 165 min into t-PA infusion [8].

Only a select group of patients were assigned to undergo immediate PTCA in most trials, with only 52% of TAMI patients, 52% of TIMI-2A patients, and 56% of patients in the Johns Hopkins trial cnsidered to be suitable candidates, while 93% of all patients were assigned to immediate PTCA in a less selective manner in the European cooperative trial, which may in part account for the higher absolute mortality rate in this study [8].

Left ventricular ejection fractions, a common end-point among the major trials were not significantly altered by immediate PTCA, or following an early, deferred approach at 3 days (Fig. 2). There was a significant increase in left ventricular performance at peak exercise noted in the early PTCA subgroup of the Johns Hopkins study, however these values were obtained prior to the delayed procedure, which might have afforded a similar improvement in coronary artery flow reserve to this group as well. It is important to note that PTCA was performed on day 3, not immediately, in the Johns Hopkins trial.

These results, while disappointing, may indicate the need for earlier intervention if significant myocardial salvage is to be achieved. The total time to 'immediate' intervention varied among the trials when considering the time from the onset of symptoms to initial angiography, (Table 1) patients could undergo the procedure as late as 4.4 h in the TAMI trial, 4.7 h in the TIMI-II pilot study, 4.6 in TIMI-IIa, 5.7 h using the mean time to angiogram in the Johns Hopkins trial, and 3.3 in the European co-operative study. With irreversible myocardial necrosis occurring between 4 and 6 h in experimental models, it is possible that an earlier approach is required to demonstrate improved outcome.

Increased morbidity was associated with PTCA immediately following thrombolytic therapy. Bleeding complications requiring transfusion were more common in patients undergoing immediate PTCA, which often occurred during a four or six hour infusion of thrombolytic agents. They were two to three times more common with this approach, compared with a deferred strategy (TAMI 22% vs 18%; TIMI-IIa 19.5 vs 7.2%; European Study 10% vs 4%). Emergency CABG was required more frequently in the setting of immediate PTCA, while more patients in the deferred group later underwent the procedure in an elective manner. Additionally, there were some patients that experienced reperfusion either from an effect of rt-PA just beyond the point of randomization or from spontaneous thrombolysis, which may occur in as many as 22% of patients [14]. These patients did not undergo the planned procedure.

The overall poor results and untoward effects of immediate PTCA following thrombolytic therapy, support a deferred procedure in the majority of patients, especially those in whom thrombolytic agents succeed in interrupting the progression of AMI. The incidence of reocclusion, reinfarction and recurrent ischemic events is higher in this setting, and mandates continued hospitalization for observation and functional testing, until optimal management of the underlying culprit coronary artery lesion can be achieved.

Influence of the thrombolytic agent

The pitfalls of combined t-PA therapy followed by coronary angioplasty may not result entirely from mechanical revascularization, but may reflect shortcomings of t-PA therapy. Since this agent does not cause fibrinogen depletion and a prolonged systemic thrombolytic state, it may be associated with a higher rate of reocclusion in the setting of coronary angioplasty. Although no synergistic, additional thrombolysis was achieved with systemic administration of urokinase with t-PA in the TAMI-II trial, the reocclusion rate following rescue PTCA was substantially reduced, with patency rates at day 7 angiography of 96% with combined therapy vs 69% among patients receiving t-PA alone (p = 0.017) [12].

Similarly, in a series of 216 patients treated with intravenous streptokinase at a mean of 3 h from symptom onset, followed by angiography within a mean 1.5 h into therapy, successful immediate PTCA with a reduction of the residual stenosis to less than 50% of the luminal diameter was achieved in 188 patients (87%) [15]. Only 53% (114/216) of the patients experienced successful thrombolysis by the time of the early angiogram; thus mechanical recanalization was performed as an immediate rescue procedure in 34% of the patients with successful PTCA results. This strategy was associated with both a high patency rate at predischarge angiography (94% of all patients enrolled), and a significant improvement in left ventricular ejection fraction (44 to 49% by the time of discharge, p < 0.0001).

Phase-5 of the ongoing TAMI trial is designed to compare clinical outcome of

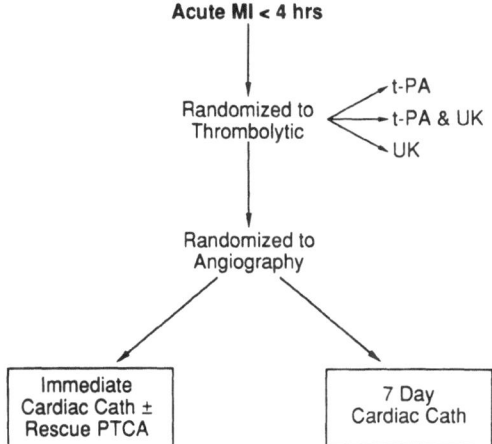

Figure 6. Thrombolysis and Angioplasty in Myocardial Infarction (TAMI) Phase-5 protocol. Outcome of angioplasty following differing thrombolytic regimens, comparing tissue-type plasminogen activator (t-PA) with urokinase (UK) or with a combination of both agents. PTCA = percutaneous transluminal coronary angioplasty.

thrombolytic therapy with t-PA, urokinase, or combination therapy (t-PA and urokinase), followed by immediate catheterization to identify patients without successful thrombolytic response who may undergo rescue PTCA, versus no angiogram until day 7 (Fig 6). The trial will not only provide information about the efficacy of combination thrombolytic therapy, but will also explore the merits of early angiography and rescue PTCA for the nearly 25% of patients who prove resistant to thrombolytic agents despite a combination of agents.

Other trials, including the SAMI and SWIFT studies are investigating combined thrombolytic therapy and PTCA using both streptokinase and its derivative, anisoylated plasminogen-streptokinase activator complex (APSAC), respectively.

Early angiography and rescue angioplasty

Lack of improvement of ventricular function following early PTCA has promoted a less aggressive approach to the patient with AMI, spawning an approach of thrombolytic therapy followed by observation alone, with a delay in all invasive evaluation [11]. The improvement in ventricular function that might accompany an earlier approach, within 3 h of symptoms, is presently unknown. Additionally, early catheterization was indispensable for identifying patients in whom thromblytic therapy was unsuccessful, who might benefit from early mechanical revascularization, or patients with critical or lethal coronary artery lesions, needing emergent CABG.

Attempts at prospective clinical identification of thrombolytic success in the

TAMI-I trial were disappointing. As many as 55% of patients with no clinical evidence of reperfusion as judged by resolution of chest pain or acute ST segment changes, or the appearance of reperfusion associated arrhythmias, were found to have patent infarct vessels despite a lack of clinically predictive indicators. Even the best clinical indicator of recanalization, complete resolution of acute ST segment elevation (96% probability) was present in only 6% of patients with patent infarct vessels at angiography. This poor correlation between clinical indicators of thrombolytic success and actual infarct vessel patency illustrates the need for early angiography identify patients who may need a complementary or alternative revascularization approach.

Rescue PTCA refers to mechanical recanalization as a backup procedure in the event of thrombolytic failure, and was employed in nearly 90% (86/96) of patients in the TAMI-I subgroup with discouraging results. Reocclusion after PTCA in this group was remarkably high at 29%. In a small subgroup of 27 patients enrolled under the combined thrombolytic protocol of TAMI Phase-II, receiving t-PA and urokinase, there was a 96% sustained patency rate after PTCA, with a 5% improvement in ejection fraction by the seventh day of the study [8]. The clinical population was similar to patients enrolled in the other TAMI protocols, but the small numbers in this group do not allow significant conclusions to be drawn.

Rescue PTCA may be more successful in the presence of a generalized fibrinolytic state; a combination of presently available agents or the employment of other primary thrombolytic agents may improve the success rate in this group. Rescue PTCA may be a useful bridge to CABG, evidenced by the lower mortality rate that was ultimately associated with successful or partially successful PTCA.

Conclusions drawn from the clinical trials

PTCA is presently an adjunct to the more important and practical consideration of early thrombolytic intervention for patients presenting with acute myocardial infarction. Mechanical revascularization is associated with both a low in-hospital and late mortality rate, but the current available clinical data demonstrates no difference in resting left ventricular performance between patients undergoing a more immediate procedure and those in whom angioplasty is deferred for several days. Although an improved response in left ventricular ejection fraction augmentation at peak exercise has been associated with early PTCA, there was no overt clinical sign of improved exercise tolerance in these patients, and whether a similar augmentation in left ventricular performance occurs after late PTCA remains unknown.

Given the safety profile of deferred PTCA following t-PA therapy, with fewer required emergency CABG surgeries and similar pre-discharge left ventricular performance characteristics, the deferred approach to PTCA in the patient with suitable coronary anatomy following systemic t-PA therapy is presently the preferred strategy. The role of angioplasty as a direct intervention in certain patients, or as a rescue procedure in the event of thrombolytic therapy failure needs further investigation.

The clinical trials demonstrate no clear benefit from immediate PTCA following t-PA treatment, but there is some mounting evidence that the use of alternative thrombolytic agents or a combination of agents may provide a more suitable post-thrombolytic environment for an immediate procedure, resulting in fewer untoward effects. The role of PTCA after thrombolytic therapy for AMI will need to be reassessed as newer thrombolytic strategies evolve, or as optimal antiplatelet and anticoagulant regimens are devised to maximize the sustained patence rate as compared with t-PA use alone.

The role of 'controlled reperfusion' of the repleting biochemical substrate prior to reperfusion and unloading of the left ventricle (16, 17) and methods designed to preserve left ventricular gometric shape AMI (18), represent new directions in therapeutic intervention for the patient presenting early with acute myocardial infarction.

References

1. The TIMI Study Group (1985) The thrombolysis in myocardial infarction (TIMI) trial: Phase I findings. *N Engl J Med* 312:932
2. The TIMI Study Group (1987) The thrombolysis in myocaridal infarction (TIMI) Phase II pilot study: Tissue plasminogen activator followed by percutaneous transluminal coronary angioplasty. *J Am Coll Cardiol* 10:51B
3. Topol EJ, O'Neill WW, Langburd AB, Walton JA et al (1987) A randomized, placebo-controlled trial of intravenous recombinant tissuetype plasminogen activator and emergency coronary angioplasty in patients with acute myocardial infarction. *Circulation* 75:420
4. Califf RM, Topol EJ, George BS et al. (1988) Characteristics and outcome of patients in whom reperfusion with intravenous tissue-type plasminogen activator fails: results of the thrombolysis and angioplasty in myocardial infarction (TAMI) I trial. *Circulation* 77:1090
5. Topol EJ, Califf RM, George BS (1987) The Thrombolysis and Angioplasty in Myocardial infarction (TAMI) group. A randomized trial of immediate versus delayed angioplasty after intravenous tissue plasminogen activator in acute myocardial infarction. *N Engl J Med* 317:581
6. Topol EJ, Califf RM (1987) The Thrombolysis and Angioplasty in Myocardial infarction (TAMI) group. Thrombolysis and angioplasty in myocardial infarction (TAMI) trial. *J Am Coll Cardiol* 10:65B
7. Guerci AD, Gerstenblith, G, Brinker JA et al. (1987) A randomized trial of intravenous tissue plasminogen activator for acute myocardial infarction with subsequent randomization to elective coronary angioplasty. *N Engl J Med* 317:1613
8. Simoons ML, The European Cooperative Study Group for Recombinant Tissue-type Plasminogen Activator (1988) Thrombolysis with tissue plasminogen activator in acute myocardial infarction: no additional benefit from immediate percutaneous coronary angioplasty. *Lancet* 197
9. The National Heart, Lung, and Blood Institute Registry (1988) Percutaneous transluminal coronary angioplasty in 1985–1986 and 1977–1981. *N Engl J Med* 318:265
10. Guerci, AD (1988) Correspondence to the editor. *N Engl J Med* 318:1617
11. Ryan TJ (1987) Angioplasty in acute myocardial infarction: Is the balloon leaking? *N Engl J Med* 317:624
12. Topol EJ, Califf RM, George BS et al (1988) Coronary arterial thrombolysis with combined infusion of recombinat tissue-type plasminogen activator and urokinase in acute myocardial infarction. *Circulation* 77:1100

13. O'Neill WW, Timmis GC, Bourdillon PD et al (1986) A prospective randomized clinical trial of intracoronary streptokinase versus coronary angioplasty for acute myocardial infarction. *N Engl J Med* 314:812

14. DeWood MA, Spores J, Hensley GR, Simpson CS et al (1983) Coronary arteriographic findings in acute transmural myocardial infarction. *Circulation* 68 (Suppl I):39

15. Stack RS, O'Connor CM, Mark DB, Hinohara T, Phillips HR, Lee MM et al (1988) Coronary perfusion during acute myocardial infarction with a combined therapy of coronary angioplasty and highdose intravenous streptokinase. *Circulation* 77:151

16. Allen BS, Okamoto F, Buckberg GD, Bugyi H, Young H, Leaf J, Beyersdorf F, Sjostrand F, Maloney JV (1986) Studies of controlled reperfusion after ischemia, XV: Immediate functional recovery after six hours of regional ischemia by careful control of conditions of reperfusion and composition of reperfusate. *J Thorac Cardiovasc Surg* 92:621

17. Allen BS, Okamoto F, Buckberg GD, Bugyi H, Leaf J (1986) Studies of controlled reperfusion after ischemia, XIII: Reperfusion conditions: critical importance of total ventricular decompression during regional reperfusion. *J Thorac Cardiovasc Surg* 92:605

18. Pfeffer MA, Lamas GA, Vaughn DE, Parisi AF, Braunwald E (1988) Effect of captopril on progressive ventricular dilitation after anterior myocardial infarction. *N Engl J Med* 319:380

Developments in Cardiovascular Medicine

Developments in Cardiovascular Medicine

Developments in Cardiovascular Medicine

43. S. Sideman and R. Beyar (eds.): [3-D] *Simulation and Imaging of the Cardiac System.* State of the Heart. Proceedings of the International Henry Goldberg Workshop, held in Haifa, Israel (1984). 1985   ISBN 0–89838–687–X

44. E. van der Wall and K.I. Lie (eds.): *Recent Views on Hypertrophic Cardiomyopathy.* Proceedings of a Symposium, held in Groningen, The Netherlands (1984). 1985
                                                                       ISBN 0–89838–694–2

45. R.E. Beamish, P.K. Singal and N.S. Dhalla (eds.), *Stress and Heart Disease.* Proceedings of a International Symposium, held in Winnipeg, Canada, 1984 (Vol. 1). 1985   ISBN 0–89838–709–4

46. R.E. Beamish, V. Panagia and N.S. Dhalla (eds.): *Pathogenesis of Stress-induced Heart Disease.* Proceedings of a International Symposium, held in Winnipeg, Canada, 1984 (Vol. 2). 1985   ISBN 0–89838–710–8

47. J. Morganroth and E.N. Moore (eds.): *Cardiac Arrhythmias.* New Therapeutic Drugs and Devices. Proceedings of the 5th Symposium on New Drugs and Devices, held in Philadelphia, Pa., U.S.A. (1984). 1985   ISBN 0–89838–716–7

48. P. Mathes (ed.): *Secondary Prevention in Coronary Artery Disease and Myocardial Infarction.* 1985   ISBN 0–89838–736–1

49. H.L. Stone and W.B. Weglicki (eds.): *Pathobiology of Cardiovascular Injury.* Proceedings of the 6th Annual Meeting of the American Section of the I.S.H.R., held in Oklahoma City, Okla., U.S.A. (1984). 1985   ISBN 0–89838–743–4

50. J. Meyer, R. Erbel and H.J. Rupprecht (eds.): *Improvement of Myocardial Perfusion.* Thrombolysis, Angioplasty, Bypass Surgery. Proceedings of a Symposium, held in Mainz, F.R.G. (1984). 1985   ISBN 0–89838–748–5

51. J.H.C. Reiber, P.W. Serruys and C.J. Slager (eds.): *Quantitative Coronary and Left Ventricular Cineangiography.* Methodology and Clinical Applications. 1986
                                                                       ISBN 0–89838–760–4

52. R.H. Fagard and I.E. Bekaert (eds.): *Sports Cardiology.* Exercise in Health and Cardiovascular Disease. Proceedings from an International Conference, held in Knokke, Belgium (1985). 1986   ISBN 0–89838–782–5

53. J.H.C. Reiber and P.W. Serruys (eds.): *State of the Art in Quantitative Cornary Arteriography.* 1986   ISBN 0–89838–804–X

54. J. Roelandt (ed.): *Color Doppler Flow Imaging and Other Advances in Doppler Echocardiography.* 1986   ISBN 0–89838–806–6

55. E.E. van der Wall (ed.): *Noninvasive Imaging of Cardiac Metabolism.* Single Photon Scintigraphy, Positron Emission Tomography and Nuclear Magnetic Resonance. 1987
                                                                       ISBN 0–89838–812–0

56. J. Liebman, R. Plonsey and Y. Rudy (eds.): *Pediatric and Fundamental Electrocardiography.* 1987   ISBN 0–89838–815–5

57. H.H. Hilger, V. Hombach and W.J. Rashkind (eds.), *Invasive Cardiovascular Therapy.* Proceedings of an International Symposium, held in Cologne, F.R.G. (1985). 1987   ISBN 0–89838–818–X

58. P.W. Serruys and G.T. Meester (eds.): *Coronary Angioplasty.* A Controlled Model for Ischemia. 1986   ISBN 0–89838–819–8

59. J.E. Tooke and L.H. Smaje (eds.): *Clinical Investigation of the Microcirculation.* Proceedings of an International Meeting, held in London, U.K. (1985). 1987
                                                                       ISBN 0–89838–833–3

Developments in Cardiovascular Medicine

60. R.Th. van Dam and A. van Oosterom (eds.): *Electrocardiographic Body Surface Mapping*. Proceedings of the 3rd International Symposium on B.S.M., held in Nijmegen, The Netherlands (1985). 1986 ISBN 0–89838–834–1
61. M.P. Spencer (ed.): *Ultrasonic Diagnosis of Cerebrovascular Disease*. Doppler Techniques and Pulse Echo Imaging. 1987 ISBN 0–89838–836–8
62. M.J. Legato (ed.): *The Stressed Heart*. 1987 ISBN 0–89838–849–X
63. M.E. Safar (ed.): *Arterial and Venous Systems in Essential Hypertension*. With Assistance of G.M. London, A.Ch. Simon and Y.A. Weiss. 1987
ISBN 0–89838–857–0
64. J. Roelandt (ed.): *Digital Techniques in Echocardiography*. 1987
ISBN 0–89838–861–9
65. N.S. Dhalla, P.K. Singal and R.E. Beamish (eds.): *Pathology of Heart Disease*. Proceedings of the 8th Annual Meeting of the American Section of the I.S.H.R., held in Winnipeg, Canada, 1986 (Vol. 1). 1987 ISBN 0–89838–864–3
66. N.S. Dhalla, G.N. Pierce and R.E. Beamish (eds.): *Heart Function and Metabolism*. Proceedings of the 8th Annual Meeting of the American Section of the I.S.H.R., held in Winnipeg, Canada, 1986 (Vol. 2). 1987 ISBN 0–89838–865–1
67. N.S. Dhalla, I.R. Innes and R.E. Beamish (eds.): *Myocardial Ischemia*. Proceedings of a Satellite Symposium of the 30th International Physiological Congress, held in Winnipeg, Canada (1986). 1987 ISBN 0–89838–866–X
68. R.E. Beamish, V. Panagia and N.S. Dhalla (eds.): *Pharmacological Aspects of Heart Disease*. Proceedings of an International Symposium, held in Winnipeg, Canada (1986). 1987 ISBN 0–89838–867–8
69. H.E.D.J. ter Keurs and J.V. Tyberg (eds.): *Mechanics of the Circulation*. Proceedings of a Satellite Symposium of the 30th International Physiological Congress, held in Banff, Alberta, Canada (1986). 1987 ISBN 0–89838–870–8
70. S. Sideman and R. Beyar (eds.): *Activation, Metabolism and Perfusion of the Heart*. Simulation and Experimental Models. Proceedings of the 3rd Henry Goldberg Workshop, held in Piscataway, N.J., U.S.A. (1986). 1987 ISBN 0–89838–871–6
71. E. Aliot and R. Lazzara (eds.): *Ventricular Tachycardias*. From Mechanism to Therapy. 1987 ISBN 0–89838–881–3
72. A. Schneeweiss and G. Schettler: *Cardiovascular Drug Therapoy in the Elderly*. 1988
ISBN 0–89838–883–X
73. J.V. Chapman and A. Sgalambro (eds.): *Basic Concepts in Doppler Echocardiography*. Methods of Clinical Applications based on a Multi-modality Doppler Approach. 1987 ISBN 0–89838–888–0
74. S. Chien, J. Dormandy, E. Ernst and A. Matrai (eds.): *Clinical Hemorheology*. Applications in Cardiovascular and Hematological Disease, Diabetes, Surgery and Gynecology. 1987 ISBN 0–89838–807–4
75. J. Morganroth and E.N. Moore (eds.): *Congestive Heart Failure*. Proceedings of the 7th Annual Symposium on New Drugs and Devices, held in Philadelphia, Pa., U.S.A. (1986). 1987 ISBN 0–89838–955–0
76. F.H. Messerli (ed.): *Cardiovascular Disease in the Elderly*. 2nd ed. 1988
ISBN 0–89838–962–3
77. P.H. Heintzen and J.H. Bürsch (eds.): *Progress in Digital Angiocardiography*. 1988
ISBN 0–89838–965–8

Developments in Cardiovascular Medicine

78. M.M. Scheinman (ed.): *Catheter Ablation of Cardiac Arrhythmias.* Basic Bioelectrical Effects and Clinical Indications. 1988   ISBN 0–89838–967–4
79. J.A.E. Spaan, A.V.G. Bruschke and A.C. Gittenberger-De Groot (eds.): *Coronary Circulation.* From Basic Mechanisms to Clinical Implications. 1987
                                                            ISBN 0–89838–978–X
80. C. Visser, G. Kan and R.S. Meltzer (eds.): *Echocardiography in Coronary Artery Disease.* 1988   ISBN 0–89838–979–8
81. A. Bayés de Luna, A. Betriu and G. Permanyer (eds.): *Therapeutics in Cardiology.* 1988   ISBN 0–89838–981–X
82. D.M. Mirvis (ed.): *Body Surface Electrocardiographic Mapping.* 1988
                                                            ISBN 0–89838–983–6
83. M.A. Konstam and J.M. Isner (eds.): *The Right Ventricle.* 1988 ISBN 0–89838–987–9
84. C.T. Kappagoda and P.V. Greenwood (eds.): *Long-term Management of Patients after Myocardial Infarction.* 1988   ISBN 0–89838–352–8
85. W.H. Gaasch and H.J. Levine (eds.): *Chronic Aortic Regurgitation.* 1988
                                                            ISBN 0–89838–364–1
86. P.K. Singal (ed.): *Oxygen Radicals in the Pathophysiology of Heart Disease.* 1988
                                                            ISBN 0–89838–375–7
87. J.H.C. Reiber and P.W. Serruys (eds.): *New Developments in Quantitative Coronary Arteriography.* 1988   ISBN 0–89838–377–3
88. J. Morganroth and E.N. Moore (eds.): *Silent Myocardial Ischemia.* Proceedings of the 8th Annual Symposium on New Drugs and Devices (1987). 1988
                                                            ISBN 0–89838–380–3
89. H.E.D.J. ter Keurs and M.I.M. Noble (eds.): *Starling's Law of the Heart Revisted.* 1988   ISBN 0–89838–382–X
90. N. Sperelakis (ed.): *Physiology and Pathophysiology of the Heart.* (Rev. ed.) 1988
                                                            ISBN 0–89838–388–9
91. J.W. de Jong (ed.): *Myocardial Energy Metabolism.* 1988   ISBN 0–89838–394–3
92. V. Hombach, H.H. Hilger and H.L. Kennedy (eds.): *Electrocardiography and Cardiac Drug Therapy.* Proceedings of an International Symposium, held in Cologne, F.R.G. (1987). 1988   ISBN 0–89838–395–1
93. H. Iwata, J.B. Lombardini and T. Segawa (eds.): *Taurine and the Heart.* 1988
                                                            ISBN 0–89838–396–X
94. M.R. Rosen and Y. Palti (eds.): *Lethal Arrhythmias Resulting from Myocardial Ischemia and Infarction.* Proceedings of the 2nd Rappaport Symposium, held in Haifa, Israel (1988). 1988   ISBN 0–89838–401–X
95. M. Iwase and I. Sotobata: *Clinical Echocardiography.* With a Foreword by M.P. Spencer. 1989   ISBN 0–7923–0004–1
96. I. Cikes (ed.): *Echocardiography in Cardiac Interventions.* 1989
                                                            ISBN 0–7923–0088–2
97. E. Rapaport (ed.): *Early Interventions in Acute Myocardial Infarction.* 1989
                                                            ISBN 0–7923–0175–7
98. M.E. Safar and F. Fouad-Tarazi (eds.): *The Heart in Hypertension.* A Tribute to Robert C. Tarazi (1925–1986). 1989   ISBN 0–7923–0197–8
99. S. Meerbaum and R. Meltzer (eds.): *Myocardial Contrast Two-dimensional Echocardiography.* 1989   ISBN 0–7923–0205–2

Developments in Cardiovascular Medicine